Additive Manufacturing Processes in Biomedical Engineering

This book covers innovative breakthroughs in additive manufacturing processes used for biomedical engineering. More and more, 3D printing is selected over traditional manufacturing processes, especially for complex designs, because of the many advantages, such as fewer restrictions, better production cost savings, higher quality control, and accuracy.

Current challenges and opportunities regarding material, design, cost savings, and efficiency are covered along with an outline of the most recent fabrication methods used for converting biomaterials into integrated structures that can fit best in anatomy while still obtaining the necessary architecture, mechanical reliability, biocompatibility, and antibacterial characteristics needed. Additional chapters also focus on selected areas of applications, such as bionics, affordable prostheses, implants, medical devices, rapid tooling, and drug delivery.

Additive Manufacturing Processes in Biomedical Engineering: Advanced Fabrication Methods and Rapid Tooling Techniques acts as a firsthand reference for commercial manufacturing organizations which are mimicking tissue organs by using additive manufacturing techniques. By capturing the current trends of today's manufacturing practices this book becomes a one-stop resource for manufacturing professionals, engineers in related disciplines, and academic researchers.

Sustainable Manufacturing Technologies: Additive, Subtractive, and Hybrid

Series Editors
Chander Prakash, Sunpreet Singh, Seeram Ramakrishna, and Linda Yongling Wu

This book series offers the reader comprehensive insights of recent research breakthroughs in additive, subtractive, and hybrid technologies while emphasizing their sustainability aspects. Sustainability has become an integral part of all manufacturing enterprises to provide various techno-social pathways toward developing environmental friendly manufacturing practices. It has also been found that numerous manufacturing firms are still reluctant to upgrade their conventional practices to sophisticated sustainable approaches. Therefore this new book series is aimed to provide a globalized platform to share innovative manufacturing mythologies and technologies. The books will encourage the eminent issues of the conventional and non-conventional manufacturing technologies and cover recent innovations.

Advances in Manufacturing Technology
Computational Materials Processing and Characterization
Edited by Rupinder Singh, Sukhdeep Singh Dhami, and B. S. Pabla

Additive Manufacturing for Plastic Recycling
Efforts in Boosting A Circular Economy
Edited by Rupinder Singh and Ranvijay Kumar

Additive Manufacturing Processes in Biomedical Engineering
Advanced Fabrication Methods and Rapid Tooling Techniques
Edited by Atul Babbar, Ankit Sharma, Vivek Jain, Dheeraj Gupta

For more information on this series, please visit: www.routledge.com/Sustainable-Manufacturing-Technologies-Additive-Subtractive-and-Hybrid/book-series/CRC SMTASH

Additive Manufacturing Processes in Biomedical Engineering
Advanced Fabrication Methods and Rapid Tooling Techniques

Edited by
Atul Babbar, Ankit Sharma,
Vivek Jain, and Dheeraj Gupta

CRC CRC Press
Taylor & Francis Group
Boca Raton London

CRC Press is an imprint of the
Taylor & Francis Group, an **informa** business

First edition published 2023
by CRC Press
6000 Broken Sound Parkway NW, Suite 300, Boca Raton, FL 33487–2742

and by CRC Press
4 Park Square, Milton Park, Abingdon, Oxon, OX14 4RN

CRC Press is an imprint of Taylor & Francis Group, LLC

Library of Congress Cataloging-in-Publication Data
Names: Babbar, Atul, editor.
Title: Additive manufacturing processes in biomedical engineering : advanced fabrication methods and rapid tooling techniques / edited by Atul Babbar, Ankit Sharma, Vivek Jain, and Dheeraj Gupta.
Description: First edition. | Boca Raton : CRC Press, [2023]
Series: Sustainable manufacturing technologies: additive, subtractive, and hybrid | Includes bibliographical references and index.
Summary: "Current challenges and opportunities regarding material, design, cost savings, and efficiency are covered along with an outline of the most recent fabrication methods used for converting biomaterials into integrated structures that can fit best in the anatomy while still obtaining the necessary architecture, mechanical reliability, biocompatibility, and anti-bacterial characteristics needed. Additional chapters will also focus on selected areas of applications such as bionics, affordable prostheses, implants, medical devices, rapid tooling and drug delivery"—Provided by publisher.
Identifiers: LCCN 2022004315 (print) | LCCN 2022004316 (ebook) | ISBN 9781032109725 (hardback) | ISBN 9781032109732 (paperback) | ISBN 9781003217961 (ebook)
Subjects: LCSH: Biomedical materials. | Additive manufacturing—Materials.
Classification: LCC R857.M3 A373 2023 (print) | LCC R857.M3 (ebook) | DDC 610.28/4—dc23/eng/20220401
LC record available at https://lccn.loc.gov/2022004315
LC ebook record available at https://lccn.loc.gov/2022004316

ISBN: 978-1-032-10972-5 (hbk)
ISBN: 978-1-032-10973-2 (pbk)
ISBN: 978-1-003-21796-1 (ebk)

DOI: 10.1201/9781003217961

Typeset in Times
by Apex CoVantage, LLC

Contents

Editors vii

List of Contributors ix

Chapter 1   Recent Advancements of Additive Manufacturing for
Patient-Specific Drug Delivery 1

*Prakash Katakam, Shanta Kumari Adiki, and
Soumya Ranjan Satapathy*

Chapter 2   Additive Manufacturing for the Development of Biological
Implants, Scaffolds, and Prosthetics 27

*Atul Babbar, Vivek Jain, Dheeraj Gupta, Ankit Sharma,
Chander Prakash, Vidyapati Kumar, and Kapil Kumar Goyal*

Chapter 3   Additive Manufacturing Process for the Development
of Orthosis of Foot 47

*Manak L. Jain, Nalinakash S. Vyas, Anil Mulewa, and
Sanjay G. Dhande*

Chapter 4   The Application of Additive Manufacturing Technology in the
Era of COVID-19 Pandemic: A State-of-the-Art Review 65

Raj Agarwal, Jaskaran Singh, and Vishal Gupta

Chapter 5   Relevance of Bio-Inks for 3D Bioprinting 81

*Bhargav Prajwal Pathri, Mohd. Shahnawaz Khan,
and Atul Babbar*

Chapter 6   Additive Manufacturing of Polymers for Biomedical
Applications 99

Subrata Mondal

Chapter 7   Additive Manufacturing for Presurgical and Postsurgical
Planning: A State-of-the-Art Review 117

Satadru Kashyap

Chapter 8   Additive Manufacturing in Biomedical Engineering: Present
and Future Applications 143

*Vidyapati Kumar, Chander Prakash, Atul Babbar, Shubham
Choudhary, Ankit Sharma and Amrinder Singh Uppal*

Chapter 9   Additive Manufacturing of Biomaterials: Classification,
Techniques, and Application 165

Sudip Dasgupta and Sambit Ray

Chapter 10 Role of 3D Printing and Chitosan-Hydrogel-Based Modifiers
in Drug Delivery 205

Lalita Chopra and Jasgurpreet Singh Chohan

Index.. 225

Editors

Dr. Atul Babbar is working as an assistant professor in the Mechanical Engineering Department of SGT University, Gurugram. He has been teaching students in academics and research fields. He is a Level 2 Non-Destructive Testing Engineer certified by the American Society of Non-Destructive Testing. His research interests include biomedical, three- and four-dimensional printing, and conventional/nonconventional machining and is not limited to these. He has authored several research articles and book chapters in various international/national Web of Science and Scopus journals. He has been granted numerous national and international patents. He has been reviewing research articles of various peer-reviewed SCI- and Scopus-indexed journals.

Dr. Ankit Sharma is currently working as an assistant professor at Chitkara College of Applied Engineering of Chitkara University. He has completed his doctoral from the Thapar Institute of Engineering and Technology. He has authored numerous national and international publications in Scopus- and Web of Science–indexed journals. His research interests include hybrid machining, additive manufacturing, and others. He has vast experience in the industry as well as academics. He has been granted with numerous national and international patents.

Dr. Vivek Jain received his PhD in 2012 from the Indian Institute of Technology Roorkee, India, M.Tech. in 2009 from Guru Nanak Dev Engineering College, Ludhiana, India with first class. He graduated in 1998 from Rajiv Gandhi College of Engineering, Research and Technology, Nagpur University, India, with first class. At present, he works as an associate professor in the Mechanical Engineering Department of Thapar Institute of Engineering & Technology, Patiala. He has vast experience, including 14 years of teaching and two years of industrial experience. His research interests include biomedical, machining, composites, and surface engineering but are not limited to these. He has published in various international/national journals. He has also filed three Indian patents. He is also handling one research project funded by DST (India).

Dr. Dheeraj Gupta is currently an associate professor in the Department of Mechanical Engineering at the Thapar Institute of Engineering & Technology, Patiala, India. He obtained his BE in mechanical engineering from Shri Govindram Seksaria Institute of Technology and Science, Indore, India, and master's and doctoral degrees from the Indian Institute of Technology Roorkee, Roorkee, India. He has more than 10 years of teaching and research experience. He has worked on a European Union–funded project in Lisbon, Portugal. He has published more than 70 articles in journals and presented at conferences. He has filed two Indian Patents on microwave processing of metals. Currently, he is a principal investigator for an Indian government–funded project.

Contributors

Shanta Kumari Adiki currently working in Sarojini Naidu Vanita Pharmacy Maha Vidyalaya, Hyderabad, Telangana, India.

Raj Agarwal received an M.Tech degree in production engineering from Thapar Institute of Engineering and Technology Patiala, Punjab, India, in 2019. He is now a research scholar in the Department of Mechanical Engineering at the Thapar Institute of Engineering and Technology Patiala. Furthermore, he has published articles in several international journals as well as papers, and book chapters in the areas of additive manufacturing and biomedical engineering. His research interests include additive manufacturing, biomechanics, biomaterials, rapid prototyping, artificial intelligence, and machine learning for advanced manufacturing. His current working focuses on the diagnosis, prediction, and treatment of diseases using machine learning.

Atul Babbar is working as an assistant professor in the Mechanical Engineering Department of SGT University, Gurugram. He has been teaching students in academics and research fields. His research interests include biomedical, three- and four-dimensional printing, and conventional/nonconventional machining and are not limited to these.

Jasgurpreet Singh Chohan has been working as an associate professor in the Department of Mechanical Engineering at Chandigarh University, India, since October 2017. Dr. Chohan performed his doctoral research on improving the surface characteristics of hip implants fabricated through a three-dimensional printing process. He has more than 12 years of experience in research and teaching at the graduate and postgraduate levels. His areas of specialization are additive manufacturing, hybrid machining, biomedical implants, advanced composites, metamaterials, human factor engineering, and multicriteria decision-making. He has filed six patents, authored four books and 12 books chapters, and published more than 52 articles in international journals and conferences.

Lalita Chopra has teaching experience of 13 years and presently works as an assistant professor in the Department of Chemistry, University Institute of Sciences, Chandigarh University, Gharuan, Mohali. Her research work includes the synthesis and characterization of biopolymer-based graft copolymers and crosslinked graft copolymers for their application as metal ion sorption from wastewater. She had published more than 30 research papers in reputed journals and attended and presented research papers in more than 20 conferences and seminars.

Shubham Choudhary is working as an assistant professor in the Department of Mechanical Engineering at Ajay Kumar Garg Engineering College. His research interests include ultraprecision finishing, computational fluid dynamics, and tribology, among others.

Sudip Dasgupta is currently working as an assistant professor in ceramic engineering at the National Institute of Technology, Rourkela, India. He obtained his PhD in materials science in 2008 from Washington State University, Pullman, USA, in the field of nanostructured calcium phosphate–based bone substitute materials and drug delivery systems. As a research associate at Central Glass and Ceramic Research Institute in India, Dr. Dasgupta worked in the field of synthesis of layered double-based organic-inorganic composite nanovector for delivering anticancerous drug molecules to tumor cells. His research interest is primarily focused on the synthesis of nanomaterials using different wet chemical and advanced synthesis routes, its processing, its characterization, and evaluation of its physical, surface, chemical, mechanical, and biological property. He has more than 15 years of research experience in mammalian cell culture, bone scaffold fabrication, and tissue engineering–related research.

Sanjay G. Dhande received his PhD from Indian Institute of Technology Kanpur. He obtained his B.Tech (Hons) from Pune, Maharashtra, in mechanical engineering. He has more than 50 years of experience, including teaching, research, and administration. After working for a couple of years as a research associate and assistant professor in the United States, he returned to IITK in 1979 and over the years served as head of the Department of Mechanical Engineering and Dean of R&D. He has many honors and awards to his credit. He has presented his research on many international platforms. He served at the Indian Institute of Technology Kanpur, India, in the capacity of director continuously for a period of 15 years. Presently he is a chairperson on the boards of governors of many industries and institutes.

Kapil Kumar Goyal is working as an assistant professor in the Department of Industrial & Production Engineering at Dr. B R Ambedkar National Institute of Technology, Jalandhar. His research interests include additive manufacturing, the Internet of Things, nature-inspired optimization algorithms, nonconventional manufacturing processes, and others.

Dheeraj Gupta is currently an associate professor in the Department of Mechanical Engineering at the Thapar Institute of Engineering & Technology, Patiala, India. He has more than 10 years of teaching and research experience. He has worked on European Union–funded project in Lisbon, Portugal. He has published articles in various international and national journals.

Vishal Gupta worked on designing and fabricating ultrasonic bone drilling during his PhD dissertation at the Indian Institute of Technology (IIT) Delhi. He has a developed novel orthopedic/trauma bone drilling process to put an end to thermal injury to bone. The developed technique has been published for an Indian Patent. He has been awarded by Gandhian Young Technological Innovation award at Rashtrapati Bhavan Delhi (GYTI, 2017) on the basis of his PhD work in the biomedical field. He has also been awarded with a grant of Rs. 15 Lacs from BIRAC SRISTI GYTI Award to develop a prototype rotary ultrasonic bone drilling setup for orthopedic/trauma-related surgery. Apart from that, during his stay at IIT Delhi, Dr. Gupta worked on the EPSRC-DST-funded project titled "Modelling of Advanced Materials for Simulation of Transformative Manufacturing Process". He has published a number of international journal papers in the biomedical field.

Manak L. Jain received his PhD in 2005, from the Indian Institute of Technology Kanpur India, M.Tech, in 1996 in biomedical engineering from the Indian Institute of Technology Madras India, BE, in 1987, in mechanical engineering from Shri G. S. Institute of Technology & Science (GSITS) Indore on July 1987. His research interests are computer-aided design/computer-aided manufacturing/computer-aided engineering, reverse engineering, biomechanics, biomodeling, medical devices, and electro-medico instrumentations. He has approximately 30 years of teaching and research experience. Presently, he is a professor in the Department of Mechanical Engineering at the Shri G. S. Institute of Technology and Science, Indore (M.P.), India.

Vivek Jain works as an associate professor in the Mechanical Engineering Department of Thapar Institute of Engineering & Technology, Patiala. He has vast experience, including 14 years of teaching and 2 years of industrial experience. His research interests include biomedical, machining, composites, surface engineering and are not limited to these. He has published articles in various international and national journals.

Satadru Kashyap is working as an assistant professor in the Department of Mechanical Engineering at Tezpur University. He has 9 years' experience in teaching and research and 4 years of industrial experience. His main research interests are in the domains of manufacturing, composites, and material science. He has completed one project from DSTSERB on composite materials (as principal investigator) and is also the co-investigator in another ongoing project on renewable resources.

Prakash Katakam currently works at the Indira College of Pharmacy, Nanded, Maharashtra, India. Prakash does research in nanotechnology, periodontics, and nanotechnology. His current project is "3D Printing Technology for Drug Delivery Challenges".

Mohd. Shahnawaz Khan currently working as an assistant professor (Sr. Grade) in the Department of Chemistry at the Institute of Engineering and Technology, JK Lakshmipat University, Jaipur. He has completed his PhD in chemistry at Dr B. R. Ambedkar University, Agra. His research interests include organic synthesis, green chemistry, heterocyclic chemistry, the development of new synthetic methodologies, and biomaterials. He has more than 24 publications in different national and international journals. He is also a reviewer for some reputed journals. He is fellow life member of the Indian Chemical Society and the Indian Council of Chemists. He also received Young Scientist Award for Best Poster Presentation & Novel Reaction Methodology.

Vidyapati Kumar is a PhD research scholar in the Mechanical Engineering Department at the Indian Institute of Technology. His research interests include biomedical, machining, composites, and surface engineering and are not limited to these.

Subrata Mondal is an associate professor at the National Institute of Technical Teachers' Training and Research Kolkata, Salt Lake City, West Bengal, India, in the Mechanical Engineering Department. Prior to this position, Dr. Mondal has worked at the Petroleum Institute, Abu Dhabi, United Arab Emirates. He has had research positions in National University of Singapore, Singapore; Colorado State University, USA; Monash University, Australia; and the University of Queensland, Australia. He got his doctoral degree in polymer science from the Hong Kong Polytechnic University, Hong Kong, SAR. His research interests are polymer composites and nanocomposites, metal matrix composites and nanocomposites, polymeric biomaterial, and polymeric membrane for water treatment, among others.

Anil Mulewa received his ME in 2016 in computer-aided design/computer-aided manufacturing/computer-aided engineering from Shri G. S. Institute of Technology and Science Indore, India, He has 5 years of teaching and 2 years of industrial experience. His areas of interest are computer-aided design/computer-aided machining/computer-aided engineering and mechatronics. Currently, he is working as an assistant professor in the Department of Mechanical Engineering.

Bhargav Prajwal Pathri is currently working as an assistant professor in the Department of Mechanical Engineering at the Institute of Engineering and Technology, JK Lakshmipat University, Jaipur. He has completed his PhD at Malaviya National Institute of Technology (MNIT), Jaipur. He received his master's in automotive engineering from Coventry University, UK. He received his bachelor's in mechanical engineering from Jawaharlal Nehru Technological University Hyderabad. His research interests include ceramic machining, tool design, advanced manufacturing processes, rapid prototyping, bioprinting, biomaterials, and computer-aided design/computer-aided manufacturing. He has published more than 25 articles in different international journals. He is also a reviewer for many reputed journals. He worked as part of the Product Design faculty at Effat University, Jeddah, Saudi Arabia.

Chander Prakash is working as a professor at the School of Mechanical Engineering, Lovely Professional University, Jalandhar, India. He has received PhD in mechanical engineering from Panjab University, Chandigarh, India. His area of research is biomaterials, rapid prototyping and three-dimensional printing, advanced manufacturing, modeling, simulation, and optimization. He has more than 12 years of teaching experience and 7 years of research experience.

Sambit Ray is currently working as a PhD scholar in the Department of Ceramic Engineering, National Institute of Technology, Rourkela, India. His research interest is primarily focused on tissue engineering and regenerative medicine for osteochondral bone defects. Mr. Ray's PhD thesis deals with osteochondral scaffolds/construct using non-mulberry silk fibroin, chitosan, and bioactive glass ceramic for bone tissue regeneration. He has research experience in cell culture, microbiology, nanomaterial synthesis, synthesis of bioactive glass, and bone scaffold fabrication

Soumya Ranjan Satapathy is currently working at DFE Pharma India Private Limited, Hyderabad, Telangana, India.

Ankit Sharma is currently working as Assistant Professor at Chitkara College of Applied Engineering of Chitkara University. He has completed his doctoral from Thapar Institute of Engineering and Technology. His research interest includes hybrid machining and additive manufacturing, among others. He has vast experience in industry as well as academics.

Jaskaran Singh has worked in the area of predictive maintenance of industrial rotating machinery components during his PhD from the India Institute of Technology Delhi, India. He further extended his research area to industrial big data analytics, Industry 4.0 manufacturing systems, and artificial intelligence (AI) during his tenure as a postdoctoral fellow at the University of Cincinnati, USA. He has a wide experience of developing and deploying AI-enabled prognostic and health management solutions for industrial machineries. He has a patent (undergoing) for his work on development of a smart rolling element bearing fault diagnosis system in collaboration with India's topmost bearing manufacturer, NBC Bearings. Furthermore, he has published articles in several international journals and presented conference papers in the areas of machine learning, deep learning, and cyber-physical systems.

Amrinder Singh Uppal is working as lead mechanical engineer in Merla Wellhead Solutions, Houston Texas. He is licensed professional engineer in Texas, USA. He has more than 10 years' industrial experience in the designing and manufacturing for the high-pressure equipment's that are used in oil and gas industry. He has co-authored national and international publications. He has been reviewing research articles of various peer review.

Nalinakash S. Vyas received his PhD and M.Tech from the Indian Institute of Technology Delhi and B.Tech from thce Indian Institute of Technology Bombay. His research areas of interest are system identification and parameter estimation, virtual instrumentation and sensor technologies, condition monitoring and neural networks. He has presented his research at many national and international platforms. He has more than 45 years of teaching and research experience; presently, he is a professor in the Department of Mechanical Engineering and the chairman of the Railway Mission, Govt. of India.

1 Recent Advancements of Additive Manufacturing for Patient-Specific Drug Delivery

Prakash Katakam[1], Shanta Kumari Adiki[2], and Soumya Ranjan Satapathy[3]

[1] Indira College of Pharmacy, Nanded, India

[2] Sarojini Naidu Vanita Pharmacy Maha Vidyalaya, Hyderabad, Telangana, India

[3] DFE Pharma India Private Limited, Hyderabad, Telangana, India

ABBREVIATIONS

3DP Three dimensional printing; 4DP Four dimensional printing; AM Additive manufacturing; API Active pharmaceutical ingredient; ASTM American Society for Testing and Materials; CAD Computer-aided design; CBER Center for Biologics Evaluation and Research; CDRH Center for Devices and Radiological Health; CLIP Continuous layer interface production; DED Directed Energy Deposition; DLP Digital light processing; DMLS Direct metal laser sintering; DOD drop-on-demand; EBM Electron beam melting; EC Ethylcellulose; FDCT fixed-dose combination therapy; FDM Fused deposition modeling; GMP Good manufacturing practice; LOM Laminated object manufacturing; MEMS Micro-electro-mechanical system; MIT Massachusetts Institute of Technology; MJ Material jetting; NHS National Health Service; NIL Nanoimprint lithography; OVJP organic vapor jet printing; PAM Pressure-assisted microsyringe; PAT Process analytical technology; PAT process analytical technology; PEG Polyethylene glycol; PEO Polyethylene oxide; PoC Point of care; PLGA polylactide-co-glycolide; PVA Polyvinyl alcohol; SDL Selective deposition lamination; SHS Selective heat sintering; SLM Selective laser melting; IJP Inkjet printing; SLA Stereolithography; SLS Selective laser sintering; SMP shape memory polymer; TIJ thermal inkjet; UAM ultrasonic additive manufacturing; US FDA U.S. Food and Drug Administration

DOI: 10.1201/9781003217961-1

CONTENTS

1.1   Introduction.. 2
1.2   AM for Driving Innovation.. 3
1.3   Trends in Patient-Specific Drug Delivery 4
      1.3.1   Patient-Centric Therapeutic Care.. 4
      1.3.2   Taking Prompts from Other Fields of Research 4
      1.3.3   Small Pharmaceutical Companies Showing an Advantage 4
      1.3.4   Decentralized Manufacturing 5
1.4   AM Technologies.. 5
      1.4.1   Vat Polymerization... 5
      1.4.2   Binder Jetting.. 7
      1.4.3   Material Jetting 9
      1.4.4   Powder Bed Fusion... 10
      1.4.5   Material Extrusion 10
      1.4.6   Direct Energy Deposition 11
      1.4.7   Sheet Lamination 12
1.5   AM in Patient-Specific Drug Delivery Systems 12
      1.5.1   Oral Dosage Formulations... 14
      1.5.2   Parenteral Devices 15
      1.5.3   Implants and Scaffolds.. 16
      1.5.4   Transdermal Devices 17
1.6   4D Drug Delivery Systems 17
1.7   Regulatory Insights... 18
1.8   Decentralization of Production Using AM 19
1.9   Challenges... 19
1.10 Conclusion 20
References.. 20

1.1   INTRODUCTION

Personalized (patient-specific) medication is one of the recent advancements and needs of the health domain. International Society for Pharmacoeconomics and Outcomes Research (ISPOR) defines *personalized medicine* as the "use of genomics to improve the safety, efficacy, and health outcome of patients through more effectively targeted risk assessment, prevention, and tailor-made medication and treatment managing approaches." According to European Commission, the term *personalized medicine* is a medical approach that intends to provide tailor-made prevention and treatments for specified groups of patients. Per the report of the National Health Service (NHS) of England, the conventional way of treatment using present methods of bulk manufacturing of medicines is found ineffective in 70% of the patients, creating a dire necessity for novel approaches in therapeutics to be tailor-made to individual patients.

Many patients have received the benefits of personalized medicine, and as a result, no less than 70 products are currently on the market [1]. The concept of personalized medicine has continuously been the aim for health care specialists; however, it is truly realizable with the current progress in technology. The emergence of the Human Genome Project, three-dimensional printing (3DP), artificial intelligence, and cutting-edge 3D scanning technology have pushed this novel idea to the forefront of medicine.

Among the various enabling technologies involved in personalized medicines, delivering therapy in a personalized way is of supreme significance. Knowing that dose adjustment or patient-specific fixed-dose recipe will serve as a foundation for improving drug delivery technologies. Various technologies such as patient-specific additive manufacturing or biomaterial-based controlled drug release will play a sheet-anchor role in personalized medicine. Tailor-made drug release tablets using 3DP have been newly initiated, with time-based drug release profiles that can be personalized [2].

The patient-specific drug delivery is a rapidly evolving area of pharmaceutical research. It is observed that patients with similar ailments may possibly have diverse complications that require diverse treatment options, such as taking medications at different times of the day. Moreover, the bioavailability profile of patients can be quite diverse, especially in adults compared to children or older adults, which questions the generally practiced concept of "one size fits all". Furthermore, patients suffering from orphan diseases sometimes cannot find medication with a suitable dose in the market because it is not commercially viable for pharmaceutical manufacturers [3–5].

Recently, "additive manufacturing" (AM), often known as the 3DP process, has gained noteworthy attention across many industries. It creates physical objects by sequential deposition of materials based on a computer-aided-design (CAD)–based geometrical model [6–8]. The dawn of 3DP technology and its application in the pharmaceutical field has led to a greater paradigm shift in the approaches of patient-centered treatment choices. The advancements of AM seen in the last decade showed a bright future of developing patient-specific oral drug delivery systems, spanning from delivering simple drug molecules to using biodegradable scaffolds for delivering protein drugs [9]. The major advantage of 3DP is to dispense medications at the point of care (PoC) in pharmacies and hospitals, where patient-specific formulations are tailored to have a specific shape, size, dose, and release profiles [4]. This is possible with 3DP, whereby a layer-by-layer deposition of materials using CAD software to achieve the desired output of products [5].

The drug delivery research has greatly progressed over the decades with a presently focusing on a targeted approach to improve the safety and efficacy aspects of the drugs [4, 10]. Drug delivery developments have gained growing attention as they can deal with highly personalized therapies via the designing of tailor-made drug release profiles. This review discusses in detail the importance of AM technologies in developing patient-specific drug delivery systems along with the current progress in patient-specific drug delivery encompassing various novel dosage formulations.

1.2 AM FOR DRIVING INNOVATION

AM technology, generally termed three-dimensional printing (3DP), uses a digital model based on CAD to build physical objects layer-by-layer. Because of its speedy fabrication process of making precise geometries of shapes, AM has gained notice-able attention in pharmaceutical and biomedical research [11].

The first 3D-printed medication, Spritam® (Aprecia Pharmaceuticals) got its first approval from the U.S. FDA in 2015, has directed augmented interest in following this platform for dosage form development. Spritam® (Levitracetam) is formulated with ZipDose® technology of Aprecia that conglomerates the precision of 3DP technology and dosage form science to create a rapid drug-releasing formulation. 3DP allows for the possibility of producing low-cost dosage forms on demand [12].

1.3 TRENDS IN PATIENT-SPECIFIC DRUG DELIVERY

The following trends are observed recently on patient-specific drug delivery, which can greatly influence on the future prospects of 3DP in the health industry [13].

1.3.1 PATIENT-CENTRIC THERAPEUTIC CARE

Recently, patient-specific medication has continued to trend the most, reflecting all aspects of therapeutics, including drug delivery. Most successful formulations for drug delivery are solid orals that can be easily swallowed and are more patient-friendly. Fast-melting, dissolving, and disintegrating tablets or gel-forming formulations are more acceptable to these special populations, such as pediatrics and geriatrics. For formulation technology, 3DP brought the versatility that is needed to rapidly develop novel dosage forms at a low cost. Now it is quite possible to formulate complex forms containing multiple active ingredients in single-dosage form and can customize the drug release profiles as per the individualized needs of the patients. The production of patient-specific dosage forms is much more flexible and can be done at a pharmacy or even at a patient's home in the future [14].

1.3.2 TAKING PROMPTS FROM OTHER FIELDS OF RESEARCH

Traditionally, pharmaceuticals and medical devices were developed for the majority of the population. Personalizing these devices offers great challenges to the pharmaceutical and medical device industries. One of the methods used by pharmaceutical companies to overcome these challenges is considering commercial manufacturers having decades of expertise in *en masse* customization, for example, automobiles, aeronautics, and others. This has been mainly made conceivable thanks to digitization and automation that can accelerate prototyping and allow small-scale manufacturing [15].

1.3.3 SMALL PHARMACEUTICAL COMPANIES SHOWING AN ADVANTAGE

Pharmaceutical and medical devices firms are the best examples of this idea. Although big manufacturing companies target general markets, small or start-up companies focusing on the personalized medicine market are better positioned to acquire the market of patient-centric treatments, and hence, bigger is not always better.

1.3.4 DECENTRALIZED MANUFACTURING

On-site or decentralized manufacturing means production at the physician's office, pharmacy, or hospital where the products will be instantly used for the benefit of the patient. The most popular examples of this concept relate to the medical devices industry, where a patient requires a customized device or a surgeon needs to make an organ tailored to a patient's body that is expected to operate. This trend is not limited to the medical field but is equally important to the pharmaceutical field. For example, Alder Hey's Children Hospital, U.K., is employing 3DP to create prototype pharmaceuticals [16]. Meanwhile, most medications are made for adult patients; it is difficult to titrate the doses for children using commercial medicines. By using 3DP, children can get accurate doses of medications.

1.4 AM TECHNOLOGIES

The term *AM* is used to designate innovative technologies to produce 3D objects rendered from CAD models. The 3DP was first initiated at the Massachusetts Institute of Technology (MIT), and later, it was licensed by various companies such as Z Corp, Soligen, Integra, Extrude Horn, Specific Surface, Therics, and TDK. The 3D models are created using the file formats with file extensions of .3ds, .ply, .stl, .wrl, and .zpr. In 2005, high-resolution 3D printers were first introduced by Z Corp, and its technology is commercially available in the market.

Popular AM technologies include, but are not limited to, the following: fused deposition modeling (FDM), inkjet printing (IJP), stereolithography (SLA), selective laser sintering (SLS), powder bed inkjet printing, electron beam direct manufacturing (EBM), and laminated object manufacturing (LOM). The American Society for Testing and Materials (ASTM) formulated the standards on AM, namely, "ASTM F42", that classify various AM processes into seven categories as shown in Table 1.1 [17–19].

1.4.1 VAT POLYMERIZATION

Vat polymerization (VP), also known as stereolithography (SLA) was invented in 1984 and patented in 1986 by Charles Hull. It uses a tank of liquid resin photopolymer, from which the 3D model is built layer by layer. The resin is cured by an ultraviolet (UV) light using motor-controlled mirrors, and a stage moves the prepared object downward once each photopolymer layer is cured and hardened. The process of the SLA (VP) technique has been demonstrated in Figure 1.1.

Micro-SLA is a variation of the conventional SLA technique in 1993 and is used in fabricating 3D tissue-engineered scaffolds to achieve biochemical and mechanical microarchitectures. This technology has become popular in preparing novel therapeutic drug carrier systems, such as microneedles, to deliver protein drugs across microporous skin structures [20]. The 3D microfabrication technology uses a composite gel and a laser beam, whereby the polymer gel layers touched by the laser beam harden the 3D object and the untreated gel is washed off [21]. Other popular technologies of vat polymerization are continuous layer interface production (CLIP)

TABLE 1.1

ASTM Standard AM Technologies [19]

AM category	Technologies	Feeding materials	Processing mechanism
Vat polymerization	Digital light processing (DLP), Stereolithography (SLA), Continuous layer interface production (CLIP)	Photopolymer fluid	UV light activated polymerization
Binder jetting (3DP)	Inkjet printing Powder bed inkjet. S-printing, ZipDose®, M-printing, Theriform™	Solid particles of polymers, metals, and ceramics	Liquid binder deposited to join solid particles
Material jetting	Drop on demand (DOD), multi-Jet, PolyJet	Solutions of photopolymers, waxy materials	Liquid polymers deposited and cured by ultraviolet light or heat
Powder bed fusion	Selective laser sintering or melting, selective heating melting, electron beam melting	Solid particles of polymers, metals, composites	Electron or Laser beam used to fuse solid particles by sintering
Material extrusion	Fused deposition modeling, syringe-based semisolid extrusion	Thermoplastic filament extrusion of polymers and composites	Heated materials selectively extrude through an orifice
Direct energy deposition	Laser-assisted direct manufacturing Direct metal tooling, laser energy net shaping, Be additive manufacturing, laser cladding, laser deposition welding	Metal or ceramic wires or particles	Laser generated thermal energy to fuse materials by melting while deposition
Sheet lamination	Laminated object manufacturing, solid foil polymerization, ultrasonic additive manufacturing, selective deposition lamination	Metal or ceramic sheets	Sheets and cut and bound to form objects

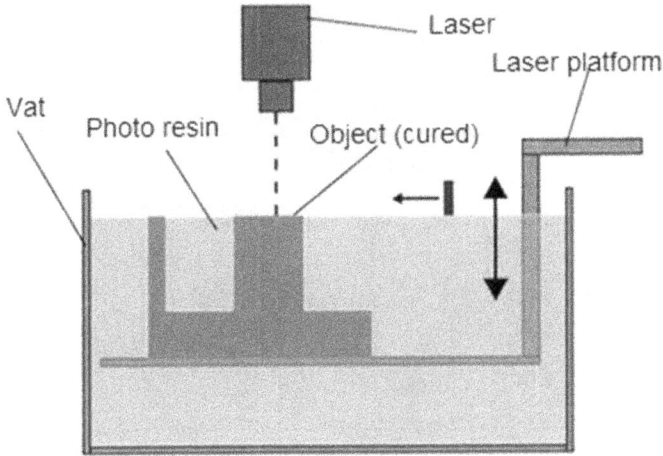

FIGURE 1.1 SLA technique showing a vat of liquid resin photopolymer from which the 3D model is built layer by layer and cured by UV light [18].

and digital light processing (DLP). VP is highly accurate, creates a fine finishing, and is a comparatively quicker process. But it is expensive, it takes a long time for post-processing, and limited photo-resins are available for use. It also requires support structures and postprocess curing for structural integrity.

1.4.2 BINDER JETTING

It is well known as "powder bed inkjet printing", the binder jetting (BJ) process employs powder materials and a binder solution. The binder is used as an adhesive for the powder layers. First, a layer of powder of a specified thickness is placed, and a print head of binder solution is moved along the X and Y axes, depositing the liquid binder onto the powder layer. This process is repetitive until a specific 3D shape is achieved. Supporting materials are not needed for BJ printing, and the powder itself is auto-supported within the powder bed. The unbound powder can be removed once the object is printed. The BJ process is shown in Figure 1.2.

IJP is a fast, simple, cost-effective, and noncontact configuration approach that has wide applications in nanobiomaterials fabrication. The IJP technique is analogous to drop-on-demand (DOD) mode, whereby it can dispense high-precision polymer (binder) solutions for therapeutic drug delivery and cell culturing. Thus, it is gaining popularity in the formulation of pharmaceutical dosage forms. Incorporating active ingredients, such as biomolecules, drugs, vitamins, and sensors, into the formulation, this technology has greatly stimulated its application in the advanced therapeutic drug delivery and the food additives industries. The resulted formulations can offer controlled release of active ingredients at the targeted site. Multiple active compounds can be incorporated into various layers of the dosage form, thus offering a pulsatile release of drugs. Additives can be introduced into the polymer layers by

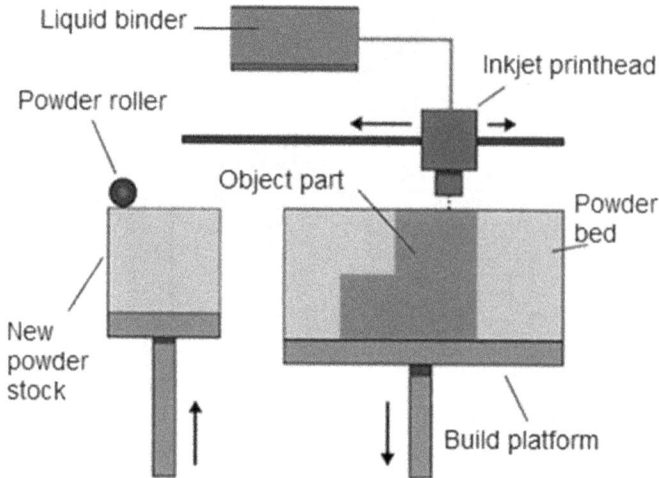

FIGURE 1.2   BJ technique showing deposition of liquid binder on the powder layer repeatedly until a specific 3D shape is achieved [18].

solvent/film-casting and injection molding [22]. The printers widely used for IJP are NanoPlotter® from GeSim and Z402® from Z Corp [11].

A novel approach to solvent-free inkjet printing is organic vapor jet printing (OVJP) recently developed by Shtein et al [23]. In contrast to conventional inkjet printing, it doesn't require liquids to dissolve the active pharmaceutical ingredients (APIs), making it attractive for direct printing of APIs without solvents [24–25]. Shalev et al. demonstrated that OVJP can deposit nanofilms of APIs, including paracetamol, fluorescein, caffeine, ibuprofen, and tamoxifen [26].

Another variation of bonding-based IJP was developed at MIT whereby a binder material is deposited over a layer of powder bed. The particles are joined by the binder, another powder layer is generated, and the binder material is deposited again in a sequential manner. After the completion of the process, the excess powder is removed, and the porous model is toughened using a sintering process. This technique finds application in porous scaffolding and tissue molding using polylactide-co-glycolide (PLGA) polymer.

The bio-IJP technique is another variant created from the idea of cell printing, which was proposed by Yan et al. [27]. This process is used for printing the living human organs. It can print cells or matrices. In this method, bio-inks, such as hydrogels and thermo-reversible smart polymers, are printed using heat-activated or piezo-electric printer heads to print living cells or proteins.

Nanoimprint lithography (NIL) is a rapid technique used to fabricate nanostructures of site-specific, enzymatically triggered smart particles for drug delivery and imaging agents [28–29]. Banu et al. employed NIL to prepare optically programmed microparticles that were used to attach molecular tags [30].

1.4.3 MATERIAL JETTING

Material jetting (MJ) creates objects in a similar manner to that of IJP. Material is jetted horizontally across a platform, where it hardens while building the object layer by layer using continuous or DOD method. The process involved in the MJ technique is shown in Figure 1.3. The material layers are cured by UV light. The availability of the materials is limited for MJ. Polymers and waxes are suitable for MJ due to their rheology and ability to form droplets. The process is highly accurate of droplet deposition and avoids wastage of materials. Thermojet® and Polyjet® are commercial technologies that use MJ [11]. Thermal inkjet (TIJ) printing uses an electrical current that is transferred to a resistor for creating heat. Small air bubbles that are produced by heating the print-head are collapsed to produce pulses of pressure to spout the ink droplets of size 10–150 pL from the nozzle. When the ink bubble impinges on the paper surface, it is converted into a solid and binds to the paper directly. This technique can't be used for structural parts, and additional postprocessing is needed. As TIJ uses high temperatures, it may degrade thermo-labile substances [31]. It is popularly used to dispense extemporaneous preparations of drugs onto 3D drug carriers such as pellets. Nanosuspensions of folic acid and rasagiline are prepared using this technique [32–33]. Polymer jetting uses a Polyjet® printer akin to an inkjet printer, which works based on PolyJet® technology. In this technique, a photopolymer is deposited in a thin layer on the substrate, and an UV lamp alongside it hardens each layer instantly.

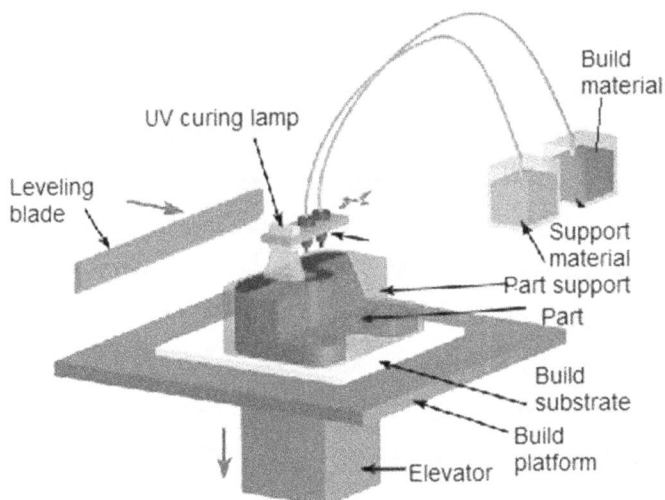

Copyright: © 2008 CustomPartNet

FIGURE 1.3 MJ technique showing material deposition layer by layer across a platform where it is solidified by UV light [34]

1.4.4 POWDER BED FUSION

The powder bed fusion (PBF) process comprises of various techniques: selective laser melting or sintering (SLM or SLS), selective heat sintering (SHS), direct metal laser sintering (DMLS), and electron beam melting (EBM) [35]. In PBF methods, an electron or laser beam in vacuum condition is employed to sinter or fuse the layers of powder materials, such as metals and alloys. The PBF technique has been demonstrated in Figure 1.4. SHS differs from other techniques in which a heated print head is used to sinter the powder material. SLM uses laser beams for melting materials to make highly dense objects formed through a layer-by-layer manner [36]. PBF is relatively less expensive, suitable for visual models. The powder itself acts as support material. However, this method is slower, has size limitations, and uses a lot of electricity, and the product finish depends on the particle size.

1.4.5 MATERIAL EXTRUSION

Material extrusion (ME), well known as fused deposition modeling (FDM) or hot-melt extrusion (HME), is a common process trademarked by Stratasys in the 1980s [11]. The material is converted into a filament and pushed through a preheated nozzle, melted, extruded, and deposited as thin continuous layers under constant pressure. The nozzle moves on X and Y axes, and the platform base moves vertically on the Z axis to deposit the material. The material layers are fused by temperature control or by chemical treatment. The process involved in the FDM technology has been shown in Figure 1.5. FDM is a popular technique, highly economical, used for making intricate models and prototypes. Critical factors are nozzle diameter, constant

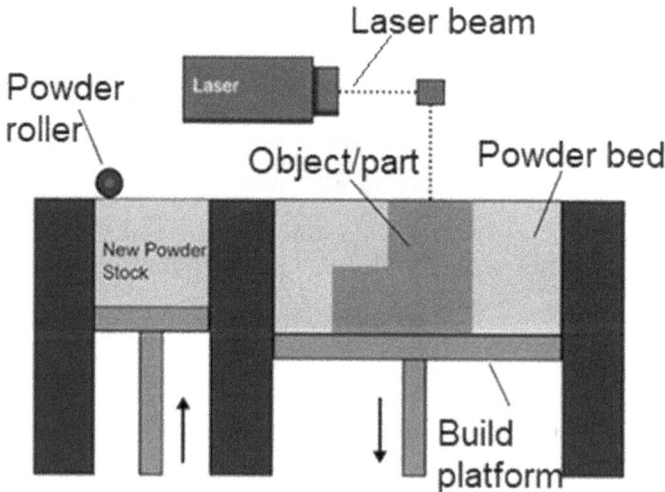

FIGURE 1.4 PBF technique showing the use of an electron beam or a laser to sinter the layers of powder materials [18].

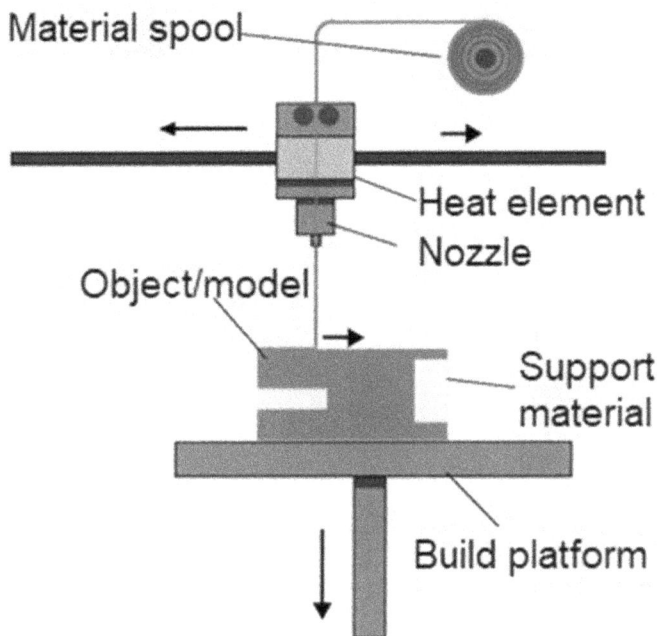

FIGURE 1.5 ME technique showing a filament of material drawn through a heated nozzle, where it is extruded and deposited as thin layers until an object is formed [18].

extrusion pressure, layer thickness, and temperature and will influence the quality and finish of the product. Other input materials used to extrude include pastes and gels, which are popularly used for drug delivery formulations. FDM is used to make various solid dosage forms, such as implants and tablets having various geometries, that are multilayered and fast-dissolving [37]. Several advantages are offered by the FDM method for fabricating patient-specific dosage forms. It is used to produce specific shapes of amorphous drugs, whereby their stability can be overcome by quick evaporation of solvent from the formulation and co-melting process of the drug with the polymer [38].

The pressure-assisted microsyringe (PAM) technique is akin to FDM but melting the materials is not required. In the PAM technique, a viscous material is passed through a syringe to create the desired 3D model [39]. Low pressure is applied to release the dissolved polymer from a viscous liquid. Drying and solidification are done subsequently to achieve sufficient strength for the prepared dosage form [40].

1.4.6 DIRECT ENERGY DEPOSITION

Directed energy deposition (DED), well known as "electron beam direct manufacturing", has various terminologies such as laser engineered net-shaping (LENS), 3D laser cladding, directed light fabrication (DLF), and direct metal deposition (DMD).

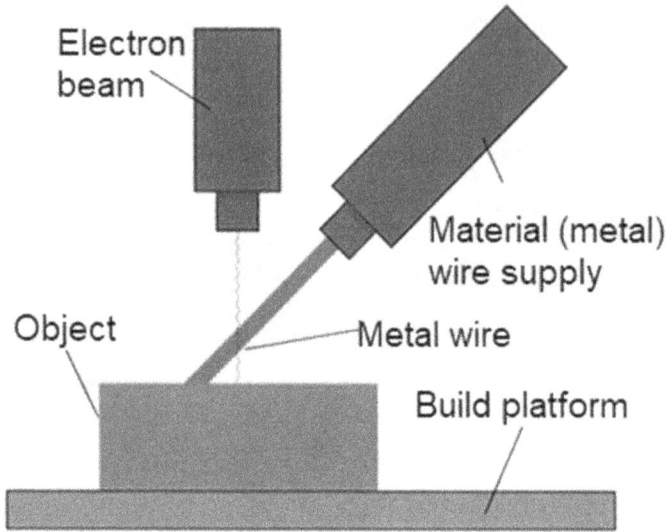

FIGURE 1.6 DED technique showing material being melted by laser beam and then deposited layer by layer to make an object [18].

DED is a complex method in which the nozzle moves in multiple directions to deliver molten materials such as polymers, metals, or ceramics using a laser beam [41]. The materials can be in the form of wire or powder. The process involved in the DED technique has been demonstrated in Figure 1.6. Other variations of this technique are Be AM (BeAM) and direct metal tooling (DMT). It has yet to be explored in the pharmaceutical field.

1.4.7 SHEET LAMINATION

The sheet lamination (SL) method includes various processes: laminated object manufacturing (LOM), ultrasonic AM (UAM), and selective deposition lamination (SDL). LOM employs a layer-by-layer sheet deposition method and often uses paper as feed material and adhesive for bonding the sheets. Figure 1.7 shows the process involved in the SL technique. Aesthetic objects are usually made using LOM and this method is not suitable for structural objects. UAM uses sheets/ribbons of various metals or paper that are bound by low-energy ultrasonic welding. This method also needs computerized numerical control postprocessing to remove unbound materials. The strength of models is dependent on the adhesive used [42].

1.5 AM IN PATIENT-SPECIFIC DRUG DELIVERY SYSTEMS

A patient-specific medication involves introducing a dosage form into a patient's body to attain a specific biological outcome to treat a certain disease. These dosage forms are classified based on the route of administration. AM has transformed the

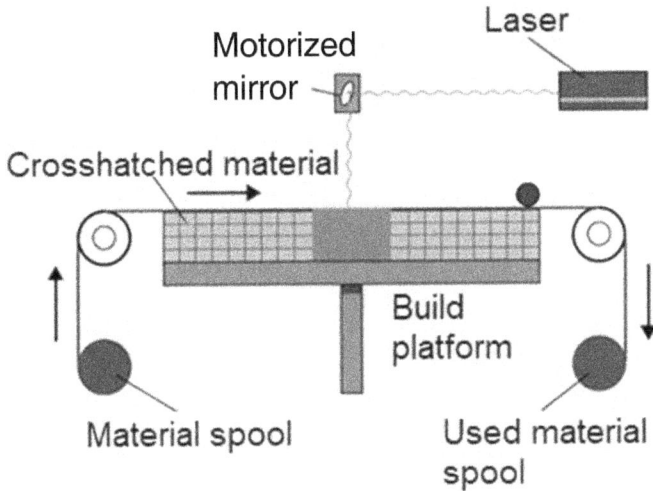

FIGURE 1.7 SL technique showing sheet metal or paper being built layer by layer using an adhesive, laser, or ultrasonic welding [18].

drug delivery towards patient-specific medication. The workflow of patient-specific drug delivery is presented in Figure 1.8 [19]. A classic patient-specific drug delivery begins with a laboratory checkup that includes a computed tomography (CT) or magnetic resonance imaging (MRI) scan that suggests information concerning the present condition of the patient and the dosage form design requirements aimed to achieve desired patient-specific therapeutics and timed-drug release parameters. Using AM technology, it is possible to provide patient-specific medication and programmed drug-release profiles. Based on these data, we can create a CAD model by which using AM the drug-loaded formulation can be administered into various routes like oral solid dosage forms, parenteral/vaginal/rectal devices, transdermal patches, implants, and scaffolds for drug delivery. Based on the patient's age, gender, weight, genetic profile, and disease condition, an optimized dose can be delivered using AM technology. Currently, there exists the unexplored potential of AM drug-delivery devices that offer patient-specific therapeutics, and there is much research is underway to materialize this process [43].

Recent research focuses on high drug loading and patient-specific medications and alternative drug delivery systems, such as buccal patches, transdermal patches, biodegradable implants, and oral delivery systems, when traditional commercial approaches can't provide such customization of medication. Much research is underway on the process of formulating oral and transdermal delivery systems using AM technologies [44]. The most prominent technologies employed in such studies are FDM, SLA, BJ, powder bed IJP, and semisolid extrusion [45–46]. Among such AM technologies, the powder extrusion method was successfully applied for formulating amorphous solid printlets of itraconazole, which can remove the necessity of the tedious and time-consuming process of FDM technology [47]. More recently,

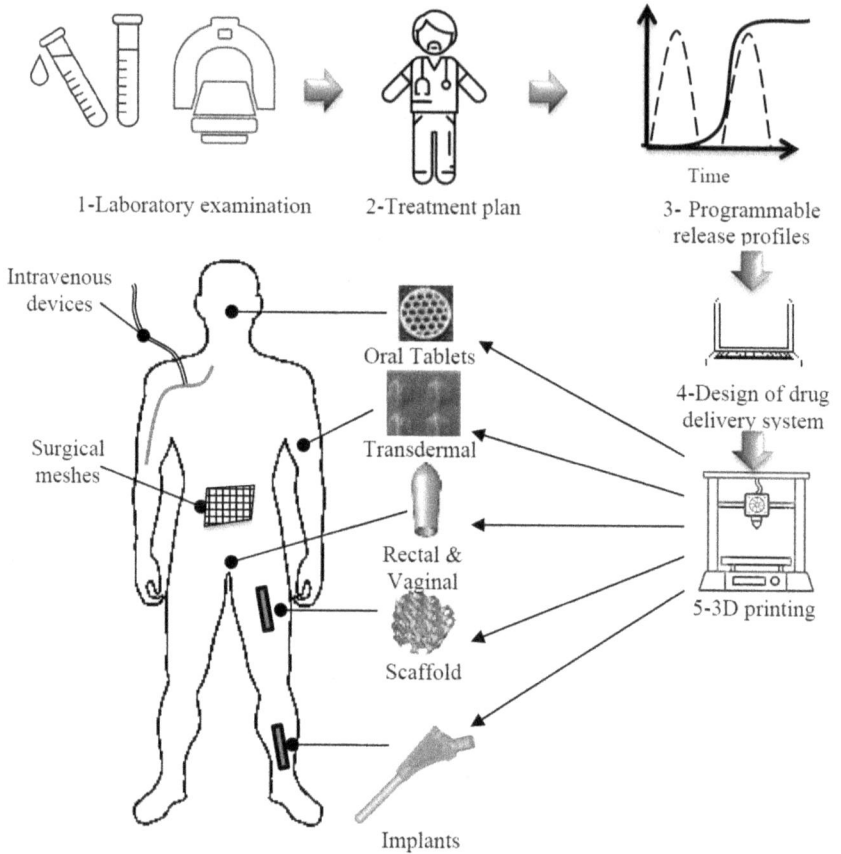

FIGURE 1.8   Workflow of AM drug delivery systems via various routes of administration [19].

Vithani *et al.* reported the ability of AM to formulate lipid-based drug delivery devices for lipophilic drugs [48]. AM has advantages of flexibility of materials selection that paves greater application in multidrug therapeutics. Recently Pereira *et al.* formulated a poly-pill of four different cardiovascular drugs [49]. Awad *et al.* made the successful formulation of 3D-printed mini-printlets that contain paracetamol and ibuprofen that are separated in the formulation [50].

1.5.1   ORAL DOSAGE FORMULATIONS

Oral solid dosage forms are considered the oldest and the most renowned drug formulations and are cheap, noninvasive, and easy to use by patients. Several dosage forms exist such as pills, tablets, capsules, lozenges, pellets, and films. However, the fixed-dose combination therapy (FDCT) in which two drugs are placed in a single tablet. This may not offer patient-specific dosage flexibility. Moreover, poly-therapy might worsen medication adherence, which may cause further deterioration of the health of patients. A single patient-specific formulation that combines all the drugs needed for patients with chronic diseases can considerably improve adherence to treatment and patient compliance. By using AM technologies, multiple drugs can be administered in a formulation of tailor-made shape, size, and desired drug release profiles by avoiding traditional methods [51–52].

Although there has been pronounced progress in drug delivery methods, oral delivery still remains the favored choice of physicians and patients because of the reason that it is quite safer, patient-compliant, and economical. Thus there is huge research under progress on oral solid dosage forms on personalization of medicines [53–54]. AM also helps in realizing multidrug recipes with complex drug release profiles [3]. On-demand formulation of tailor-made patient-specific drug delivery systems having selective geometry, design, and shape can be easily achieved using AM, which until has been now very difficult to achieve using conventional manufacturing technologies. There are some limitations of AM technologies, including producing porous structures and uneven shapes in dosage forms [55]. The FDM technology can only produce dosage forms for thermostable drugs using few compatible excipients till today. When using SLA, there is a chance of drug degradation when exposed to UV light, which is used to induce the polymerization reaction [56].

AM was successful in formulating sublingual, orodispersible, fast-disintegrating/dissolving, and immediate-release dosage forms [57–60]. Flexible therapeutic dosage forms that offer tailored recipes of drugs, doses, and preferred release kinetics have attracted the attention of researchers because of the advantages offered by these patient-specific dosage forms. Many researchers have fabricated modified-release patient-specific dosage forms employing AM technologies. In a study, HME and FDM were employed to produce various shapes, such as cylinders, spheres, tori, cubes, and pyramids, of paracetamol tablet formulations. It was noticed that the drug release was independent of the surface area of the tablet and dependent on "surface area–to–volume ratio", showing influence of different shapes on the drug-dissolution kinetics, and the controlled drug release was mediated by erosion mechanism [61]. This shows how various shapes of tablets modify the drug release kinetics and thereby assist in designing novel dosage forms with precise pharmacokinetic characteristics directed to different absorption sites of gastrointestinal tract (GIT). Thus, AM is proving to be the most promising technology for patient-specific drug delivery.

1.5.2 Parenteral Devices

Parenteral devices are used to deliver drugs via an intravenous (IV) route of administration using a catheter or a needle. AM research on IV devices was focused on customized catheters for local delivery of drugs. Drug-coated catheters are being manufactured to prevent infections. Antimicrobial coatings have been proved to prevent bacterial adherence on to the surface of catheters [62]. In conventional coating processes, an antimicrobial agent at 2% w/w concentration prevents a bacterial attack, whereas the 3DP catheter tips showed antimicrobial effect at low concentrations of 1% w/w, thereby proving the technological advantage of AM [63]. As the medical devices and pharmaceutical industries are aimed at patient-specific devices and medications, the future road map of AM can use medical imaging techniques to design patient-specific devices for 3DP purposes. Based on published data, FDM technology has gained prominence in catheter manufacturing with a promising future [64]. Nevertheless, the use of SLS technology could be possible in future research

HME is also a favored method due to the advantage of reducing waste of organic solvents and its environmentally friendly nature [65]. Alhijjaj *et al.* explored the potential of HME using an FDM printer for formulating modified drug release objects of polymer blends of Eudragit and polyvinyl alcohol (PVA) with polyethylene oxide (PEO), polyethylene glycol (PEG), and Tween 80 [66]. In another study, patient-specific wound dressings of antibacterial metal ions were formulated showing the potential of HME technology [67]. Furthering its advantage, Melocchi *et al.* successfully extruded the filaments of PEO, EC, Eudragit RL100, and PVA and subsequently printed them as discs using an FDM printer [68]. The HME method can be employed for a spectrum of polymers to make filaments with different physical properties for suitable pharmaceutical applications [69]. A detailed review on patient-specific drug delivery related to 3DP dosage form design, and several novel applications have recently reviewed by Dumpa *et al.* [70].

1.5.3 IMPLANTS AND SCAFFOLDS

Since the dawn of AM technologies, research in dentistry has been revolutionized by focusing on fabricating patient-specific dental prosthetics, artificial teeth, and fractured bones [71–72]. AM is also being explored to fabricate tissue scaffolds for bone-graft procedures. In periodontology, AM is used for making patient-specific bioabsorbable fiber-guided scaffolds, sinus and bone augmentation, socket preservation, implant placement, and maintenance in periodontal defects [73]. Lei *et al.* prepared a guided tissue regeneration (GTR) membrane embedded with platelet-rich fibrin that was intended for severe bone defects [74]. Rasperini *et al.* fabricated bioresorbable scaffolds for periodontal repairs [75]. PLGA is the most prospective polymer in scaffold fabrication for guided bone regeneration.

Stents coated with biocompatible and biodegradable scaffolds containing drugs can serve as drug delivery systems, especially for antimicrobials. For the past few years, significant research is going on for tailor-made patient-specific biocompatible scaffolds loaded with antimicrobials, which are designed to be used to stimulate bone recovery and avoid infections [76].

Surgical meshes are woven structures to form sheets that are made from inorganic biocompatible materials. They can be temporary or permanent (biodegradable). Hence, investigators are working on developing innovative surgical meshes recently [77]. Cox *et al.* used AM to fabricate titanium-based antibiotic-eluting implants [78]. Hassanin *et al.* chose the SLM process for titanium drug-delivery implants that release the drug through micro-channels [79]. Drug coated implants, scaffolds, and meshes were fabricated using AM technology to add clinical functionality of preventing or healing an infection or to lessen the pain [80].

Rectal administration of medications has been in practice for centuries, especially as a recommended route of administration for children, older adults, and comatose and dysphagic patients. Various rectal dosage forms are present such as suppositories, creams, ointments, and gels. Similarly, vaginal local drug delivery systems, like pessaries, tablets, gels, solutions, and vaginal rings, are available in the market for various etiologies [81]. Recent research has shown the fabrication of several patient-specific rectal and vaginal rectal devices with different shapes and tailored drug-eluting mechanisms employing AM [82–83].

1.5.4 TRANSDERMAL DEVICES

Transdermal patches are used to deliver drugs systemically through the skin. Traditional manufacturing methods to achieve high-throughput production compete with the requirements of patient-specific doses [84]. In other words, transdermal dosage forms can be manufactured in a faster and continuous way while addressing patient-specific dosages simultaneously. Transdermal thin-film patches and microneedles are used to deliver the drugs systemically [85], whereas local drug delivery is achieved by coatings on drug delivery vehicles, such as wafers and rods [72]. Film-forming drug delivery devices are also used for both oral and transmucosal drug delivery and for facilitating rapid drug release and absorption into the systemic circulation. Conventionally the films are prepared by dispersing drug in polymer matrix and followed by extrusion or film-casting methods. General approaches of film formation suffer from limitations of stability and drug loading. Microneedle patches are potential formulations used to deliver drugs through the transdermal route. The SLA microfabrication technique has been used to fabricate microneedle patches with high resolution (1–25 µm) [86], although it has been primarily employed to fabricate micro parts using ceramics and polymers and ceramics [87–88]. However, SLA needs various fabrication steps and customized equipment to make micro objects. Drug-coated and drug-eluting microneedles were fabricated using AM, which offers several advantages over conventional microfabrication methods [89–90].

1.6 4D DRUG DELIVERY SYSTEMS

New research is under progress in the area of 3DP on novel materials that are capable to alter their properties influenced by external factors with respect to time. Such structural modification of 3D objects over time, which is known as the fourth dimension, led to new technology, termed "4D printing" [91]. Thus, a fourth dimension, called time, has been introduced in the 4DP methods. The 4DP products have the capability of self-fold or unfold by altering their configurations such as shape, property, or functionality. In pharmaceutical applications of drug delivery, the well-timed drug release profiles could be activated by stimuli, such as body temperature, time, pH, and/or enzymatic action [92].

Intelligent, responsive, or smart materials elicit a programmed change in physicochemical properties when exposed to specific external stimuli. Two types of smart materials are employed in 4DP for pharmaceuticals, such as hydrogels and shape memory polymers (SMPs). SMPs are already being used in conventional pharmaceutical research for drug delivery. Hydrogels swell and change their morphology when exposed to solvents such as water by the diffusion process, causing swelling, whereas SMPs react to certain stimuli, such as pH, UV light, or temperature. SMPs adopt a short-term configuration until their exposure to external stimuli and recover to permanent shapes. When a smart material is exposed to a stimulus, the temperature rises to glass transition temperature (Tg). Below Tg, the polymer is in glassy state, and above Tg, it transforms into a flexible rubbery state by causing alterations in structural morphology. The polymer recovers to its relaxed state if the temperature falls below Tg. Taking advantage of this behavior of SMPs, dynamic stents capable of deforming at physiological temperature when inserted into the body of the patient are fabricated [93]. Hence, 4DP offers the fabrication of patient-specific customized stents of precise shapes and sizes can be prepared timely and cost-effectively. Yi *et al.* fabricated an AM local drug delivery membrane aimed for growth suppression in pancreatic cancer [94].

In another interesting study, remote-controllable 3DP stents with magnetically responsive iron oxide and thermo-responsive PLA. These thermo-responsive SMP-magnetic stents offer patient-specific application and have the ability to be remotely controlled [95–96]. While programming a 4DP object, certain critical issues, such as the structure orientation of SMPs within the product, should be carefully considered [93].

Based on the drug delivery mechanism, SMP objects can be classified as bio-adhesive and encapsulating devices. A trilayered mucoadhesive device was fabricated that has a pH-sensitive outer hydrogel layer. At pH 6.5, this device fixes onto the intestinal wall and releases the drug into mucosal layers in a controlled manner [97]. Another research study showed the fabrication of thermo-responsive drug-eluting devices called "theragrippers". These devices having multiple arms get spontaneously attached onto the tissues when the temperature reaches above 32 °C and can release the drug constantly up to 7 days [98]. Magnetic-responsive hydrogels were prepared that could be controlled remotely to reach the target site and can be useful for site-specific drug delivery and guided surgical procedures [99]. Self-folding micro containers were fabricated in which yeast cells and pancreatic β-cells and fibroblasts are entrapped [100]. These containers release the contents when exposed to programmed temperatures [101]. The lithography technique was used to fabricate bilayered micro-robots, having a pH-sensitive layer and a magnetic iron oxide-polymeric layer for anticancer therapy [102].

4DP is still in a growing stage in pharmaceutical research due to its novelty. Recently, intravesical bladder retentive devices using SMPs were fabricated [103]. The SMPs are programmed to have temporary configuration until introduced into the bladder. When the devices reach the bladder, they transform back to permanent shape, thus permitting them to be retained in the bladder and provide localized, prolonged drug delivery. Although 4DP is in its primitive stage, pharmaceutical scientists can revive it by creating devices that were hitherto challenging to fabricate.

1.7   REGULATORY INSIGHTS

The U.S. FDA has published guidance on pharmacogenomic data submissions, which will allow medications to be patient-specific, thereby maximizing therapeutic benefits and minimizing potential risks for every patient [104].

There is a need to develop policies on patient-specific medicine involving the Center for Devices and Radiological Health and the Center for Biologics Evaluation and Research, and many obstacles should be aligned with the U.S. FDA [105]. While the U.S. FDA is interested in revising regulatory structures, certain uncertainties in regulations are dragging the financial investments in the 3DP field. Personalized medicine labeling requires several experts to develop a robust knowledge base [106]. The European Union regulatory framework is working on several tools and guidelines toward the commercialization of personalized medication [107]. The clinical trials regulations are being simplified to conduct clinical trials and thereby facilitating research on personalized medicines. University College London has partnered with UK-based company FabRx, which is working on patient-specific medicines and devices using 3DP technologies. They recently conducted the world's first clinical trials, in which 3DP was incorporated in hospital pharmacy to fabricate patient-specific isoleucine formulations for children suffering from rare metabolic maple syrup urine disease [108]. These advancements demonstrate the potential benefits of AM, and there is a need for advancing this technology from the academic world to real-world benefits for the patients.

1.8 DECENTRALIZATION OF PRODUCTION USING AM

Currently, patient-specific compounding and dispensing are in practice in hospital and community pharmacies across the world. The same way 3DP technology can be easily introduced into compounding, thus making decentralized production of patient-specific formulations is not a difficult task. Using the right quality API-loaded filaments and patient-specific CAD, the FDM technology can be successfully used to achieve pharmaceutical compounding in hospitals and pharmacies. Pharmacists can take advantage of AM technologies to print patient-specific dosage forms with complex shapes and predefined architecture in a cost-effective manner [109].

1.9 CHALLENGES

Self-printing of dosage forms by a pharmacist is clinically beneficial to patients in many aspects. FDM 3D printers are economical, available as open sources, and can be easily built at a cheaper cost. Thermoplastic filaments made from pharmaceutical-grade polymers, such as PLA, PVA, EVA, and cellulose derivatives, can offer printing of patient-specific dosage forms using several drugs [100, 110–111].

Presently, commercial 3DPs do not follow global manufacturing practices (GMP) requirements. Furthermore, regulating the use of 3DP in clinical settings, such as hospitals or local pharmacies, remains an unmet need. The quality and safety issues of drugs printed at home are two important challenges to implementing 3DP. To minimize this risk, proper training should be given to implement this technology in remote settings.

Furthermore, there is a risk of combining multiple APIs within a single formulation can lead to adverse effects of poly-pills. In order to develop ideal 3DP for formulations, there is a need for greater collaboration among excipient suppliers, printer manufacturers, and scientist and pharmaceutical regulators [111]. Other challenges that can be addressed by 3DP is counterfeit medicines. To overcome this issue, researchers have developed a computerized track-and-trace system in which QR codes using smart inks are used to print directly on acetaminophen-loaded tablets [112].

Numerous production facilities add technological and logistics challenges to ensure the uniformity of dosage forms due to multiple variables that influence the processing such as 3DPs, the source of raw materials, and operation conditions [4]. Hence, there is a necessity for suitable quality control measurements, such as using PAT, colorimetry [113–114], NIR spectroscopy [115–116], and Raman spectroscopy [117], to screen the performance of dosage forms in order to fulfill the regulatory requirements.

1.10 CONCLUSION

Although 3DP is today in the developmental stage in the pharmaceutical field, the transformation to 4D may be possible in near future. Using smart polymers can offer a novel targeted drug delivery that can be used for patient-specific needs, stimulating the digital revolution in health care, more specifically for drug delivery applications. With complementary support from U.S. FDA, funding agencies, and research collaborations, developing cutting-edge complex formulations using AM will accelerate innovations in the health care industry. Presently, there are few technical and quality control challenges, which may delay the advancement of AM technologies for patient-specific drug delivery. AM will soon come out with the proof-of-concept stage and prove to be a widely accepted manufacturing tool for patient-specific drug delivery with a multitude of prospective benefits. It is expected that after establishing the ideal 3DP platform, the time will come very soon to commence a new era in health care, and we can see 3DP occupying every pharmacy in the future.

REFERENCES

1. M.A. Hamburg and F.S. Collins, The path to personalized medicine, *N. Engl. J. Med.* 363 (2010), pp. 301–304.
2. Y. Sun and Soh. S, Printing tablets with fully customizable release profiles for personalized medicine, *Adv. Mater.* 27 (2015), pp. 7847–7853.
3. N. Sandler and M. Preis, Printed drug-delivery systems for improved patient treatment, *Trends Pharmacol. Sci.* 37 (2016), pp. 1070–1080.
4. S.J. Trenfield, A. Awad, A. Goyanes, S. Gaisford and A.W. Basit, 3D printing pharmaceuticals: Drug development to frontline care, *Trends Pharmacol. Sci.* 39 (2018), pp. 440–451.
5. F.M. Mwema and E.T. Akinlabi, Basics of fused deposition modelling (FDM), in *Fused Deposition Modeling, SpringerBriefs in Applied Sciences and Technology*, Springer, Cham, 2020. https://doi.org/10.1007/978-3-030-48259-6_1
6. V.R. Kulkarni, A. Lu and M. Maniruzzaman, 3D printing in personalized drug delivery, *American Pharmaceutical Review* (2021). www.americanpharmaceuticalreview.com/Featured-Articles/573677-3D-Printing-in-Personalized-Drug-Delivery/
7. N. Shahrubudin, T.C. Lee and R. Ramlan, An overview on 3D printing technology: Technological, materials, and applications, *Procedia Manuf.* 35 (2019), pp. 1286–1296.

8. A. Radhakrishnan, G. Kuppusamy, S. Ponnusankar and N.K. Shanmukhan, Pharmacogenomic phase transition from personalized medicine to patient-centric customized delivery, *Pharmacogenomics J.* 20 (2020), pp. 1–8.

9. R. Thakkar, A.R. Pillai, J. Zhang, Y. Zhang, V. Kulkarni and M. Maniruzzaman, Novel on-demand 3-dimensional (3-d) printed tablets using fill density as an effective release-controlling tool, *Polymers (Basel).* 12 (2020), 1–21.

10. K. Liang, S. Carmone, D. Brambilla and J-C. Leroux, 3D printing of a wearable personalized oral delivery device: A first-in-human study. *Sci. Adv.* 4 (2018), p. eaat2544. https://doi.org/10.1126/sciadv.aat2544.

11. P. Katakam, B. Dey, F.H. Assaleh, N.T. Hwisa, S.K. Adiki, B.R. Chandu and A. Mitra, Top-down and bottom-up approaches in 3d printing technologies for drug delivery challenges, *Crit. Rev. Ther. Drug Carrier Syst.* 32 (2015), pp. 61–87.

12. E. Mathew, G. Pitzanti, E. Larrañeta and D.A. Lamprou, 3D printing of pharmaceuticals and drug delivery devices, *Pharmaceutics* 12 (2020), p. 266.

13. S. Beale, 3 Personalized medicine trends for 2020, 2020. www.mastercontrol.com/gxp-lifeline/3-personalized-medicine-trends-for-2020/

14. F. Thomas, Demand for custom dosage forms fuels innovation, *Pharm. Tech.* 44 (2020) pp. 16–20.

15. V. Holt, Five expert insights into digital manufacturing and mass customization, *Industry Week*, 2018. www.industryweek.com/technology-and-and-iiot/article/22025978/five-expert-insights-into-digital-manufacturing-and-mass-customization

16. 3D printed pills could enable doctors to tailor medication for children, *Alder Hey Children's Hospital, UK*, 2018. https://alderhey.nhs.uk/contact-us/press-office/latest-news/3d-printed-pills-could-enable-doctors-tailor-medication-children

17. ISO/ASTM52900–15, *Standard Terminology for Additive Manufacturing—General Principles—Terminology*, ASTM International, West Conshohocken, PA, 2015. www.astm.org/Standards/ISOASTM52900.htm

18. The 7 categories of additive manufacturing, *Additive Manufacturing Research Group*, Loughborough University, UK, 2012. www.lboro.ac.uk/research/amrg/about/the7categoriesofadditivemanufacturing/

19. A. Mohammed, A. Elshaer, P. Sareh, M. Elsayed and H. Hassanin, Additive manufacturing technologies for drug delivery applications, *Int. J. Pharm.* 580 (2020), p. 119245.

20. F.P.W. Melchels, J. Feijen and D.W. Grijpma, A review on stereolithography and its applications in biomedical engineering, *Biomaterials* 31 (2010), pp. 6121–6130.

21. A. Nishiguchi, A. Mourran, H. Zhang and M. Möller, In-gel direct laser writing for 3d-designed hydrogel composites that undergo complex self-shaping, *Adv. Sci.* 5 (2018), p. 1700038.

22. A. Pimpin and W. Srituravanich. Review on micro and nano lithography techniques and their applications, *Eng. J.* 16 (2011), pp. 37–56.

23. M. Shtein, P. Peumans, J.B. Benziger and S.R. Forrest, Direct mask-free patterning of molecular organic semiconductors using organic vapor jet printing, *J. Appl. Phys.* 96 (2004), p. 4500.

24. N. Sandler, A. Määttänen, P. Ihalainen, L. Kronberg, A. Meierjohann, T. Viitala *et al.*, Inkjet printing of drug substances and use of porous substrates-towards individualized dosing, *J. Pharm. Sci.* 100 (2011), pp. 3386–3395.

25. R. Daly, T.S. Harrington, G.D. Martin and I.M. Hutchings, Inkjet printing of pharmaceuticals – a review of research and manufacturing, *Int. J. Pharm.* 494 (2015), pp. 554–567.

26. S. Raghavan, J.M. Mazzara, N. Senabulya, P.D. Sinko, E. Fleck, C. Rockwell *et al.*, Printing of small molecular medicines from the vapor phase, *Nat. Commun.* 8 (2017), p. 711.

27. K.C. Yan, K. Paluch, K. Nair and W. Sun, Effects of process parameters on cell damage in a 3d cell printing process, Proceedings of the ASME International Mechanical Engineering Congress and Exposition, 2009 November 13–19. Lake Buena Vista, FL. New York: ASME, 2009, pp. 75–81.

28. X.F. Cui, T. Boland, D.D. D'Lima and M.K. Lotz, Thermal inkjet printing in tissue engineering and regenerative medicine, *Recent Pat. Drug. Deliv. Formul.* 6 (2012), pp. 149–155.

29. K.R. Kam and T.A. Desai, Nano- and microfabrication for overcoming drug delivery challenges, *J. Mater. Chem. B Mater. Biol. Med.* 1;14 (2013), pp. 1878–1884.

30. S. Banu, S. Birtwell, G. Galitonov, Y. Chen, N. Zheludev and Y. Morgan, Fabrication of diffraction encoded micro-particles using nano-imprint lithography, *J. Micromech. Microeng.* 17 (2007), pp. S116–S121.

31. A.B.M. Buanz, M.H. Saunders, A.W. Basit and S. Gaisford, Preparation of personalized-dose salbutamol sulphate oral films with thermal inkjet printing, *Pharm. Res.* 28 (2011), pp. 2386–2392.

32. N. Genina, E.M. Janßen, A. Breitenbach, J. Breitkreutz and N. Sandler, Evaluation of different substrates for inkjet printing of rasagiline mesylate, *Eur. J. Pharm. Biopharm.* 85 (2013), pp. 1075–1083.

33. J. Pardeike, D.M. Strohmeier, N. Schrödl, C. Voura, M. Gruber, J.G. Khinast *et al.*, Nanosuspensions as advanced printing ink for accurate dosing of poorly soluble drugs in personalized medicines, *Int. J. Pharm.* 420 (2011), pp. 93–100.

34. Additive fabrication, CustomPartNet, Olney. www.custompartnet.com/wu/additive-fabrication

35. Q. Yang, H. Li, Y. Zhai, X. Li and P. Zhang, The synthesis of epoxy resin coated Al2O3 composites for selective laser sintering 3D printing, *Rapid Prototyp. J.* 24 (2018), pp. 1059–1066.

36. R. Singh, S. Singh and M.S.J. Hashmi. Implant materials and their processing technologies, in *Reference Module in Materials Science and Materials Engineering*, Elsevier, 2016. https://doi.org/10.1016/B978-0-12-803581-8.04156-4.

37. M. Bansal, V. Sharma, G. Singh and S.L. Harikumar, 3D printing for the future of pharmaceuticals dosages forms, *Int. J. Appl. Pharm.* 10 (2018), pp. 1–7.

38. S. Qi and D. Craig, Recent developments in micro- and nanofabrication techniques for the preparation of amorphous pharmaceutical dosage forms, *Adv. Drug. Deliv. Rev.* 100 (2016), pp. 67–84.

39. J. Goole and K. Amighi, 3D printing in pharmaceutics: A new tool for designing customized drug delivery systems, *Int. J. Pharm.* 499 (2016), pp. 376–394.

40. H. Wen, B. He, H. Wang, F. Chen, P. Li, M. Cui *et al.*, Structure-based gastro-retentive and controlled-release drug delivery with novel 3D printing, *AAPS PharmSciTech.* 20 (2019) p. 68.

41. I. Gibson, R. David and S. Brent, Directed energy deposition processes, in *Additive Manufacturing Technologies*, Springer, New York, 2015, pp. 245–268.

42. D. Li, A review of microstructure evolution during ultrasonic additive manufacturing, *Int. J. Adv. Manuf. Technol.* 113 (2021), pp. 1–19.

43. M. Pandey, H. Choudhury, J.L.C. Fern, A.T.K. Kee, J. Kou, J.L.J. Jing *et al.*, 3D printing for oral drug delivery: A new tool to customize drug delivery, *Drug. Deliv. Transl. Res.* 10 (2020), pp. 986–1001.

44. Y.J. Sun and S. Soh, Printing tablets with fully customizable release profiles for personalized medicine, *Adv. Mater.* 27 (2015), pp. 7847–7853.

45. S.H. Lim, H. Kathuria, J.J.Y. Tan and L. Kang, 3D printed drug delivery and testing systems-a passing fad or the future? *Adv. Drug. Deliv. Rev.* 132 (2018), pp. 139–168.

46. C. Li, D. Pisignano, Y. Zhao and J. Xue, Advances in medical applications of additive manufacturing, *Engineering* 6 (2020), pp. 1222–1231.

47. A. Goyanes, N. Allahham, S.J. Trenfield, E. Stoyanovd, S. Gaisford and A.W. Basit, Direct powder extrusion 3D printing: Fabrication of drug products using a novel single-step process, *Int. J. Pharm.* 567 (2019), p. 118471.

48. K. Vithani, A. Goyanes, V. Jannin, A.W. Basit, S. Gaisford and B.J. Boyd, An overview of 3D printing technologies for soft materials and potential opportunities for lipid-based drug delivery systems, *Pharm. Res.* 36 (2018), p. 4.

49. B.C. Pereira, A. Isreb, R.T. Forbes, F. Dores, R. Habashy, J.B. Petit *et al.*, Temporary Plasticiser: A novel solution to fabricate 3D printed patient-centred cardiovascular '*polypill*' architectures, *Eur. J. Pharm. Biopharm.* 135 (2019), pp. 94–103.

50. A. Awad, F. Fina, S.J. Trenfield, P. Patel, A. Goyanes, S. Gaisford *et al.*, 3D printed pellets (miniprintlets): A novel, multi-drug, controlled release platform technology, *Pharmaceutics* 11 (2019), p. 148.

51. J. Norman, R.D. Madurawe, C.M.V. Moore, M.A. Khan and A. Khairuzzaman, A new chapter in pharmaceutical manufacturing: 3Dprinted drug products, *Adv. Drug Deliv. Rev.* 108 (2017), pp. 39–50.

52. M.A. Alhnan, T.C. Okwuosa, M. Sadia, K.W. Wan, W. Ahmed and B. Arafat, Emergence of 3D printed dosage forms: Opportunities and challenges. *Pharm. Res.* 33 (2016), pp. 1817–1832.

53. S. Angeliki, T. Eleni, D.M. Rekkas and V. Marilena, 3D-printed modified-release tablets: A review of the recent advances, in *Molecular Pharmacology*, IntechOpen, London, 2020. www.intechopen.com/chapters/70777

54. A. Goyanes, H. Chang, D. Sedough, G.B. Hatton, J. Wang, A. Buanz *et al.*, Fabrication of controlled-release budesonide tablets via desktop (FDM) 3D printing, *Int. J. Pharm.* 496 (2015), pp. 414–420.

55. S. Pravin and A. Sudhir, Integration of 3D printing with dosage forms: A new perspective for modern healthcare, *Biomed. Pharmacother.* 107 (2018), pp. 146–154.

56. L.K. Prasad and H. Smyth, 3D printing technologies for drug delivery: A review, *Drug Dev. Ind. Pharm.* 42 (2015), pp 1019–1031. DOI: 10.3109/ 03639045.2015.1120743

57. W. Jamróz, M. Kurek, E. Łyszczarz, J. Szafraniec, J. Knapik-Kowalczuk, K. Syrek *et al.*, 3D printed orodispersible films with aripiprazole, *Int. J. Pharm.* 533 (2017), pp. 413–420.

58. U.M. Musazzi, F. Selmin, M.A. Ortenzi, G.K. Mohammed, S. Franzé, P. Minghetti *et al.*, Personalized orodispersible films by hot melt ram extrusion 3D printing, *Int. J. Pharm.* 551 (2018), pp. 52–59.

59. W. Kempin, V. Domsta, G. Grathoff, I. Brecht, B. Semmling, S. Tillmann *et al.*, Immediate release 3D-printed tablets produced via fused deposition modeling of a thermosensitive drug, *Pharm. Res.* 35 (2018), p. 124.

60. N.G. Solanki, M. Tahsin, A.V. Shah and A.T.M. Serajuddin, Formulation of 3D printed tablet for rapid drug release by fused deposition modeling: Screening polymers for drug release, drug polymer miscibility and printability, *J. Pharm. Sci.* 107 (2018), pp. 390–401.

61. A. Goyanes, P.R. Martinez, A. Buanz, A.W. Basit and S. Gaisford, Effect of geometry on drug release from 3D printed tablets, *Int. J. Pharm.* 494 (2015), pp. 657–663.

62. E. Mathew, J. Domínguez-Robles, E. Larrañeta and D.A. Lamprou, Fused deposition modelling as a potential tool for antimicrobial dialysis catheters manufacturing: New trends vs. conventional approaches, *Coatings* 9 (2019), p. 515.

63. J.A. Weisman, D.H. Ballard, U. Jammalamadaka, K. Tappa, J. Sumerel, H.B. D'Agostino, D.K. Mills and P.K. Woodard, 3D printed antibiotic and chemotherapeutic eluting catheters for potential use in interventional radiology: In vitro proof of concept study, *Acad. Radiol.* 26 (2019), pp. 270–274.

64. J.A. Weisman, J.C. Nicholson, K. Tappa, U. Jammalamadaka, C.G. Wilson and D.K. Mills, Antibiotic and chemotherapeutic enhanced three-dimensional printer filaments and constructs for biomedical applications, *Int. J. Nanomed.* 10 (2015), pp. 357–370.

65. A.V. Keating, J. Soto, C. Tuleu, C. Forbes, M. Zhao and D.Q.M. Craig, Solid state characterisation and taste masking efficiency evaluation of polymer based extrudates of isoniazid for paediatric administration, *Int. J. Pharm.* 536 (2018), pp. 536–546.

66. M. Alhijjaj, P. Belton and S. Qi, An investigation into the use of polymer blends to improve the printability of and regulate drug release from pharmaceutical solid dispersions prepared via fused deposition modeling (FDM) 3D printing, *Eur. J. Pharm. Biopharm.* 108 (2016), pp. 111–125.

67. Z. Muwaffak, A. Goyanes, V. Clark, A.W. Basit, S.T. Hilton and S. Gaisford, Patient-specific 3D scanned and 3D printed antimicrobial polycaprolactone wound dressings, *Int. J. Pharm.* 527 (2017), pp. 161–170.

68. A. Melocchi, F. Parietti, A. Maroni, A. Foppoli, A. Gazzaniga and L. Zema, Hot-melt extruded filaments based on pharmaceutical grade polymers for 3D printing by fused deposition modelling, *Int. J. Pharm.* 509 (2016), pp. 255–263.

69. K. Tappa and U. Jammalamadaka, Novel biomaterials used in medical 3D printing techniques, *J. Funct. Biomater.* 9 (2018), p. 17.

70. N. Dumpa, A. Butreddy, H. Wang, N. Komanduri, S. Bandari and M.A. Repka, 3D printing in personalized drug delivery: An overview of hot-melt extrusion-based fused deposition modelling, *Int. J. Pharm.* 600 (2021), p. 120501.

71. A. Barazanchi, K.C. Li, B. Al-Amleh, K. Lyons, J.N. Waddell, Additive technology: Update on current materials and applications in dentistry, *J. Prosthodont.* 26 (2017), pp. 156–163.

72. R. Patel, T. Sheth, S. Shah, M. Shah, A new leap in periodontics: Three-dimensional (3D) printing, *J. Adv. Oral Res.* 8 (2017), pp. 1–7.

73. M. Gul, A. Arif and R. Ghafoor, Role of three-dimensional printing in periodontal regeneration and repair: Literature review, *J. Indian Soc. Periodontol.* 33 (2019), pp. 504–510.

74. L. Lei, Y. Yu, T. Ke, W. Sun and L. Chen, The application of three-dimensional printing model and platelet-rich fibrin technology in guided tissue regeneration surgery for severe bone defects, *J. Oral Implantol.* 45 (2019), pp. 35–43.

75. G. Rasperini, S.P. Pilipchuk, C.L. Flanagan, C.H. Park, G. Pagni, S.J. Hollister, *et al.*, 3D-printed bioresorbable scaffold for periodontal repair, *J. Dent. Res.* 94 (2015), pp. 153S–157S.

76. M. Elsayed, M. Ghazy, Y. Youssef and K. Essa, Optimization of SLM process parameters for Ti6Al4V medical implants, *Rapid Prototyp. J.* 25 (2019), pp. 433–447.

77. K. Baylón, P. Rodríguez-Camarillo, A. Elías-Zúñiga, J.A. Díaz-Elizondo, R. Gilkerson and K. Lozano, Past, present and future of surgical meshes: A review, *Membranes* 7 (2017), p. 47.

78. S.C. Cox, P. Jamshidi, N.M. Eisenstein, M.A. Webber, H. Hassanin, M.M. Attallah, *et al.*, Adding functionality with additive manufacturing: Fabrication of titanium-based antibiotic eluting implants, *Mater. Sci. Eng. C* 64 (2016), pp. 407–415.

79. H. Hassanin, L. Finet, S.C. Cox, P. Jamshidi, L.M. Grover, D.E.T. Shepherd *et al.*, Tailoring selective laser melting process for titanium drug-delivering implants with releasing micro-channels, *Addit. Manuf.* 20 (2018), pp. 144–155.

80. S. Mohanty, L.B. Larsen, J. Trifol, P. Szabo, H.V.R. Burri, C. Canali *et al.*, Fabrication of scalable and structured tissue engineering scaffolds using water dissolvable sacrificial 3D printed moulds, *Mater. Sci. Eng. C* 55 (2015), pp. 569–578.

81. K.K. Jain, Current status and future prospects of drug delivery systems, in *Drug Delivery System*, Springer, New York, 2014, pp. 1–56.

82. J. Fu, X. Yu and Y. Jin, 3D printing of vaginal rings with personalized shapes for controlled release of progesterone, *Int. J. Pharm.* 539 (2018), pp. 75–82.

83. S. Krezić, E. Krhan, E. Mandžuka, N. Kovač, D. Krajina, A. Marić et al., Fabrication of rectal and vaginal suppositories using 3D printed moulds: The challenge of personalized therapy, *IFMBE Proceedings*, 2020, pp. 729–734.

84. A. Adamo, R.L. Beingessner, M. Behnam, J. Chen, T.F. Jamison, K.F. Jensen, *et al.*, On-demand continuous-flow production of pharmaceuticals in a compact, reconfigurable system, *Science* 352 (2016), pp. 61–67.

85. K. Ita, Transdermal delivery of drugs with microneedles—potential and challenges, *Pharmaceutics* 7 (2015), pp. 90–105.

86. F.S. Iliescu, S. Paunica, D. Vrtacnik and A.R. Bobei, A double softlithography method for processing of nono microneedles arrays, *UPB Sci. Bull. B: Chem. Mater. Sci.* 79 (2017), pp. 121–132.

87. H. Hassanin and K. Jiang, Multiple replication of thick PDMS micropatterns using surfactants as release agents, *Microelectron. Eng.* 88 (2011), pp. 3275–3277.

88. Z. Zhu, H. Hassanin and K. Jiang, A soft moulding process for manufacture of net-shape ceramic microcomponents, *Int. J. Adv. Manuf. Technol.* 47 (2010), pp. 147–152.

89. C.L. Caudill, J.L. Perry, S. Tian, J.C. Luft and J.M. DeSimone, Spatially controlled coating of continuous liquid interface production microneedles for transdermal protein delivery, *J. Control. Release* 284 (2018), pp. 122–132.

90. M.J. Uddin, N. Scoutaris, S.N. Economidou, C. Giraud, B.Z. Chowdhry, R.F. Donnelly *et al.*, 3D printed microneedles for anticancer therapy of skin tumours, *Mater. Sci. Eng. C* 107 (2020), p. 110248.

91. Z.X. Khoo, J.E.M. Teoh, Y. Liu, C.K. Chua, S. Yang, J. An *et al.*, 3D printing of smart materials: A review on recent progresses in 4D printing, *Virtual Phys. Prototyp.* 10 (2015), pp. 103–122.

92. Y.S. Lui, W.T. Sow, L.P. Tan, Y. Wu, Y. Lai, H. Li, 4D printing and stimuli-responsive materials in biomedical aspects, *Acta Biomater.* 92 (2019), pp. 19–36.

93. Q. Ge, A.H. Sakhaei, H. Lee, C.K. Dunn, N.X. Fang, M.L. Dunn. Multimaterial 4D printing with tailorable shape memory polymers, *Sci. Rep.* 6 (2016), p. 31110.

94. H-G. Yi, Y-J. Choi, K.S. Kang, J.M. Hong, R.G. Pati, M.N. Park *et al.*, A 3D-printed local drug delivery patch for pancreatic cancer growth suppression, *J. Control. Release* 238 (2016), pp. 231–241.

95. H. Wei, Q. Zhang, Y. Yao, L. Liu, Y. Liu and J. Leng, Direct-write fabrication of 4D active shape-changing structures based on a shape memory polymer and its nanocomposite, *ACS Appl. Mater. Interfaces* 9 (2016), pp. 876–883.

96. M. Zarek, N. Mansour, S. Shapira and D. Cohn, 4D printing of shape memory based personalized endoluminal medical devices, *Macromol. Rapid Commun.* 38 (2017). https://doi.org/10.1002/marc.201600628

97. H. He, J. Guan and J.L. Lee, An oral delivery device based on self-folding hydrogels, *J. Control. Release* 110 (2006), pp. 339–346.

98. K. Malachowski, J. Breger, H.R. Kwag, M.O. Wang, J.P. Fisher, F.M. Selaru *et al.*, Stimuli-responsive theragrippers for chemomechanical controlled release, *Angew. Chem.* 53 (2014), pp. 8045–8049.

99. J.C. Breger, C. Yoon, R. Xiao, H.R. Kwag, M.O. Wang, J.P. Fisher *et al.*, Self-folding thermo-magnetically responsive soft microgrippers, *ACS Appl. Mater. Interfaces* 7 (2015), pp. 3398–3405.

100. C. Yoon, R. Xiao, J. Park, J. Cha, T.D. Nguyen, D.H. Gracias *et al.*, Functional stimuli responsive hydrogel devices by self-folding, *Smart Mater. Struct.* 23 (2014), p. 094008.

101. G. Stoychev, N. Puretskiy and L. Ionov, Self-folding all-polymer thermoresponsive microcapsules, *Soft Matter* 7 (2011), pp. 3277–3279.

102. H. Li, G. Go, S.Y. Ko, J-O. Park and S. Park, Magnetic actuated pH-responsive hydrogel based soft micro-robot for targeted drug delivery, *Smart Mater. Struct.* 25 (2016), p. 027001.

103. A. Melocchi, N. Inverardi, M. Uboldi, F. Baldi, A. Maroni, S. Pandini *et al.*, Retentive device for intravesical drug delivery based on water-induced shape memory response of poly(vinyl alcohol): Design concept and 4D printing feasibility. *Int. J. Pharm.* 559 (2019), pp. 299–311.

104. US FDA pharmacogenomic data submissions guide brings personalized medicine closer, *The Pharma Letter*, 2005. www.thepharmaletter.com/article/us-fda-pharmaco genomic-data-submissions-guide-brings-personalized-medicine-closer?__cf_chl_ jschl_tk__=pmd_306238e8927861004ff0439c7ce1e09e58600b05–1627539738–0-gq NtZGzNAnijcnBszQii

105. Personalized medicine: A biological approach to patient treatment. US Foods and Drugs Administration, 2016. www.fda.gov/drugs/news-events-human-drugs/personalized-medicine-biological-approach-patient-treatment

106. D. Greenbaum, Regulation and the fate of personalized medicine, *Virtual Mentor* 14 (2012), pp. 645–652.

107. Personalised medicine, Legal framework, *European Commission*, 2015. https://ec.europa.eu/health/human-use/personalised-medicine_en

108. A. Goyanes, C.M. Madla, A. Umerji, G. Duran Piñeiro, J.M.G. Montero, M.J.L. Diaz *et al.*, Automated therapy preparation of isoleucine formulations using 3D printing for the treatment of MSUD: First single-centre, prospective, crossover study in patients, *Int. J. Pharm.* 567 (2019), p. 118497.

109. W. Jamróz, J. Szafraniec, M. Kurek and R. Jachowicz, 3D printing in pharmaceutical and medical applications—recent achievements and challenges, *Pharm. Res.* 35 (2018), p. 176.

110. N. Genina, J. Holländer, H. Jukarainen, E. Mäkilä, J. Salonen, N. Sandler, Ethylene vinyl acetate (EVA) as a new drug carrier for 3D printed medical drug delivery devices, *Eur. J. Pharm. Sci.* 90 (2016), pp. 53–63.

111. K. Osouli-Bostanabad and K. Adibkia, Made-on-demand, complex and personalized 3D-printed drug products, *Bioimpacts* 8 (2018), pp. 77–79.

112. S.J. Trenfield, H. Xian Tan, A. Awad, A. Buanz, S. Gaisford, A.W. Basit *et al.*, Track-and-trace: Novel anticounterfeit measures for 3D printed personalised drug products using smart material inks, *Int. J. Pharm.* 567 (2019), p. 118443.

113. H. Vakili, J.O. Nyman, N. Genina, M. Preis and N. Sandler, Application of a colorimetric technique in quality control for printed pediatric orodispersible drug delivery systems containing propranolol hydrochloride, *Int. J. Pharm.* 511 (2016), pp. 606–618.

114. H. Wickström, J.O. Nyman, M. Indola, H. Sundelin, L. Kronberg, M. Preis *et al.*, Colorimetry as quality control tool for individual inkjet-printed pediatric formulations, *AAPS PharmSciTech.* 18 (2017), pp. 293–302.

115. H. Vakili, H. Wickstrom, D. Desai, M. Preis and N. Sandler, Application of a hand-held NIR spectrometer in prediction of drug content in inkjet printed orodispersible formulations containing prednisolone and levothyroxine, *Int. J. Pharm.* 524 (2017), pp. 414–423.

116. M. Edinger, L-D Iftimi, D. Markl D, M. Al-Sharabi, D. Bar-Shalom, J. Rantanen and N. Genina, Quantification of inkjet-printed pharmaceuticals on porous substrates using Raman spectroscopy and near-infrared spectroscopy, *AAPS PharmSciTech.* 20 (2019), p. 207.

117. M. Edinger, D. Bar-Shalom, J. Rantanen and N. Genina, Visualization and nondestructive quantification of inkjet-printed pharmaceuticals on different substrates using Raman spectroscopy and Raman chemical imaging, *Pharm. Res.* 34 (2017), pp. 1023–1036.

2 Additive Manufacturing for the Development of Biological Implants, Scaffolds, and Prosthetics

Atul Babbar[1], Vivek Jain[2], Dheeraj Gupta[2], Ankit Sharma[3], Chander Prakash[4], Vidyapati Kumar[5], and Kapil Kumar Goyal[6]

[1] Department of Mechanical Engineering, Shree Guru Gobind Singh Tricentenary University, Gurugram 122505, India

[2] Department of Mechanical Engineering, Thapar Institute of Engineering and Technology, Patiala, India

[3] Chitkara College of Applied Engineering, Chitkara University, Rajpura 140401, India

[4] School of Mechanical Engineering, Lovely Professional University, Phagwara 144001, India

[5] Department of Mechanical Engineering, Indian Institute of Technology, Kharagpur 721302, India

[6] Department of Industrial and Production Engineering, Dr B R Ambedkar National Institute of Technology, Jalandhar

CONTENTS

2.1   Introduction to Additive Manufacturing 28
2.2   Biomaterials and Applications 29
2.3   Role of Implants in Biomedical Engineering 29
2.4   Scaffolds in Biomedical Engineering 34
2.5   Prosthetics in Biomedical Engineering 35
2.6   Conclusion and Future Possibilities 37
References 38

DOI: 10.1201/9781003217961-2

2.1 INTRODUCTION TO ADDITIVE MANUFACTURING

Modern three-dimensional (3D) printing technology has gained broad popularity in the contemporary environment owing to its several benefits over conventional and nontraditional manufacturing methods, such as cost reduction, speed, design flexibility, one-step production, and sustainable development. Additive manufacturing (AM) is the layer-by-layer production of a 3D component from a computer-aided-designed (CAD) or digitalized 3D layout, which streamlines the machining process and eliminates extraneous material from a more extensive stock. This technology is unique in that it instantly changes the material to its final shape with little material waste while maintaining the necessary geometric proportions. Due to the accessibility to broader types of 3D printing techniques [1–4], this AM process is utilized for a particular material and application, making determining the suitable AM technology a problematic task. Various techniques provide varied surface finishes, high-dimensional accuracy, and postprocessing requirements depending on the printing medium. AM has applications in a wide range of industries, including aerospace, structural, biomedical, and complex component manufacturing. Moreover, different processes and machining techniques have been used in various designing and manufacturing stages [5–31].

Furthermore, AM has piqued many people's curiosity owing to its adaptability in manufacturing cost-effective, rapid surgical devices and patient-centered biological implants [32–35]. Dental implants, artificial livers, and synthetic cardiovascular systems have all been successfully repaired or manufactured using AM, but it is not restricted to orthopedic implants and may also be used to produce medical electronic microfluidic devices. In this case, stress shielding develops due to a mechanical mismatch between metal implants and native biological parts or organs, leading to organ or portion resorption failure and implant failure. This kind of implant failure is more prevalent in implants manufactured using traditional methods. Consequently, it is vital to develop an additive printing technology that appears to be a viable choice for creating prostheses with regulated permeability and durability that mimic the characteristics of the natural skeleton and organs, hence lowering the danger of stress shielding. The potential to use 3D-printing technology to make highly personalized medical implants has created a once-in-a-lifetime opportunity to treat specific body component issues [36–37]. Rapid prototyping and rapid production are two important uses of AM technology, as seen in Figure 2.1.

AM's capacity to make complicated shaped implants as a demand-based manufacturing strategy has made the process far more economical and cost-efficient. AM does not need tools for product fabrication, resulting in an exact cost per component in this method; nevertheless, in conventional machining, the cost of tooling plays a significant part in determining the cost of AM components. The economic analysis provided a case for 3D printing to manufacture body implants [38]. Using AM methods, it is possible to produce items with complicated architecture in a short time. The modeling of machining technology processes, tool and mold design, specific machining equipment, distribution and warehousing activities, and so on is not required for AM methods. All that is necessary are the foundations of production processes and how the machine applies a material.

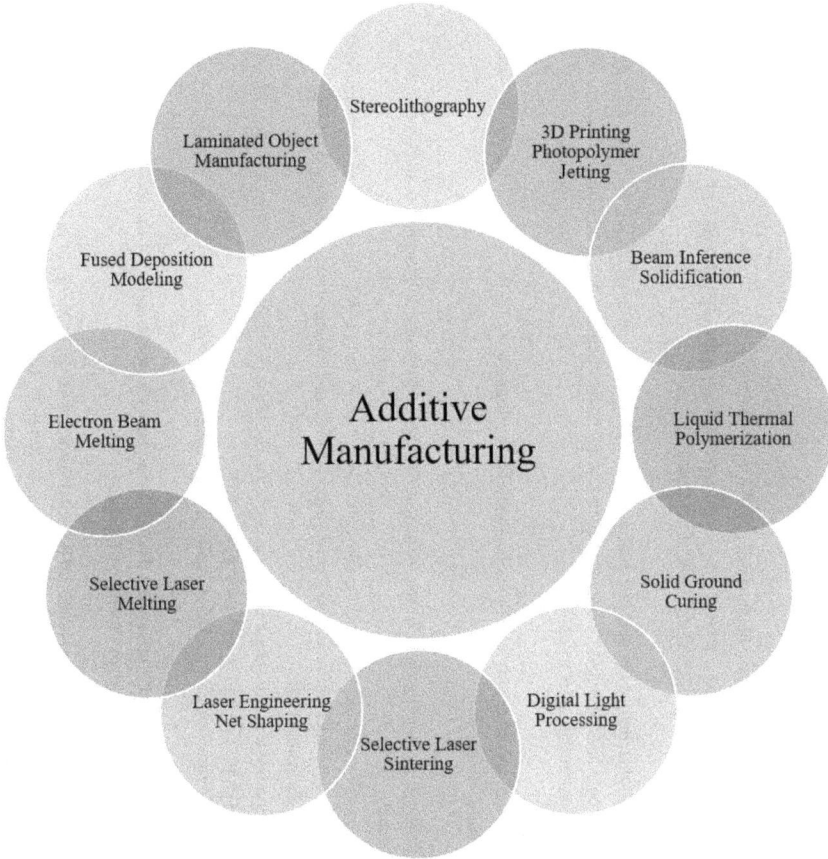

FIGURE 2.1 Classification of AM process.

2.2 BIOMATERIALS AND APPLICATIONS

Biomaterials have been employed in regulated pharmaceutical delivery techniques, sutures and adhesives, cardiac bypass, rehabilitative and orthopedic devices, ocular devices including corneas and corrective lenses, and dentistry. Several components, including titanium, have indeed been utilized to generate therapeutic implants. Bioceramics, polymers, metals, and composites are just a handful of the materials accessible. Table 2.1 outlines the current biological applications for biomaterials.

2.3 ROLE OF IMPLANTS IN BIOMEDICAL ENGINEERING

Implants are artificial equipment designed to be implanted into the body to supplant or maintain a biological structure and supply medications and supervise physiological processes. Sensory equipment [73]; cerebral and neurological equipment, such as neuronal, cochlear, and retinal implants [74–75]; subcutaneous implants [76];

TABLE 2.1

Biomedical Applications of Different Biomaterials

References	Biomaterial	Applications
[39]	Silicones, hydrogels	Advances in ophthalmology such as intraocular lenses (IOL), contact lenses.
[40–44]	Polymeric component, Metallic component, ceramic material, PU, PE, PBE, PP, SS	Vascular prostheses, mechanical gates, stents, cardiovascular pumping systems, blood bags, and catheters are all examples of products that may be used in the field of cardiology.
[45–50]	PCL, silk, collagen	Nerve regeneration scaffolds are used in both the central and peripheral nervous systems.
[45, 51–53]	PLLA, PDLA	Medication transmission, vascular bypass, skeletal fasteners, stabilization pegs, and dermal filler for facial atrophy are all used in the treatment of facial atrophy.
[53–56]	PLGA	Pharmaceutical delivery
[45, 57]	PCL	Everlasting implantation; medication release; maxillo-cranial facial implant
[58–60]	PCL_gelatin, PCL–chitosan, PCL–collagen	Rejuvenation of tissues
[61–63]	PPD	Intrinsic rupture fixation, medical implants in the form of films, foaming agents, and molded scaffolds are all possible applications.
[64–66]	LDPE, HDPE	Rhinoplasty surgeries, comprehensive hip arthroplasty, and osteolysis therapy using polymer-ceramic composites
[67–68]	PMMA	Dentistry implantation for rehabilitation and aesthetics, orbital medicinal implantation, rhinoplasty, cranioplasty, bone cement in hip joint restoration.
[69–70]	PDMS	Implantable electrical equipment and sensors, clinical implants, esophageal analogues, catheters, shunts, blood pumps, and pacemakers are all included inside this enclosure.
[71]	PA such as nylon and nylon-composites	Sutures, denture manufacture, bone regeneration scaffold material, and nanofillers
[72]	CNT and composite material	Metallic sealants for musculoskeletal implantable devices to increase the permeability of the substrate, minimize metallic ionization, and enhance hydroxyapatite production

Note: PU, polyurethane, PE, polyesters, PBE, polybutesters, PP, polypropylene, SS, stainless steel, PCL, polycaprolactone, UHMWPE, ultra-high-molecular-weight polyethylene (UHMWPE), PLLA, poly(l-lactic acid), PLA, poly(l-lactic acid), PLGA, poly(lactic-co-glycolic acid), PCL, polycaprolactone, PDLA, poly(d-lactic acid), PPD, poly-para-dioxanone, LDPE, low-density polyethylene, HDPE, high-density polyethylene, PMMA, poly(methyl methacrylate), PDMS, poly-dimethylsiloxane, PAs, polyamides, CNTs, carbon nanotubes and composites.

and cardiological systems, such as vascular bypass, stents, mechanical heart gates, and pacemakers [74], are all illustration of biomedical implants. Sutures and wound dressings [77], vertebral and dentistry implants [78], aesthetic [79], and structural implants [80], such as rods, braces, craniofacial, and hip and knee replacements, are all examples of biomedical implants. Biomedical implants are also utilized as ophthalmic equipment, such as spectacles, contact lenses, and insulin delivery [77].

Bioactive materials may be used to manufacture these biomedical implants. The word *bioactive* refers to a material's ability to biological effect on its surroundings. Compounds that encourage scaffolds include compounds that enhance a physiological action in the location where they are implanted. Furthermore, since cells naturally produce growth hormones and cytokines, these scaffolds might be used to stimulate repair and regeneration [19]. Jardini et al. [81] proffered AM methods for designing and fabricating a bio-model in the form of an implant for the surgical rehabilitation of a significant cranial defect, as shown in Figure 2.2.

According to research and experience, dental implants' success depends on a well-designed and meticulous treatment plan. Previously, panoramic radiographs and clinical judgment were used to determine implant size and angulation during surgery. Almog et al. [82] described the surgical guide fabrication process in this context illustrated in Figure 2.3.

An invasive primary bone tumor is a benign fibrous histiocytoma (BFH). Because the risk of recurrence is high when the local excision is incomplete, one-piece resection is required. Clinicians face a significant challenge in reconstructing the bone after the tumor has been removed. As shown in Figure 2.4, Dong et al. [83] investigated the efficacy of 3D printing in treating BFH of the scapula.

Infection and implant failure, such as dental implants shown in Figure 2.5, are among the hazards associated with the operation during implant insertion or removal. It is also necessary to examine the material's inflammatory response or rejection.

Implants are constructed of biomaterials that stimulate cell and tissue development via cell adhesion, proliferation, and differentiation; restrict undesirable cell

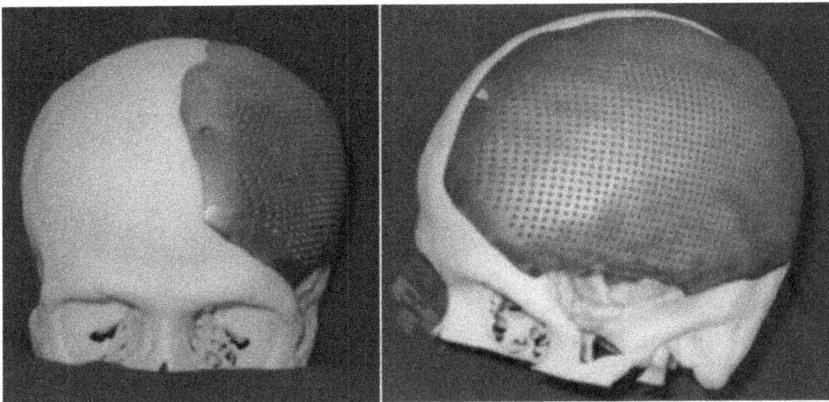

FIGURE 2.2   Bio-model and prosthesis for cranial reconstruction surgery [81].

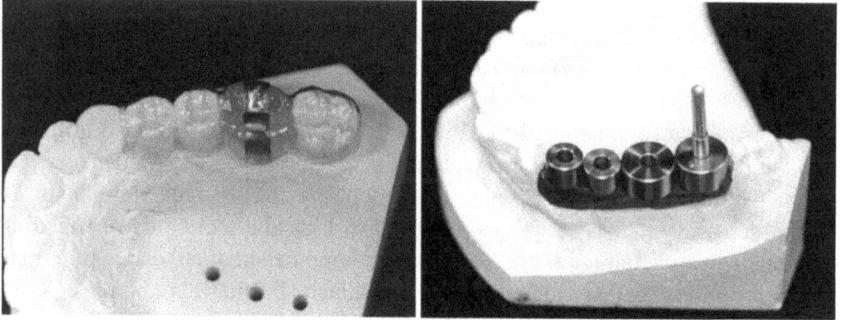

FIGURE 2.3   Surgical guide [82].

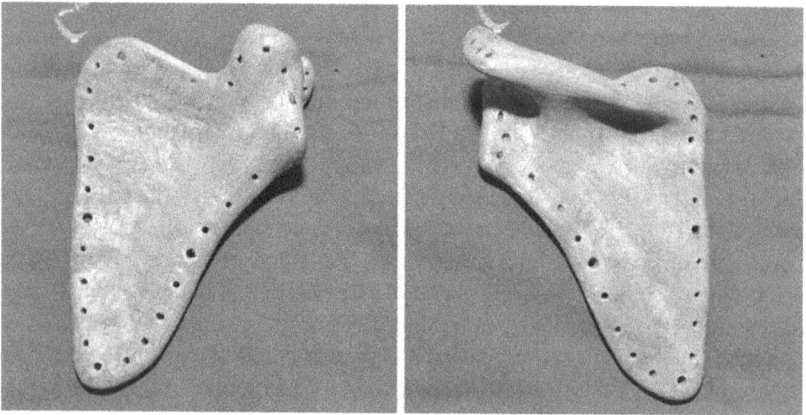

FIGURE 2.4   Scapula prosthesis [83].

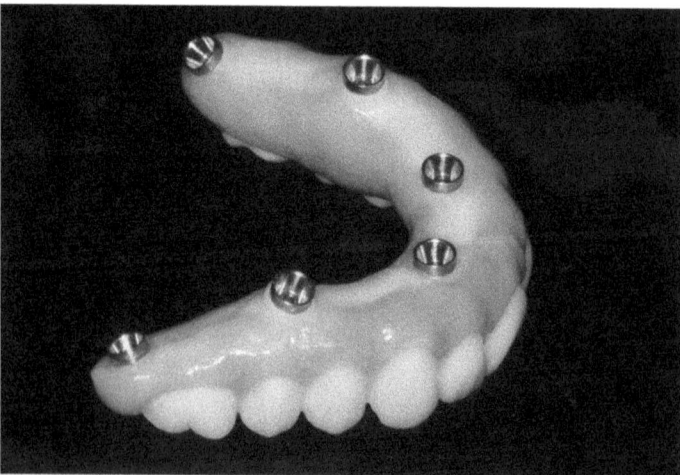

FIGURE 2.5   Dental implants [84].

and tissue growth; tune tissue response; and limit immunological reactions to aid in native tissue regeneration and replacement [85–86]. The malposition of the acetabular cup in large-diameter metal-on-metal prosthetic hip designs is linked to high wear, metal debris reaction, and early failure in clinical studies. Saikko et al. [87] used a hip-joint simulator to investigate the effect of a steep angle of the acetabular cup position on the wear of a large-diameter metal-on-metal prosthesis illustrated in Figure 2.6.

Matsushita et al. [88] utilized chemical and heat treatments to induce bioactivity in Titanium foams for spinal interbody fusion, as shown in Figure 2.7.

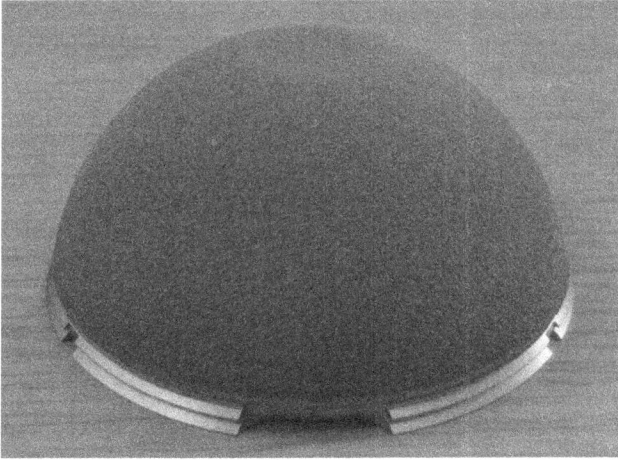

FIGURE 2.6   Acetabular cup [87].

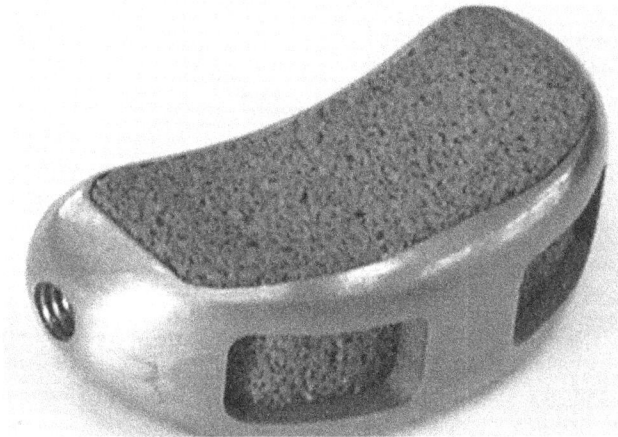

FIGURE 2.7   Interbody fusion cage [88].

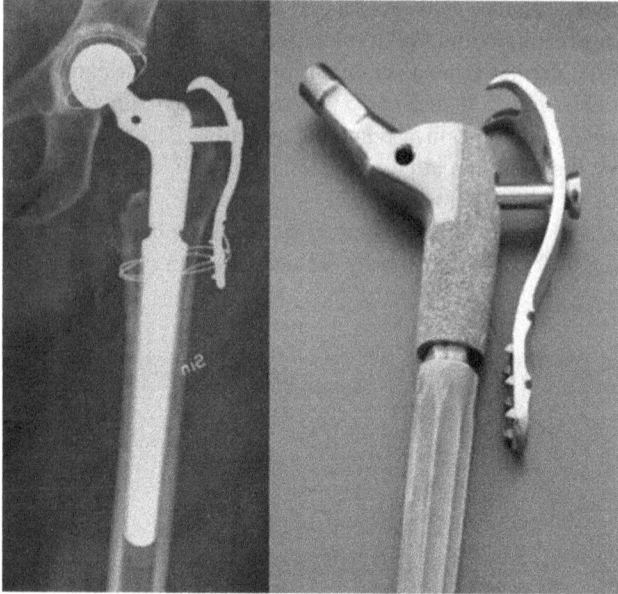

FIGURE 2.8 Hip prosthesis [89].

Hedlundh et al. [89] examined a pivotal case of total hip arthroplasty using an advanced method that combined the stem system's trochanteric attachment bolt and a locking plate with polyaxial screws shown in Figure 2.8.

2.4 SCAFFOLDS IN BIOMEDICAL ENGINEERING

Scaffolds composed of synthesized or natural polymers have been designed in recent decades to heal injured or deteriorating tissues and deliver medications to particular areas. Scaffolds are constructions that are 3D structures that replicate the tissue's original ECM (extracellular matrix) and serve as cell adhesion and development platform.

Bone tissue may undergo biological remodeling through a dynamic process of osteoclast absorption and subsequent osteoblast-induced bone formation [68, 90–91]. Nonetheless, when a big segmental bone defect reaches a crucial size of roughly 10 mm [31], the body is typically unable to complete the self-repairing function. External intervention is necessary to help self-repair by constructing bridges on the bone defect site [92]. As a result, bone transplants are often used in clinical procedures to help mend significant segmental bone lesions. According to the Centers for Disease Control and Prevention statistics, bone is the second-most used grafting tissue, having almost 2 million bone transplantations done each year [93]. The gold standard for bone restoration is autografts derived from the patient [94]. The autograft's size, however, is quite restricted.

Furthermore, removing the autograft adds to the surgical stress and increases the chance of morbidity at the source location. Allografts from different persons are a more abundant choice than autografts. They almost always result in disease transmission and immunological rejection [95]. As a consequence, bone replacement is in great demand for regenerating bone tissues in anticipation of surgery.

The intended bone replacements must have an exterior to minimize excessive bone tissue removal in problem areas. More crucially, they must have a porous and linked pore structure to establish a microenvironment favorable to cell activity and reproduction [96–97]. Several methods have been suggested to create porous scaffolds for bone repair, including the pore-forming assistive technique [98–99], the gas foaming system [100–101], sol-gel processes [102–103], and the freeze-drying technique [104–105]. Although these approaches may create porous structures, they have several drawbacks, such as incorrect pore structure management and limited customization capacity for particular fault sites [106–107]. Furthermore, some of these techniques will certainly leave some organic pore-forming agent residues, which will impair the biological characteristics of the scaffolds and compromise the quality of bone healing. Exploring a construction approach for scaffolds that obtains the particular exterior form and precisely controls the pore structure is thus critical for their future orthopedic use. Various optimization techniques are used to improve additive manufacturing process parameters for appropriate scaffold and implant design [108–127].

AM may create a porous scaffold with a unique outward form and a porous interior structure. A 3D scaffold framework with the appropriate layout is often developed using CAD software before the AM process. The 3D scaffold model is split into a series of 2D slices prior to being converted to typical stereolithography (STL) files with exact 2D slice characteristics. An AM machine executes the appropriate toolpath along with the 2D directions for directly creating 2D layers based on these STL files. To create a 3D component, each layer is constructed on top of the preceding one. This manufacturing technology is called AM because of the production technique of putting one layer on top of the previous one. Currently, researchers around the globe are working hard to develop porous implants for bone healing using AM methods. Poukens [128], for example, used AM to effectively create a porous mandible implant, which was then placed in a patient. Jardini et al. [129] from Brazil employed a tailored porous scaffold made from AM technology to treat a significant cranial lesion, while an Australian biomedical team used AM-derived porous titanium implants to treat a 71-year-old patient who was facing amputation of the heel bone. All these accomplishments point to a bright future for AM methods in bone tissue restoration. As shown schematically in Figure 2.9, a conventional deployment of scaffolds synthesized using AM techniques.

2.5 PROSTHETICS IN BIOMEDICAL ENGINEERING

Prosthetics are often intended to have the same or lighter weights as the lost limb or body parts in order to reduce fatigue and enhance the flexibility of usage. Prosthetic devices have evolved much more sophisticated as a result of ongoing technical advancements [131]. Practically, it can potentially execute activities previously

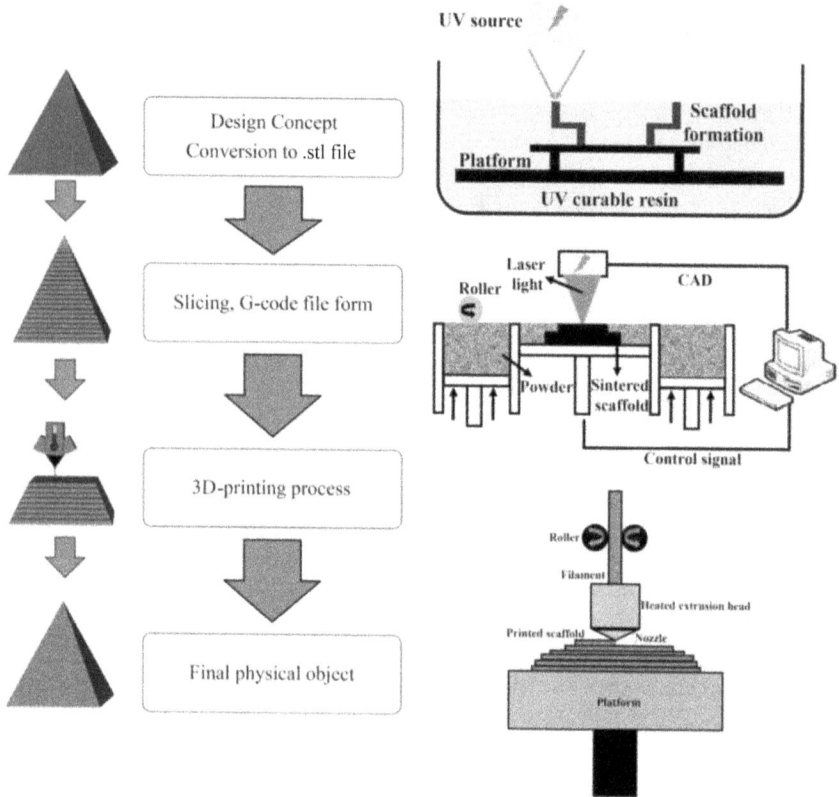

FIGURE 2.9 A conceptual illustration depicting the scaffold manufactured using AM [130].

considered challenging or impossible. Unfortunately, due to the increased expense of modern prostheses, it is out of access for many individuals. 3D printing is a way for lowering the exorbitant costs of modern prostheses. Three-dimensional printers employ a CAD layout to produce the element in consecutive stages. For a better fit, the CAD model may be utilized in combination with the wearer's anatomic data. Three-dimensional printing technology allows for highly customized, more ergonomic prostheses that can be completely produced. As a result, the patients feel higher confidence while wandering around. This innovation enables researchers to transform the approach prostheses are devised, produced, and fitted to bodily parts. The manufacturing process of the prosthesis commences with scanning the patient's preferred portions using a 3D scanner.

Personalized designs of certain body parts may be created using any 3D CAD program based on the scanned pictures. Electronics, mechanics, and software are major components of the sophisticated 3D-printed prosthesis, allowing for the production of an all-in-one solution. Biosensors enable the prostheses for contractions and mobility detecting, as well as driving the bodily components. Numerous prostheses now include Wireless and cellular communication. Several researchers revealed the

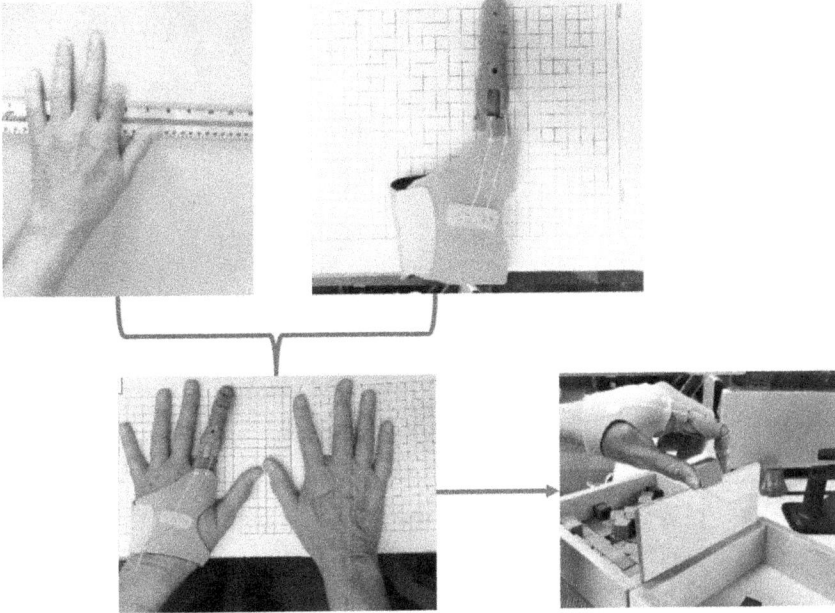

FIGURE 2.10 3D-printed finger prosthetic [132].

creation of high-quality, low-cost prostheses utilizing various thermoplastic components [83]. Figure 2.10 depicts the patient conducting the box-and-block assessment after the 3D-printed finger prosthesis has been attached. Bone-anchored prostheses, such as a transfemoral bone-anchored prosthesis and a transtibial bone-anchored prosthesis, are also widely used during patients' recovery after an amputation. Figure 2.11 also demonstrates a lower limb prosthesis and its proper alignment.

2.6 CONCLUSION AND FUTURE POSSIBILITIES

AM is a rapidly evolving technology used to build individualized and customized biomedical implants, scaffolds, and prosthetic devices in a range of sectors. In the realm of biomedical engineering, several types of AM technologies have been discussed, as well as their relevant production techniques and procedures. According to the proposal, future dental and clinical research on AMs and industrial research should utilize a standardized nomenclature. This would allow for a more systematic comparison of the utilization of different AM approaches. More medical and dental applications will be possible because of current and future improvements in additive manufacturing processes, devices, and materials. In this context, recent literature on bioactive biomedical implants, scaffolds, and prostheses employed in regenerative treatments, drug delivery, and other fields has been reviewed. Biomaterials are continually being

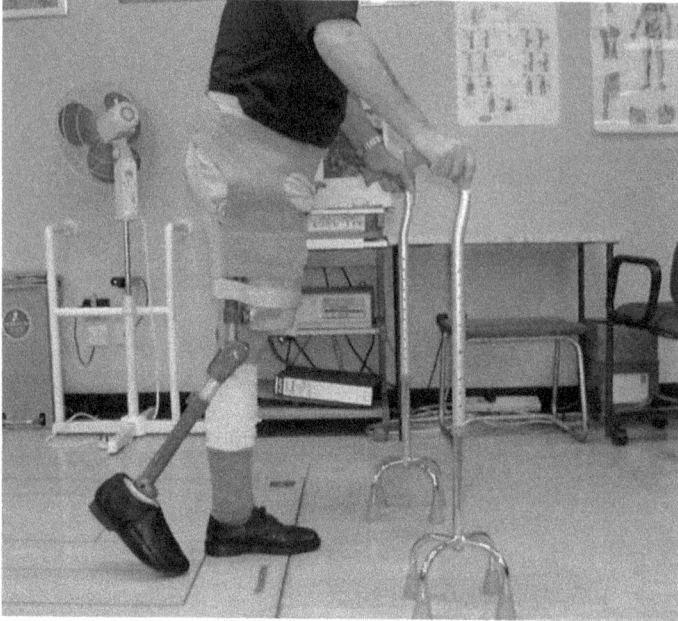

FIGURE 2.11   Bone-anchored prosthesis [133].

developed to give innovative biomedical implants, either entirely original or by blending advantageous properties of popular and safer biomaterials to improve implant implementation and effectiveness. As a result, materials that increase the body's natural reaction while supporting cell adhesion and proliferation are necessary. Bioactivity produced by cells, in which implants with cells are used to regenerate tissue and treat illnesses, is another subject that has emerged in recent years.

While there are a variety of manufacturing processes for developing bioactive implants that are tailored to a given application, emerging techniques, like additive layer manufacturing, provide the sector with benefits and adaptability. Prospects for medical AM research utilizing different approaches may be seen in the following areas: Medical components, notably tools, instruments, and parts for clinical equipment may be repaired using directed energy deposition. In medicine, sheet lamination may be used to make multimetal components, particularly for equipment and instruments. The extrusion of materials may also comprise composite and multimaterial components employed in medical aids and medical rehabilitation equipment like prostheses. Implants and tools, appliances, medical models, and biomanufacturing may all benefit from binder jetting and material jetting.

REFERENCES

1. Labonnote N, Rønnquist A, Manum B, Rüther P. Additive construction: State-of-the-art, challenges and opportunities. *Automation in Construction*. 2016:347–66.

2. Bose S, Ke D, Sahasrabudhe H, Bandyopadhyay A. Additive manufacturing of biomaterials. *Progress in Materials Science*. 2018;93:45–111.
3. Wang X, Jiang M, Zhou Z, Gou J, Hui D. 3D printing of polymer matrix composites: A review and prospective. *Composites Part B: Engineering*. 2017:442–58.
4. Singh D, Babbar A, Jain V, Gupta D, Saxena S, Dwibedi V. Synthesis, characterization, and bioactivity investigation of biomimetic biodegradable PLA scaffold fabricated by fused filament fabrication process. *Journal of the Brazilian Society of Mechanical Sciences and Engineering*. 2019;41.
5. Sharma A, Kumar V, Babbar A, Dhawan V, Kotecha K. Experimental investigation and optimization of electric discharge machining process parameters using grey-fuzzy-based hybrid techniques. *Materials*. 2021;14(19):5820.
6. Sharma A, Kalsia M, Uppal AS, Babbar A, Dhawan V. Machining of hard and brittle materials: A comprehensive review. *Materials Today: Proceedings* [Internet]. Elsevier Ltd.; 2021;1–5. Available from: https://doi.org/10.1016/j.matpr.2021.07.452
7. Kumar R, Ranjan N, Babbar A. On investigations of 3D printed nylon 6 parts prepared by fused filament fabrication. *Materials Today: Proceedings* [Internet]. Elsevier Ltd; 2021;92–5. Available from: https://doi.org/10.1016/j.matpr.2021.08.103
8. Babbar A, Rai A, Sharma A. Latest trend in building construction: Three-dimensional printing. *Journal of Physics: Conference Series*. 2021;1950:012007.
9. Babbar A, Jain V, Gupta D. Thermo-mechanical aspects and temperature measurement techniques of bone grinding. *Materials Today: Proceedings* [Internet]. Elsevier Ltd; 2019;33:1458–62. Available from: https://doi.org/10.1016/j.matpr.2020.01.497
10. Babbar A, Sharma A, Kumar R, Pundir P, Dhiman V. Functionalized biomaterials for 3D printing: An overview of the literature. *Additive Manufacturing with Functionalized Nanomaterials* [Internet]. Elsevier; 2021:87–107. Available from: www.sciencedirect.com/science/article/pii/B9780128231524000053
11. Singh G, Babbar A, Jain V, Gupta D. Comparative statement for diametric delamination in drilling of cortical bone with conventional and ultrasonic assisted drilling techniques. *Journal of Orthopaedics* [Internet]. Elsevier B.V.; 2021;25:53–8. Available from: https://doi.org/10.1016/j.jor.2021.03.017
12. Babbar A, Sharma A, Singh P. Multi-objective optimization of magnetic abrasive finishing using grey relational analysis. *Materials Today: Proceedings* [Internet]. Elsevier Ltd; 2021;1–6. Available from: https://doi.org/10.1016/j.matpr.2021.01.004
13. Singh S, Prakash C, Pramanik A, Basak A, Shabadi R, Królczyk G, et al. Magneto-rheological fluid assisted abrasive nanofinishing of β-Phase Ti-Nb-Ta-Zr alloy: Parametric appraisal and corrosion analysis. *Materials* [Internet]. 2020;13:5156. Available from: www.mdpi.com/1996-1944/13/22/5156
14. Babbar A, Jain V, Gupta D, Prakash C, Singh S, Sharma A. 3D Bioprinting in pharmaceuticals, medicine, and tissue engineering applications. In *Advanced Manufacturing and Processing Technology* [Internet]. First edition. Boca Raton, FL: CRC Press, 2021, pp. 147–61. Available from: www.taylorfrancis.com/books/9781000193169/chapters/10.1201/9780429298042-7
15. Sharma A, Jain V, Gupta D, Babbar A. A review study on miniaturization. In *Advanced Manufacturing and Processing Technology* [Internet]. First edition. Boca Raton, FL: CRC Press, 2021, p. 111–31. Available from: www.taylorfrancis.com/books/9781000193169/chapters/10.1201/9780429298042-5
16. Babbar A, Jain V, Gupta D, Prakash C, Sharma A. Fabrication and machining methods of composites for aerospace applications. In *Characterization, Testing, Measurement, and Metrology* [Internet]. First edition. Boca Raton, FL: CRC Press, 2020, pp. 109–24. Available from: www.taylorfrancis.com/books/9781000193336/chapters/10.1201/9780429298073-7

17. Babbar A, Jain V, Gupta D, Prakash C, Singh S, Sharma A. Effect of process parameters on cutting forces and osteonecrosis for orthopedic bone drilling applications. In *Characterization, Testing, Measurement, and Metrology* [Internet]. First edition. Boca Raton, FL: CRC Press, 2020, pp. 93–108. Available from: www.taylorfrancis.com/books/9781000193336/chapters/10.1201/9780429298073-6

18. Babbar A, Jain V, Gupta D, Sharma A. Fabrication of microchannels using conventional and hybrid machining processes. In *Non-Conventional Hybrid Machining Processes* [Internet]. First edition. Boca Raton, FL: CRC Press, 2020, pp. 37–51. Available from: www.taylorfrancis.com/books/9780429642746/chapters/10.1201/9780429029165-3

19. Sharma A, Grover V, Babbar A, Rani R. A Trending nonconventional hybrid finishing/machining process. In *Non-Conventional Hybrid Machining Processes* [Internet]. First edition. Boca Raton, FL: CRC Press, 2020, pp. 79–93. Available from: www.taylorfrancis.com/books/9780429642746/chapters/10.1201/9780429029165-5

20. Sharma A, Babbar A, Jain V, Gupta D. Influence of cutting force and drilling temperature on glass hole surface integrity during rotary ultrasonic drilling. *Advances in Production and Industrial Engineering* [Internet]. 2021:369–78. Available from: http://link.springer.com/10.1007/978-981-15-5519-0_28

21. Babbar A, Sharma A, Chugh M. Application of flexible sintered magnetic abrasive brush for finishing of brass plate. *Optimization in Engineering Research*. 2020;1:36–47.

22. Babbar A, Prakash C, Singh S, Gupta MK, Mia M, Pruncu CI. Application of hybrid nature-inspired algorithm: Single and bi-objective constrained optimization of magnetic abrasive finishing process parameters. *Journal of Materials Research and Technology* [Internet]. Korea Institute of Oriental Medicine; 2020;9:7961–74. Available from: https://doi.org/10.1016/j.jmrt.2020.05.003

23. Babbar A, Sharma A, Bansal S, Mago J, Toor V. Potential applications of three-dimensional printing for anatomical simulations and surgical planning. *Materials Today: Proceedings* [Internet]. Elsevier Ltd; 2020;33:1558–61. Available from: https://doi.org/10.1016/j.matpr.2020.04.123

24. Singh D, Babbar A, Jain V, Gupta D, Saxena S, Dwibedi V. Synthesis, characterization, and bioactivity investigation of biomimetic biodegradable PLA scaffold fabricated by fused filament fabrication process. *Journal of the Brazilian Society of Mechanical Sciences and Engineering* [Internet]. 2019;41:121. Available from: http://link.springer.com/10.1007/s40430-019-1625-y

25. Babbar A, Kumar A, Jain V, Gupta D. Enhancement of activated tungsten inert gas (A-TIG) welding using multi-component TiO2-SiO2-Al2O3 hybrid flux. *Measurement* [Internet]. Elsevier Ltd; 2019;148:106912. Available from: https://doi.org/10.1016/j.measurement.2019.106912

26. Kumar M, Babbar A, Sharma A, Shahi AS. Effect of post weld thermal aging (PWTA) sensitization on micro-hardness and corrosion behavior of AISI 304 weld joints. *Journal of Physics: Conference Series* [Internet]. 2019;1240:012078. Available from: https://iopscience.iop.org/article/10.1088/1742-6596/1240/1/012078

27. Sharma A, Jain V. Experimental investigation of cutting temperature during drilling of float glass specimen. *IOP Conference Series: Materials Science and Engineering*. 2020;715:012050.

28. Sharma A, Jain V, Gupta D. A novel investigation study on float glass hole surface integrity & tool wear using chemical assisted rotary ultrasonic machining. *Materials Today: Proceedings* [Internet]. 2020;26:632–7. Available from: https://linkinghub.elsevier.com/retrieve/pii/S2214785319342324

29. Sharma A, Jain V, Gupta D. Effect of pre and post tempering on hole quality of float glass specimen: For rotary ultrasonic and conventional drilling. *Silicon*. 2021;13:2029–39.

30. Sharma A, Jain V, Gupta D. Characterization of chipping and tool wear during drilling of float glass using rotary ultrasonic machining. *Measurement: Journal of the International Measurement Confederation*. 2018;128:254–63.

31. Sharma A, Jain V, Gupta D. Comparative analysis of chipping mechanics of float glass during rotary ultrasonic drilling and conventional drilling: For multi-shaped tools. *Machining Science and Technology*. 2019;23:547–68.

32. Zuback JS, DebRoy T. The hardness of additively manufactured alloys. *Materials*. 2018;11:2070.

33. Chen Y, Xu Z, Smith C, Sankar J. Recent advances on the development of magnesium alloys for biodegradable implants. *Acta Biomaterialia*. 2014:4561–73.

34. Yang HG. Numerical simulation of the temperature and stress state on the additive friction stir with the smoothed particle hydrodynamics method. *Strength of Materials*. 2020;52:24–31.

35. Pandey A, Awasthi A, Saxena KK. Metallic implants with properties and latest production techniques: A review. *Advances in Materials and Processing Technologies*. 2020:167–202.

36. Ni J, Ling H, Zhang S, Wang Z, Peng Z, Benyshek C, et al. Three-dimensional printing of metals for biomedical applications. *Materials Today Bio*. 2019;3:100024.

37. Babbar A, Jain V, Gupta D. Thermo-mechanical aspects and temperature measurement techniques of bone grinding. *Materials Today: Proceedings*. 2019:1458–62.

38. Bandyopadhyay A, Bose S, Das S. 3D printing of biomaterials. *MRS Bulletin*. 2015;40:108–14.

39. ASM International. Overview of biomaterials and their use in medical devices. *ASM International*. 2003;1–11.

40. Zdrahala RJ, Zdrahala IJ. Biomedical applications of polyurethanes: A review of past promises, present realities, and a vibrant future. *Journal of Biomaterials Applications*. 1999;14:67–90.

41. Babbar A, Sharma A, Kumar R, Pundir P, Dhiman V. Functionalized biomaterials for 3D printing: An overview of the literature. *Additive Manufacturing with Functionalized Nanomaterials*. 2021:87–107.

42. Zhu Y, Gao C, He T, Shen J. Endothelium regeneration on luminal surface of polyurethane vascular scaffold modified with diamine and covalently grafted with gelatin. *Biomaterials*. 2004;25:423–30.

43. Yuan Y, Ai F, Zang X, Zhuang W, Shen J, Lin S. Polyurethane vascular catheter surface grafted with zwitterionic sulfobetaine monomer activated by ozone. *Colloids and Surfaces B: Biointerfaces*. 2004;35:1–5.

44. Chakraborty S, Kumar V. Development of an intelligent decision model for non-traditional machining processes. *Decision Making: Applications in Management and Engineering*. 2021;4:194–214.

45. Stratton S, Shelke NB, Hoshino K, Rudraiah S, Kumbar SG. Bioactive polymeric scaffolds for tissue engineering. *Bioactive Materials*. 2016:93–108.

46. Horner PJ, Gage FH. Regenerating the damaged central nervous system. *Nature*. 2000:963–70.

47. Kumar V, Diyaley S, Chakraborty S. Teaching-learning-based parametric optimization of an electrical discharge machining process. *Facta Universitatis, Series: Mechanical Engineering*. 2020;18:281–300.

48. Scheib J, Höke A. Advances in peripheral nerve regeneration. *Nature Reviews Neurology*. 2013:668–76.

49. Cao J, Xiao Z, Jin W, Chen B, Meng D, Ding W, et al. Induction of rat facial nerve regeneration by functional collagen scaffolds. *Biomaterials*. 2013;34:1302–10.

50. Kumar V, Das PP, Chakraborty S. Grey-fuzzy method-based parametric analysis of abrasive water jet machining on GFRP composites. *Sādhanā*. 2020;45:106.

51. Liu Z, Liu X, Ramakrishna S. Surface engineering of biomaterials in orthopedic and dental implants: Strategies to improve osteointegration, bacteriostatic and bactericidal activities. *Biotechnology Journal*. 2021;16:2000116.
52. Karst D, Yang Y. Molecular modeling study of the resistance of PLA to hydrolysis based on the blending of PLLA and PDLA. *Polymer*. 2006;47:4845–50.
53. Kadambi P, Luniya P, Dhatrak P. Current advancements in polymer/polymer matrix composites for dental implants: A systematic review. *Materials Today: Proceedings*. 2021:740–5.
54. Jin S, Xia X, Huang J, Yuan C, Zuo Y, Li Y, et al. Recent advances in PLGA-based biomaterials for bone tissue regeneration. *Acta Biomaterialia*. 2021:56–79.
55. Tan F, Zhu Y, Ma Z, Al-Rubeai M. Recent advances in the implant-based drug delivery in otorhinolaryngology. *Acta Biomaterialia*. 2020:46–55.
56. Babbar A, Jain V, Gupta D. Neurosurgical bone grinding. *Biomanufacturing*. 2019:137–55.
57. Jędzierowska M, Binkowski M, Koprowski R, Wróbel Z. Evaluation of the effect of a PCL/NaNoSiO2 implant on bone tissue regeneration using X-ray micro-computed tomography. *Advances in Intelligent Systems and Computing*. 2021:107–17.
58. Hernandez JL, Park J, Yao S, Blakney AK, Nguyen H V., Katz BH, et al. Effect of tissue microenvironment on fibrous capsule formation to biomaterial-coated implants. *Biomaterials*. 2021;273.
59. Dong Q, Zhang M, Zhou X, Shao Y, Li J, Wang L, et al. 3D-printed Mg-incorporated PCL-based scaffolds: A promising approach for bone healing. *Materials Science and Engineering C*. 2021;129.
60. Hu B, Guo Y, Li H, Liu X, Fu Y, Ding F. Recent advances in chitosan-based layer-by-layer biomaterials and their biomedical applications. *Carbohydrate Polymers*. 2021;271:118427.
61. Pérez-Merino P, Dorronsoro C, Llorente L, Durán S, Jiménez-Alfaro I, Marcos S. In vivo chromatic aberration in eyes implanted with intraocular lenses. *Investigative Ophthalmology and Visual Science*. 2013;54:2654–61.
62. Terrada C, Julian K, Cassoux N, Prieur AM, Debre M, Quartier P, et al. Cataract surgery with primary intraocular lens implantation in children with uveitis: Long-term outcomes. *Journal of Cataract and Refractive Surgery*. 2011;37:1977–83.
63. Sharma A, Kumar V, Babbar A, Dhawan V, Kotecha K, Prakash C. Experimental investigation and optimization of electric discharge machining process parameters using grey-fuzzy-based hybrid techniques. *Materials*. 2021;14:5820.
64. Teo AJT, Mishra A, Park I, Kim YJ, Park WT, Yoon YJ. Polymeric biomaterials for medical implants and devices. *ACS Biomaterials Science and Engineering*. 2016:454–72.
65. Zhou J, Huang X, Zheng D, Li H, Herrler T, Li Q. Oriental nose elongation using an L-shaped polyethylene sheet implant for combined septal spreading and extension. *Aesthetic Plastic Surgery*. 2014;38:295–302.
66. Prakash C, Kumar V, Mistri A, Uppal AS, Babbar A, Pathri BP, et al. Investigation of functionally graded adherents on failure of socket joint of FRP composite tubes. *Materials*. 2021;14:6365.
67. Peltola MJ, Vallittu PK, Vuorinen V, Aho AAJ, Puntala A, Aitasalo KMJ. Novel composite implant in craniofacial bone reconstruction. *European Archives of Oto-Rhino-Laryngology*. 2012;269:623–8.
68. Gao C, Peng S, Feng P, Shuai C. Bone biomaterials and interactions with stem cells. *Bone Research*. 2017;5:1–33.
69. Tayyaba S, Ashraf MW, Ahmad Z, Wang N, Afzal MJ, Afzulpurkar N. Article fabrication and analysis of polydimethylsiloxane (PDMS) microchannels for biomedical application. *Processes*. 2021;9:1–31.

70. Babbar A, Jain V, Gupta D, Prakash C, Singh S, Sharma A. 3D Bioprinting in pharmaceuticals, medicine, and tissue engineering applications. *Advanced Manufacturing and Processing Technology*. 2020:147–61.

71. Kubyshkina G, Zupančič B, Štukelj M, Grošelj D, Marion L, Emri I. Sterilization effect on structure, thermal and time-dependent properties of polyamides. *Conference Proceedings of the Society for Experimental Mechanics Series*. 2011:11–19.

72. Li X, Liu X, Huang J, Fan Y, Cui F zhai. Biomedical investigation of CNT based coatings. *Surface and Coatings Technology*. 2011;206:759–66.

73. Huang Y, Van Dessel J, Martens W, Lambrichts I, Zhong WJ, Ma GW, et al. Sensory innervation around immediately vs. delayed loaded implants: A pilot study. *International Journal of Oral Science*. 2015;7:49–55.

74. Arsiwala A, Desai P, Patravale V. Recent advances in micro/nanoscale biomedical implants. *Journal of Controlled Release*. 2014;189:25–45.

75. Takmakov P, Ruda K, Scott Phillips K, Isayeva IS, Krauthamer V, Welle CG. Rapid evaluation of the durability of cortical neural implants using accelerated aging with reactive oxygen species. *Journal of Neural Engineering*. 2015;12.

76. Guo R, Merkel AR, Sterling JA, Davidson JM, Guelcher SA. Substrate modulus of 3D-printed scaffolds regulates the regenerative response in subcutaneous implants through the macrophage phenotype and Want signaling. *Biomaterials*. 2015;73:85–95.

77. Li J, Stachowski M, Zhang Z. Application of responsive polymers in implantable medical devices and biosensors. *Switchable and Responsive Surfaces and Materials for Biomedical Applications*. 2015:259–98.

78. Klein M, Schiegnitz E, Al-Nawas B. Systematic review on success of narrow-diameter dental implants. *The International Journal of Oral & Maxillofacial Implants*. 2014;29:43–54.

79. Yahyavi-Firouz-Abadi N, Menias CO, Bhalla S, Siegel C, Gayer G, Katz DS. Imaging of cosmetic plastic procedures and implants in the body and their potential complications. *American Journal of Roentgenology*. 2015;204:707–15.

80. Silva V V., Domingues RZ, Lameiras FS. Microstructural and mechanical study of zirconia-hydroxyapatite (ZH) composite ceramics for biomedical applications. *Composites Science and Technology*. 2001;61:301–10.

81. Jardini AL, Larosa MA, Macedo MF, Bernardes LF, Lambert CS, Zavaglia CAC, et al. Improvement in cranioplasty: Advanced prosthesis biomanufacturing. *Procedia CIRP*. 2016:203–8.

82. Almog DM, Torrado E, Meitner SW. Fabrication of imaging and surgical guides for dental implants. *Journal of Prosthetic Dentistry*. 2001;85:504–8.

83. Liu D, Fu J, Fan H, Li D, Dong E, Xiao X, et al. Application of 3D-printed PEEK scapula prosthesis in the treatment of scapular benign fibrous histiocytoma: A case report. *Journal of Bone Oncology*. 2018;12:78–82.

84. Tischler M, Patch C, Bidra AS. Rehabilitation of edentulous jaws with zirconia complete-arch fixed implant-supported prostheses: An up to 4-year retrospective clinical study. *Journal of Prosthetic Dentistry*. 2018;120:204–9.

85. Francis R, Kumar DS, editors. *Biomedical Applications of Polymeric Materials and Composites*. Weinheim, Germany: John Wiley & Sons. Dec 19, 2016.

86. Babbar A, Jain V, Gupta D, Agrawal D. Finite element simulation and integration of CEM43 °C and Arrhenius models for ultrasonic-assisted skull bone grinding: A thermal dose model. *Medical Engineering and Physics*. 2021;90:9–22.

87. Saikko V, Ahlroos T, Revitzer H, Ryti O, Kuosmanen P. The effect of acetabular cup position on wear of a large-diameter metal-on-metal prosthesis studied with a hip joint simulator. *Tribology International*. 2013;60:70–6.

88. Matsushita T, Fujibayashi S, Kokubo T. Titanium foam for bone tissue engineering. *Metallic Foam Bone: Processing, Modification and Characterization and Properties*. 2017:111–30.

89. Hedlundh U, Karlsson L. Combining a hip arthroplasty stem with trochanteric reattachment bolt and a polyaxially locking plate in the treatment of a periprosthetic fracture below a well-integrated implant. *Arthroplasty Today*. 2016;2:141–5.
90. Currey JD. The structure and mechanics of bone. *Journal of Materials Science*. 2012:41–54.
91. Babbar A, Jain V, Gupta D, Prakash C. Experimental investigation and parametric optimization of neurosurgical bone grinding under bio-mimic environment. *Surface Review and Letters*. July 28, 2021:2141005.
92. Yang Y, Wu P, Wang Q, Wu H, Liu Y, Deng Y, et al. The enhancement of Mg corrosion resistance by alloying Mn and laser-melting. *Materials*. 2016;9.
93. Hoover S, Tarafder S, Bandyopadhyay A, Bose S. Silver doped resorbable tricalcium phosphate scaffolds for bone graft applications. *Materials Science and Engineering C*. 2017;79:763–9.
94. Faroni A, Mobasseri SA, Kingham PJ, Reid AJ. Peripheral nerve regeneration: Experimental strategies and future perspectives. *Advanced Drug Delivery Reviews*. 2015:160–7.
95. Shau D, Patton R, Patel S, Ward L, Guild G. Synthetic mesh vs. allograft extensor mechanism reconstruction in total knee arthroplasty—A systematic review of the literature and meta-analysis. *Knee*. 2018:2–7.
96. Wang Z, Wang C, Li C, Qin Y, Zhong L, Chen B, et al. Analysis of factors influencing bone ingrowth into three-dimensional printed porous metal scaffolds: A review. *Journal of Alloys and Compounds*. 2017:271–85.
97. Kumar A, Mandal S, Barui S, Vasireddi R, Gbureck U, Gelinsky M, et al. Low temperature additive manufacturing of three dimensional scaffolds for bone-tissue engineering applications: Processing related challenges and property assessment. *Materials Science and Engineering R: Reports*. 2016:1–39.
98. Chevalier E, Chulia D, Pouget C, Viana M. Fabrication of porous substrates: A review of processes using pore forming agents in the biomaterial field. *Journal of Pharmaceutical Sciences*. 2008:1135–54.
99. Pia G, Casnedi L, Ionta M, Sanna U. On the elastic deformation properties of porous ceramic materials obtained by pore-forming agent method. *Ceramics International*. 2015;41:11097–105.
100. Moghadam MZ, Hassanajili S, Esmaeilzadeh F, Ayatollahi M, Ahmadi M. Formation of porous HPCL/LPCL/HA scaffolds with supercritical CO2 gas foaming method. *Journal of the Mechanical Behavior of Biomedical Materials*. 2017;69:115–27.
101. Costantini M, Colosi C, Mozetic P, Jaroszewicz J, Tosato A, Rainer A, et al. Correlation between porous texture and cell seeding efficiency of gas foaming and microfluidic foaming scaffolds. *Materials Science and Engineering C*. 2016;62:668–77.
102. Theodorou GS, Kontonasaki E, Theocharidou A, Bakopoulou A, Bousnaki M, Hadjichristou C, et al. Sol-Gel Derived Mg-based ceramic scaffolds doped with zinc or copper ions: Preliminary results on their synthesis, characterization, and biocompatibility. *International Journal of Biomaterials*. 2016;2016.
103. Ros-Tárraga P, Murciano A, Mazón P, Gehrke SA, De Aza PN. New 3D stratified Si-Ca-P porous scaffolds obtained by sol-gel and polymer replica method: Microstructural, mineralogical and chemical characterization. *Ceramics International*. 2017;43:6548–53.
104. Abd-Khorsand S, Saber-Samandari S, Saber-Samandari S. Development of nanocomposite scaffolds based on TiO2 doped in grafted chitosan/hydroxyapatite by freeze drying method and evaluation of biocompatibility. *International Journal of Biological Macromolecules*. 2017;101:51–8.
105. Fereshteh Z, Fathi M, Bagri A, Boccaccini AR. Preparation and characterization of aligned porous PCL/zein scaffolds as drug delivery systems via improved unidirectional freeze-drying method. *Materials Science and Engineering C*. 2016;68:613–22.

106. Janik H, Marzec M. A review: Fabrication of porous polyurethane scaffolds. *Materials Science and Engineering C.* 2015:586–91.

107. Babbar A, Jain V, Gupta D, Singh S, Prakash C, Pruncu C. Biomaterials and fabrication methods of scaffolds for tissue engineering applications. *3D Printing in Biomedical Engineering.* 2020 (pp. 167–86), Springer, Singapore.

108. Kumar V, Chakraborty S. Analysis of the surface roughness characteristics of EDMed components using GRA method. *Proceedings of the International Conference on Industrial and Manufacturing Systems (CIMS-2020)* 2022 (pp. 461–78), Springer, Cham.

109. Chakraborty S, Das PP, Kumar V. A grey fuzzy logic approach for cotton fibre selection. *Journal of The Institution of Engineers (India): Series E.* 2017;98.

110. Chakraborty S, Kumar V, Ramakrishnan KR. Selection of the all-time best world XI test cricket team using the TOPSIS method. *Decision Science Letters.* 2019;8:95–108.

111. Chakraborty S, Das PP, Kumar V. Application of grey-fuzzy logic technique for parametric optimization of non-traditional machining processes. *Grey Systems: Theory and Application.* 2018;8:46–68.

112. Babbar A, Jain V, Gupta D, Agrawal D, Prakash C, Singh S, et al. Experimental analysis of wear and multi-shape burr loading during neurosurgical bone grinding. *Journal of Materials Research and Technology.* 2021;12:15–28.

113. Singh S, Singh G, Prakash C, Ramakrishna S. Current status and future directions of fused fi lament fabrication. *Journal of Manufacturing Processes* [Internet]. Elsevier; 2020;55:288–306. Available from: https://doi.org/10.1016/j.jmapro.2020.04.049

114. Prakash C, Kansal HK, Pabla BS, Puri S, Prakash C, Kansal HK, et al. Experimental investigations in powder mixed electric discharge machining of Ti—35Nb—7Ta—5Zr β—titanium alloy. *Materials and Manufacturing Processes* [Internet]. Taylor & Francis; 2017;32:274–85. Available from: http://dx.doi.org/10.1080/10426914.2016.1198018

115. Prakash C, Kansal HK, Pabla BS, Puri S. On the influence of nanoporous layer fabricated by PMEDM on β-Ti implant: Biological and computational evaluation of bone-implant interface. *Materials Today: Proceedings.* 2017;4:2298–307.

116. Prakash C, Kansal HK, Pabla BS, Puri S. To optimize the surface roughness and microhardness of β-Ti alloy in PMEDM process using non-dominated sorting genetic algorithm-II. 2015 2nd International Conference on Recent Advances in Engineering and Computational Sciences, RAECS, 2015.2016.

117. Prakash C, Kansal HK, Pabla BS, Puri S. Multi-objective optimization of powder mixed electric discharge machining parameters for fabrication of biocompatible layer on β-Ti alloy using NSGA-II coupled with Taguchi based response surface methodology. *Journal of Mechanical Science and Technology.* 2016;30:4195–204.

118. Prakash C, Singh S, Farina I, Fraternali F, Feo L. Physical-mechanical characterization of biodegradable Mg-3Si-HA composites. *PSU Research Review.* 2018;2:152–74.

119. Prakash C, Kansal HK, Pabla BS, Puri S. Potential of silicon powder-mixed electro spark alloying for surface modification of β-phase titanium alloy for orthopedic applications. *Materials Today: Proceedings.* 2017:10080–3.

120. Prakash C, Kansal HK, Pabla BS, Puri S. Experimental investigations in powder mixed electric discharge machining of Ti—35Nb—7Ta—5Zrβ-titanium alloy. *Materials and Manufacturing Processes.* 2017;32:274–85.

121. Prakash C, Kansal HK, Pabla BS, Puri S. Powder mixed electric discharge machining: An innovative surface modification technique to enhance fatigue performance and bioactivity of β-Ti implant for orthopedics application. *Journal of Computing and Information Science in Engineering.* 2016;16:1–9.

122. Singh S, Singh N, Gupta M, Prakash C, Singh R. Mechanical feasibility of ABS/HIPS-based multi-material structures primed by low-cost polymer printer. *Rapid Prototyping Journal* [Internet]. 2019;25:152–61. Available from: www.emeraldinsight.com/doi/10.1108/RPJ-01-2018-0028

123. Prakash C, Singh S, Pabla BS, Uddin MS. Synthesis, characterization, corrosion and bioactivity investigation of nano-HA coating deposited on biodegradable Mg-Zn-Mn alloy. *Surface and Coatings Technology* [Internet]. Elsevier B.V; 2018;346:9–18. Available from: https://doi.org/10.1016/j.surfcoat.2018.04.035

124. Prakash C, Singh S, Ramakrishna S, Królczyk G, Le CH. Microwave sintering of porous Ti—Nb-HA composite with high strength and enhanced bioactivity for implant applications. *Journal of Alloys and Compounds.* 2020;824.

125. Prakash C, Singh S, Verma K, Sidhu SS, Singh S. Synthesis and characterization of Mg-Zn-Mn-HA composite by spark plasma sintering process for orthopedic applications. *Vacuum* [Internet]. Elsevier; 2018;155:578–84. Available from: https://doi.org/10.1016/j.vacuum.2018.06.063

126. Prakash C, Kansal HK, Pabla BS, Puri S, Aggarwal A. Electric discharge machining—A potential choice for surface modification of metallic implants for orthopedic applications: A review. *Proceedings of the Institution of Mechanical Engineers, Part B: Journal of Engineering Manufacture.* 2016:331–53.

127. Prakash C, Singh S, Pabla BS, Sidhu SS, Uddin MS. Bio-inspired low elastic biodegradable Mg-Zn-Mn-Si-HA alloy fabricated by spark plasma sintering. *Materials and Manufacturing Processes* [Internet]. Taylor & Francis; 2019;34:357–68. Available from: https://doi.org/10.1080/10426914.2018.1512117

128. Parthasarathy J. 3D modeling, custom implants and its future perspectives in craniofacial surgery. *Annals of Maxillofacial Surgery.* 2014;4:9.

129. Jardini AL, Larosa MA, de Carvalho Zavaglia CA, Bernardes LF, Lambert CS, Kharmandayan P, et al. Customised titanium implant fabricated in additive manufacturing for craniomaxillofacial surgery. *Virtual and Physical Prototyping.* 2014;9:115–25.

130. Ghorbani F, Li D, Ni S, Zhou Y, Yu B. 3D printing of acellular scaffolds for bone defect regeneration: A review. *Materials Today Communications.* 2020;22.

131. Rosicky J, Grygar A, Chapcak P, Bouma T, Rosicky J. Application of 3D scanning in prosthetic and orthotic clinical practice. *Proceedings of the 7th International Conference on 3D Body Scanning Technologies.* Nov 30, 2016, pp. 88–97.

132. Zuniga J. 3D Printed antibacterial prostheses. *Applied Sciences.* 2018;8:1651.

133. Devinuwara K, Dworak-Kula A, O'Connor RJ. Rehabilitation and prosthetics postamputation. *Orthopaedics and Trauma.* 2018;32:234–40.

3 Additive Manufacturing Process for the Development of Orthosis of Foot

Manak L. Jain[1], Nalinakash S. Vyas[2], Anil Mulewa,[3] and Sanjay G. Dhande[4]

[1] Professor, Dept. of mechanical engineering, Shri G. S. Institute of Technology and Science Indore, India

[2] Professor, Dept. of Mechanical Engineering, Indian Institute of Technology Kanpur, India

[3] Assistant Professor, Dept. of Mechanical Engineering, Shri G. S. Institute of Technology and Science Indore, India

[4] Ex. Professor, Dept. of mechanical engineering, Dept. of Computer Science & Engineering, Indian Institute of Technology Kanpur, India)

E-mail: mljain_iitk@rediffmail.com, vyas@iitk.ac.in, anilmulewa89@gmail.com, sgdhande@gmail.com

CONTENTS

3.1 Overview of Rapid Prototyping 48
    3.1.1 Fused Deposition Modeling RP system 48
3.2 What Is Orthosis and Reverse Engineering 48
3.3 Development of an Ankle–Foot Orthosis 50
    3.3.1 Conventional Manufacturing Process 50
    3.3.2 Advance Indigenous Approach for AFO Design 51
    3.3.3 Mechanical Design Consideration 53
3.4 Methodology 53
    3.4.1 CAD Manufacturing Process 53
        3.4.1.1 Extracting Features and Segmenting Point Cloud 54
    3.4.2 Solid Modeling of AFO 55
3.5 Prototyping of AFO 56
    3.5.1 Clubfoot Model Making with Silicone Material 57
    3.5.2 Testing of AFO 60

3.6   Result and Discussion.. 61
3.7   Conclusion 61
References.. 62

3.1   OVERVIEW OF RAPID PROTOTYPING

The additive manufacturing process is a manufacturing process for building a physical prototype in which the three-dimensional (3D) physical part is built by the deposition of physical materials layer over layer. The process is also known as the rapid prototype (RP) system. Here, initially, a computer-aided-design (CAD) model is created virtually on a system and then is imported into an RP system, where a virtual model is converted into a physical prototype 3D model. The goal of RP is to quickly fabricate complex-shaped 3D parts directly from CAD models. Several RP techniques exist, and all employ the same basic five steps; these steps constitute the principle of working with an RP system, in which each physical layer will be placed over the previous one. These five steps follow:

1. Create a CAD model of the design.
2. Convert the CAD model to stereolithography (STL) format.
3. Slice the STL file into thin cross-sectional layers.
4. Construct the model one layer atop another.
5. Clean and finish the model.

3.1.1   FUSED DEPOSITION MODELING RP SYSTEM

In the fused deposition modeling (FDM) process, a spool of filament 1.27 mm in diameter feeds into the unit's extruding head. The extruder head moves in the X–Y plane (Figure 3.1). There is a choice of materials, including different colors and medical-grade acrylonitrile butadiene styrene (ABS), that can be gamma-sterilized [1]. The filament is melted to liquid inside the extruder head at 270 °C by a resistance heater [2]. Initially, the model is converted to an STL format in the CAD system and sent to the FDM slicing software [3]. There the STL file is sliced into thin cross sections of a desired thickness. Supports are created for overhanging parts and are sliced as well. The sliced model and supports are converted into a machine language file that contains actual instructions for the FDM machine [4]. A toolpath is generated which is followed by the numerically controlled extruder head [5]. It has been observed that postcuring is not required [6].

3.2   WHAT IS ORTHOSIS AND REVERSE ENGINEERING

An orthosis is an assistive device that not only provides immobilization, support, correction, or protection but also treats musculoskeletal injuries [8]. A radical change in manufacturing orthotic devices has already happened due to the exponential growth of the additive manufacturing process. The development of individualized devices able to adapt properly the patient's anatomical shapes, due to these devices,

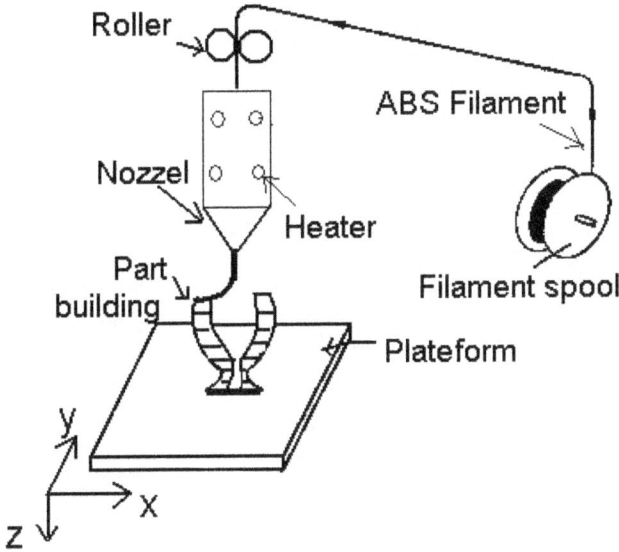

FIGURE 3.1 Schematic sketch of FDM RP system [7].

accomplish their rehabilitative function. With RP, the individualized orthotic devices have been already applied to the manufacturing of spinal braces and exoskeleton parts and in the medical and dental industries. In the present chapter, we restrict this to foot orthosis only [9].

The types of foot orthosis normally depend on the types of abnormality for which it is used, such as flatfoot orthosis, drop-foot orthosis, and clubfoot orthosis, among others. Foot and ankle orthoses are normally used (1) to correct the shape of the foot; (2) to control, guide, limit, and/or immobilize the foot and ankle; and (3) to aid rehabilitation from the fractures after the removal of a cast. Medically, there are many types of foot abnormalities, but some that normally use orthotics devices are (1) flatfoot, (2) cavus foot, and (3) clubfoot, among others. If the technology applied improves the quality of life of people suffering from disabilities with products by designing, testing, applying, and evaluating solutions, then this technology is known as rehabilitation engineering. In rehabilitation engineering, it is possible to develop custom prosthetics/orthotics/equipment and devices for the betterment of human life. Custom devices are usually developed by using reverse engineering (RE), technology in which the physical part's geometry is represented from its discrete point cloud data. In RE, the basic steps involved are (1) data acquisition, (2) preprocessing of acquired data, (3) solid model creation, and, finally, (4) physical prototype building. To improve personalize fitting (customization) and thereby increase the patient's health success rate, RE and additive manufacturing play a great role in the health care of patients. In this chapter, we mainly focus on abnormal foot conditions of babies, specifically clubfoot orthosis design [9–10] [5, 11].

3.3 DEVELOPMENT OF AN ANKLE–FOOT ORTHOSIS

Traditionally, ankle–foot orthosis (AFO) design and manufacturing have been a matter of skill and experience, and even until now, there has not been a proper scientific methodology for designing and manufacturing AFO [7]. Using CAD, a designer is able to conceive and render the geometry of a shoe or a car or an airplane in an effective and efficient manner. Designing the shoe, nesting cut pieces, and developing curved surfaces are some of the activities that are now carried out using CAD software systems, such as Imageware surfacer, Unigraphics, Catia, Proe, and others. Using an RP system in computer-aided manufacturing (CAM), a designer is not only able to render a shoe last on a computer screen but is also able to realize or make a physical full-scale model in a polymer material. These RP models are very useful for evaluating the form, fit, and function of a design. Developments in CAD/CAM technology have been successfully demonstrated in foot orthotics, particularly for the comfort of athletes and adults. It is a commercially viable method for replacing most normal manufacturing stages [10, 12].

This section deals with the traditional method of AFO, the mechanical design considerations of AFO, the proposed mechanism for a corrective procedure, and our approach to AFO design, with an Indigenously developed unique technique based on the geometrical modeling and prototyping of an AFO solid model.

3.3.1 CONVENTIONAL MANUFACTURING PROCESS

The traditional manufacturing process of AFO takes place according to the design flow chart as shown in Figure 3.2.

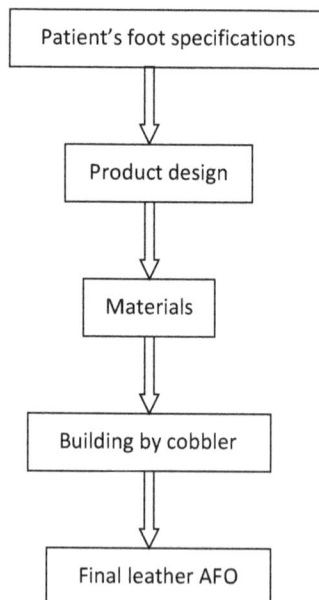

FIGURE 3.2 Conventional manufacturing of AFO [6].

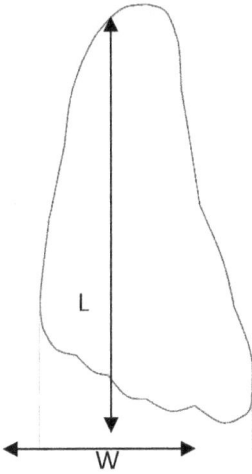

FIGURE 3.3A Foot profile of baby [6].

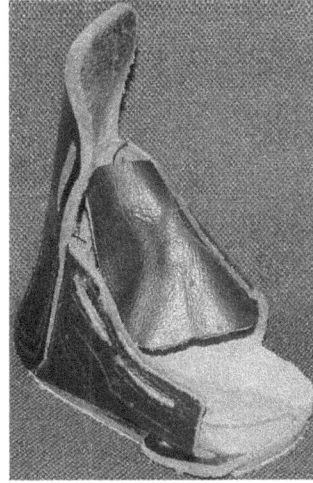

FIGURE 3.3B Traditional leather AFO [6].

Initially, the foot of the baby is placed on a cardboard paper, and then, with the help of a marker pen, the foot boundary is plotted on this paper. Based on this plot, the minimum and maximum sizes of the foot are determined. According to the obtained foot profile (Figure 3.3a), a flat, stiff wood material about 2 mm thick is taken and finished so as to match the foot profile, but about 10–15% more is kept more in order to give clearance. On the outer top surface (lateral side) of this wood strip, a wedge shape (30–35 degree) leather piece, depending on the nature of deformity, is glued with adhesive to the finished wood piece. This wedge should be fixed in such a way so that it helps reduce the equines of the forefoot and heel varus of clubfoot. After this, a soft padding about 1 mm thick is glued to the top surface of both this wood strip and the wedge. Because of its strength and stretchability properties, we used leather as the material for fixing to the upper side surface of the wood profile, which will help in fixing the foot. After marking on it the different shape and size for each foot, the leather patches are cut and stitched together by the cobbler, which gives an approximate leather envelope. This upper leather envelope is fixed and glued to the previously developed wooden profile. This will give traditional leather AFO shown in Figure 3.3b, which will be fitted to the baby's abnormal foot for its correction.

The method has limitations, because it is time-consuming and involves experience and skill, and a designer is not able to visualize clearly how the AFO will come up when it is actually placed and fitted over the abnormal foot.

3.3.2 ADVANCE INDIGENOUS APPROACH FOR AFO DESIGN

This section introduces a new technique for the customized design of AFO, which fits properly to the baby's clubfoot and gives a nice and more comfortable feel. Some suitable joints, which resemble the anatomic foot joints, are kept in its design. Hence, the AFO becomes flexible and helps in moving the clubfoot for correction with the help of a mechanism fitted to it. The point cloud data of a patient's clubfoot, which is exported from MIMICS software, is the basic input for design. The technique is based on clubfoot point cloud analysis, curve design, composite surface design, solid model creation, and prototyping of AFO. The techniques utilized one given in the flow chart shown in Figure 3.4. This section deals with the adopted methodology for the current research work. The section mainly describes the acquisition of medical imaging data of patients, CAD, RP, and silicon modeling (rapid tooling) of clubfoot. The flow diagram in Figure 3.4 represents the main sequence of operations to be performed for conducting the present development. Initially, we scan the adult foot

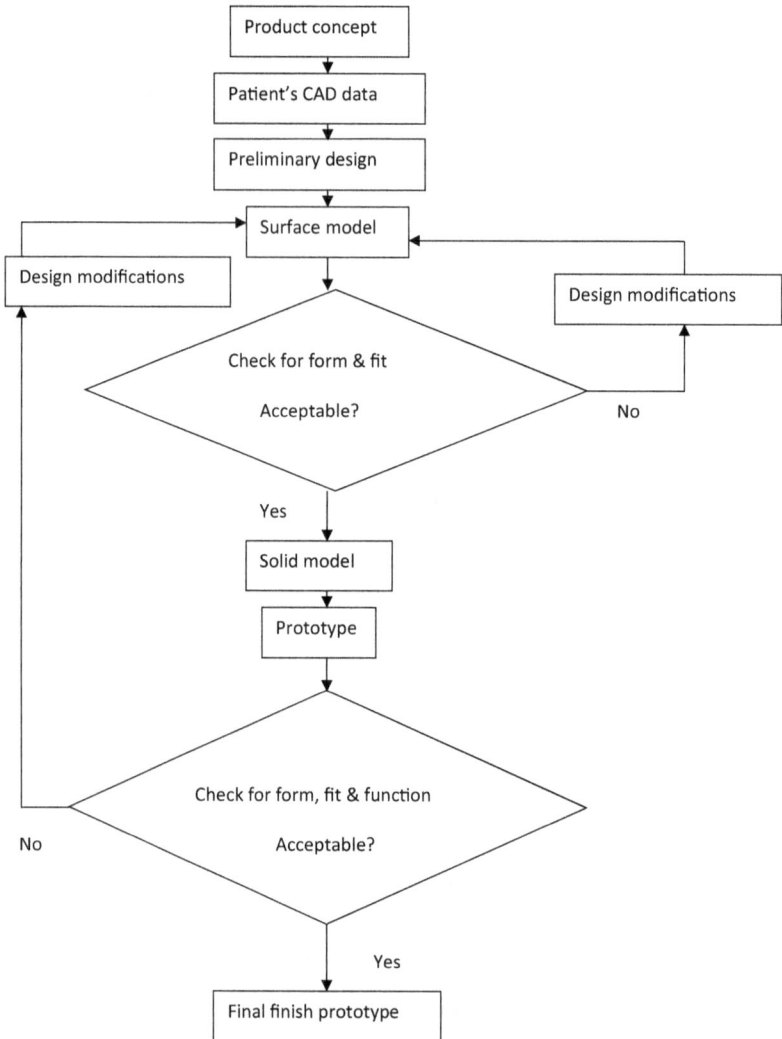

FIGURE 3.4   CAD manufacturing of AFO [6].

with computed tomography (CT), and after successful integration of the CT with RP, we extend the techniques to magnetic resonance imaging (MRI) of a baby's clubfoot [5, 12].

3.3.3 MECHANICAL DESIGN CONSIDERATION

An AFO, like any other product, has four aspects: (1) function, (2) strength, (3) ergonomics, and (4) aesthetic. All these aspects are equally important. Functionally, an AFO provides protection, as well as grip, to the clubfoot. It should rotate the clubfoot as per the required degree of rotation so as to achieve the normal foot geometry in a given time period. It should be plane at forefoot and sufficiently hard so as to prevent the wrong deformation of clubfoot during its timely growth. The design should be such that the patient feels comfortable and happy while wearing it. It should not act as an obstacle while the patient performs their daily normal activities. The AFO should have an adequate ergonomic design with proper ventilation, required padding, and so on that allows plenty of room for growth, because babies' feet continue to take shape during the initial period of their growth. Aesthetics for AFO are also a major factor as people like an AFO that adds beauty and style to their baby. The primary purpose of AFO is to correct clubfoot, and in order to do so, it must have a corrective load applying mechanism and must fit the foot well. Poorly designed and fitted AFO can cause discomfort and other foot problems and will not correct the deformity. The design of AFO should conform to the shape of a normal foot; on wearing it, the clubfoot should be forced to conform to the shape of AFO.

Apart from the previously mentioned four major design considerations, the following recommendations for the design of AFO should also be kept in mind. This recommendation helps evaluate the performance of AFO during its fit on the foot.

3.4 METHODOLOGY

3.4.1 CAD MANUFACTURING PROCESS

If traditional techniques are employed, each new design takes a considerable amount of time, as the method is based on skill, as well as on trial and error, and the product may not be competitive any longer, thus, a need exists for adopting modern technologies to reduce this lead time and decrease development cost. We utilize CAD/CAM modern tools for effectively designing and manufacturing AFO. Initially, the point cloud data of the baby's foot is acquired through an MRI scan, and before segmenting the cloud and creating the surface model, it is important to decide the strategy for surface fitting [5]. Hence, outlined strategy is as follows:

- Sample the point cloud and remove noise, if any.
- Segment the point cloud.
- Create cross sections.
- Create curves from the cross section and modify they.
- Create surfaces from the curves.
- Check the quality of the final surface.

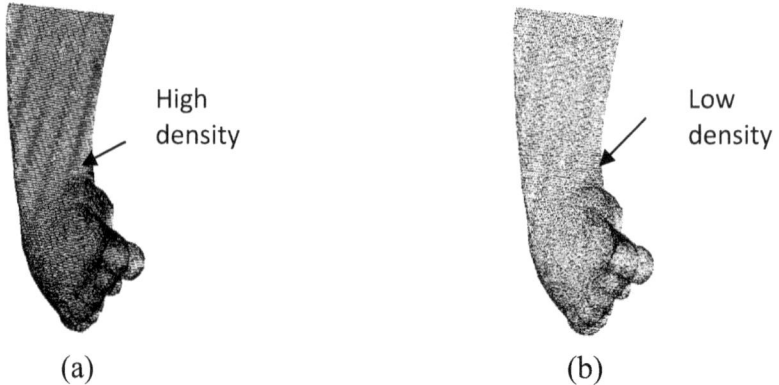

FIGURE 3.5   Point cloud data of clubfoot: (a) Dense cloud; (b) sampled cloud [6].

Keeping the preceding strategy in the mind, we proceeded on the acquired point clouds and developed the AFO prototype as shown in Figure 3.5.

3.4.1.1   Extracting Features and Segmenting Point Cloud

The data are broken into meaningful portions by identifying points along feature lines, based on angular, curvature, and edge in the original object as observed in its RP model. All point clouds must be readjusted to create the digital image of the complete clubfoot in one coordinate system. This is called registration. Figures 3.6a and 3.6b show extracted clouds and their segmentation into the three interested regions of the shank, heel, and foot.

After point cloud processing, the curves are created in an interrogated way, which are modified and edited on point networks. The curve fitting is done piecewise, and the individual curves should satisfy the required constraints of tangency and position. For simplicity and accuracy, we need normalized cubic spline curves. A provision is also made on the curves so that their tangency factor can be manipulated by the designer because the shape of a cubic curve is dependent, to a large extent, on the magnitude of tangent vectors at the end points. A step-by-step procedure of curve designing in unigraphics CAD software is adopted, and a correct curves model, ready for processing of surface fitting next, is obtained and is shown in Figure 3.7.

After curve modeling, the surface modeling is planned with surfacing strategies to fit a surface (refer to Figure 3.8). The decision is dependent on many criteria like downstream application (solid modeling, finite element analysis (FEA), RP, etc.) requirements. A surface can be created in the surfacer version of the unigraphics software by fitting to multiple surface patches joined along their boundaries with C^0 (position) and C^1 (Tangent) continuity, with the following strategies:

- Point data
- Lofting and blending
- Bounding with curves
- Revolving
- Offsetting and mirroring

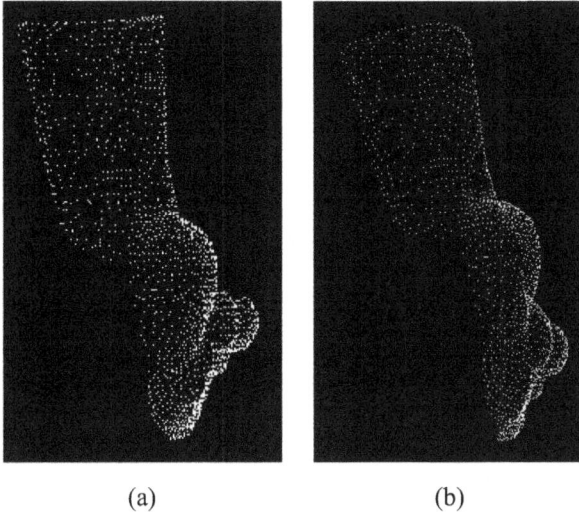

(a)   (b)

FIGURE 3.6   Segmentation of point cloud: (a) Single segment; (b) three segments [6].

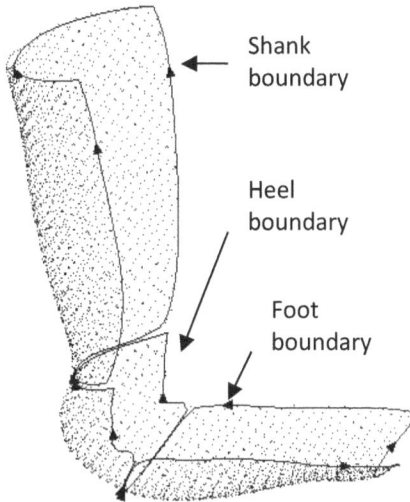

Shank boundary

Heel boundary

Foot boundary

FIGURE 3.7   Curves model of proposed AFO [6].

A step-by-step surface-fitting procedure for AFO is adopted as shown in Figure 3.8.

3.4.2   SOLID MODELING OF AFO

The AFO design deals with converting ideas into reality and aims at fulfilling AFO functional requirements. In this section, a systemic approach is discussed for the design and development of its solid model. The solid modeling is done keeping in consideration its functionality and strength. Our research is related to a baby's

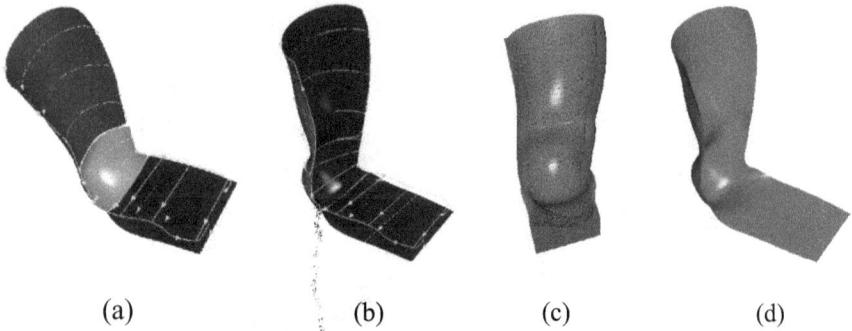

FIGURE 3.8   Surface models of AFO: (a) Three patches; (b) matched single patch; (c) form and fit check; (d) final surface model of AFO [6].

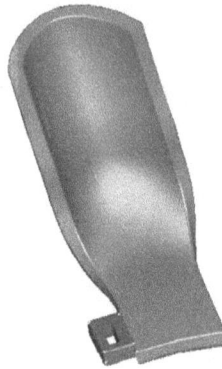

FIGURE 3.9   Simple one-piece AFO [6].

deformed foot, and hence, an ABS polymeric material, which is a tough plastic, is chosen for the design consideration [5, 10]. It is lighter in weight and nontoxic, and it has a good look. Hence, the chosen material fulfills the design requirements. A step-by-step procedure for solid modeling of AFO to fulfill the previously discussed design requirements is adapted as shown in Figure 3.9.

3.5   PROTOTYPING OF AFO

The third step after model study is the design of AFO and its prototyping (refer to Figure 3.10). As our research at this stage is limited to customization and hence after proper AFO design strategy, its surface model using deformed foot point cloud data is created. The surface model is then converted into a solid model and is fabricated in FDM, whose testing is done on a silicone foot model, and after its success, actual testing is extended to the patient [13].

The SML file contains the actual instruction code for the FDM hardware. The SML file orders the FDM to take a specific toolpath at each Z level. The file also has

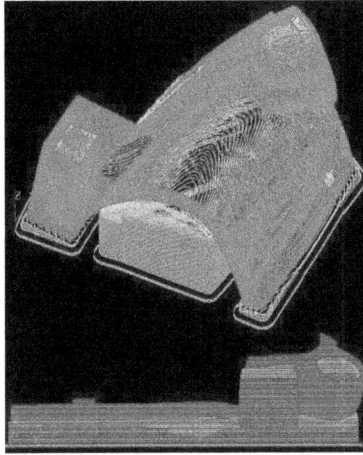

FIGURE 3.10   File showing slices, base, and support of AFO [6].

TABLE 3.1
Properties of P400-ABS Plastic

S. No.	Particular	Value
1.	Tensile Strength	34.5 MPa
2.	Flexural Strength	65.5 MPa
3.	Tensile Modulus	2482.8 Mpa
4.	Flexural Modulus	2620.7 Mpa
5.	Melting Point	270 °C
6.	Softening Point	104.4 °C
7.	Specific Gravity	1.05 gm/cc

information about the model and support material consumption and build time of the job. The created SML file is sent to the FDM hardware, where it builds the part with ABS, which is a nontoxic and tough plastic having the properties of P400-ABS plastic [13], as shown in Table 3.1

After the AFO is built, its postprocessing, that is, finalizing of the part, is done, which mainly involves removing support material from the model and its surface finishing by mechanical means.

3.5.1   Clubfoot Model Making with Silicone Material

A much-anticipated application of RP is rapid tooling, the automatic fabrication of production-quality machine tools. The RP parts are used as patterns for making molds and dies. In the simplest and oldest rapid tooling technique, an RP-positive pattern is suspended in a vat of liquid silicone rubber. When the rubber hardens, it is cut into half and the RP pattern is removed. The resulting rubber mold can be used to cast replicas of the original RP pattern with different materials. Tools often have complex geometries, yet they must be dimensionally accurate; the molds and dies in our case are made using the RP polymeric clubfoot model as a master pattern and then using plaster of paris (POP) cast silicon clubfoot are made.

The ABS clubfoot model is rigid in nature and does not deform because of the applied corrective load, so we cannot perform an experimental study on it, and hence, the need for a silicone foot model arises. The silicone clubfoot model plays an important role in understanding the behavior of the foot model due to physiotherapy. This model has also been found to be very useful for doing the experiment on it due to applied corrective load. The entire process begins with a pattern (usually one created from an RP system), and the mold-making and duplication processes proceed following the block diagram of Figure 3.11.

For making the silicone rubber foot model, the RP foot model, which we built in FDM, is used as a master pattern for making the mold. To eliminate any difficulties when trying to remove the ABS master pattern from mold, a single lap of white petroleum jelly is applied over the whole surface of an RP foot model. The plaster of Paris bandage (P-400) of 4″ in length is used as a mold material. This bandage is cut into patches of suitable length. Each patch, after being immersed in water, is carefully wrapped over the Vaseline RP foot model, and the process is repeated until the whole surface of the foot model is covered in a thickness of about 4 mm. This wrapped model is left as is for about 10 minutes. Once the P-400 bandage is set, a suitable parting line with a marker pen is drawn, it is cut with a surgeon's blade, and the RP foot model is carefully removed. The parting edges of this mold are matched again, joined, and lapped with a new POP bandage strip, which gives us the foot mold.

This mold is dried in an oven at 35 °C for about 24 hours, which removes all the moisture and it becomes hard. The surface finishing on the interior of this mold is very important, as the surface finish and tolerance will be faithfully reproduced in the finished cast. For a better surface finish, the inside cloth textures of the POP mold are covered completely by solid lubrication and painting. For solid lubrication, one-fourth volume of the mold is filled with fine boric powder, shaken thoroughly, and the powder lubricant taken out completely. The inside surface of the mold is then evenly spray-painted with Royal Luxury Acrylic Emulsion paint, which gives a very smooth wall finish. The painted mold is backed in oven at 40 °C for about 25 hr. This gives us a mirror-like mold surface finish, and it is sprayed evenly with a silicon-release agent spray S3 (for MCP vacuum casting).

After completing the mold, silicone rubber and a catalyst are mixed in the proper proportion for creating the cast. The amount of silicone to be used is determined by multiplying the volume of the mold by a constant factor of 1.1, the specific gravity

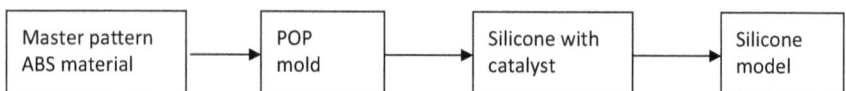

| Master pattern ABS material | → | POP mold | → | Silicone with catalyst | → | Silicone model |

FIGURE 3.11 Flow chart of silicone foot integrated process [6].

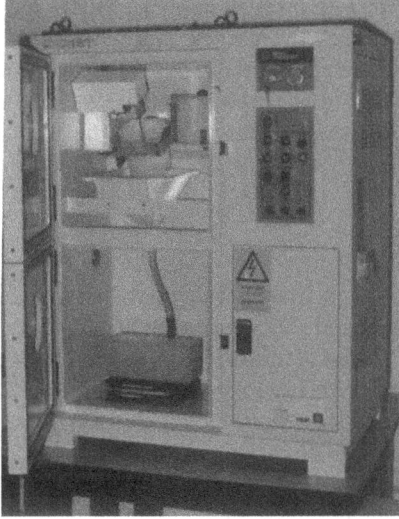

FIGURE 3.12   MCP vacuum casting machine [14].

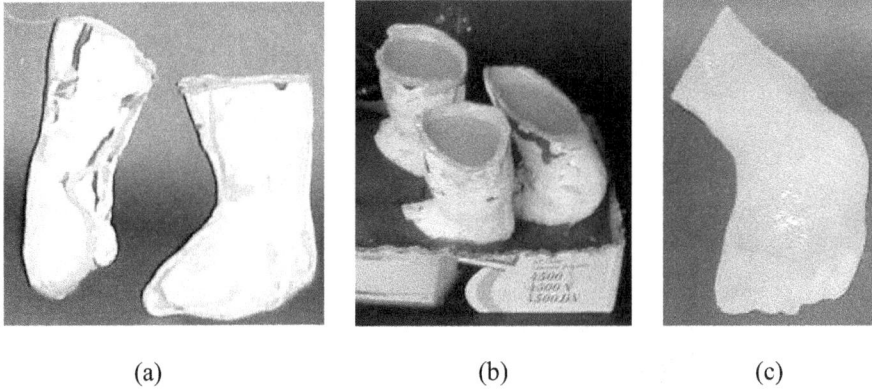

(a)   (b)   (c)

FIGURE 3.13   Process of silicone clubfoot making: (a) POP mold; (b) silicone casting; (c) silicone clubfoot model [6].

of the silicone. The required amount of catalyst is 10% by weight of the silicone. The two materials are poured into a glass jar and mixed thoroughly. After mixing, the container is placed inside the vacuum chamber of the MCP System equipment (Figure 3.12), and the vacuum was started. This is the de-gassing stage and is completed in approximately 10 minutes. The resulting de-gassed silicone mixture is then removed from the chamber and poured under the mold very slowly and steadily. During this stage, it is important to maintain the steadiness and to avoid sudden rushes of rubber in the mold to prevent bubbles and damage to the mold setup. Figure 3.13 illustrates the pouring of the silicone into the POP clubfoot mold.

Next the mold is cured in an oven set at 40 °C. Molds may be cured at room temperature; however, curing in an oven accelerates the process, which is completed in 4–8 hours depending on the size of the mold. When the curing process was completed, the mold is removed from the oven, and the mold bandages are taken out by immersing the whole unit in water. This gives us a finished silicone clubfoot model ready for experimental use.

3.5.2   TESTING OF AFO

An experimental setup with a silicone rubber clubfoot model for a corrective load application was fabricated and is shown in Figure 3.14. Per the medical literature [10], the origin of the clubfoot deformity is considered to be in the hindfoot region; hence, three strain gauges (Make: Tokyo Sokki Kenkyujo Co. Ltd Made in Japan with Gauge Factor 2.11) are placed in the region of the clubfoot silicone model as follows:

The first is placed at the posterior bottom side of the calcaneus.
The second is positioned near the contact zone of the fibula and the talus on the extreme lateral side.

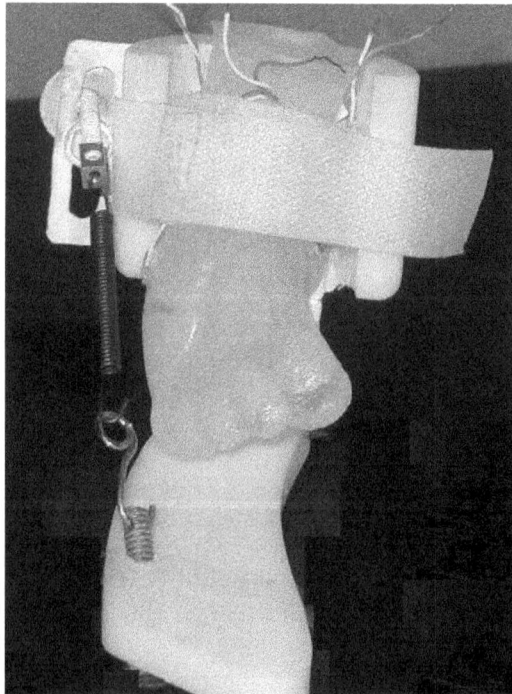

FIGURE 3.14   Experimental setup for applying corrective load to the silicone clubfoot model and inserted transducer at places of interest [6].

The third is positioned above the cuboid anterior side.

All the strain gauges are positioned inside the mold during the silicone rubber casting, and their orientations are shown in Figure 3.14.

3.6   RESULT AND DISCUSSION

During the early stages of this research, we have prototyped many AFOs whose solid models were shown in an earlier section of this chapter. Those AFOs are of two types: rigid and flexible. The rigid AFOs (fix, shape, size) have the provision of holding and keeping the foot statically, as equivalent to a normal foot. This AFO does not have any provision of dynamically quantitative load applying arrangements and hence does not meet the requirements of AFO. The designing and prototyping of this type of AFO give feedback on how to proceed. One such prototype is shown in Figure 3.15. After prototyping of this rigid AFO, in the next step, a flexible AFO is prototyped by providing a rubber joint to the double-dowel section as shown in Figure 3.16. This AFO does not give enough degree of freedom for correction, and both the rigid and the flexible AFO fail in form, fit, and function tests.

3.7   CONCLUSION

RP offers to be a significant clinical tool for customized orthosis building for a patient's deformed foot. Using FDM models can be enormously helpful in planning

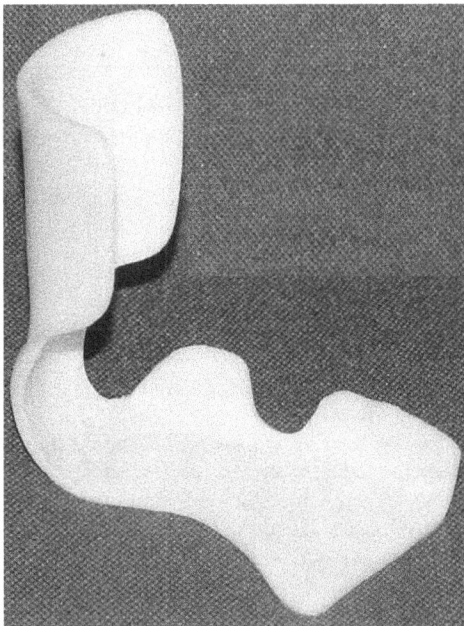

FIGURE 3.15   Prototype of a rigid AFO [6].

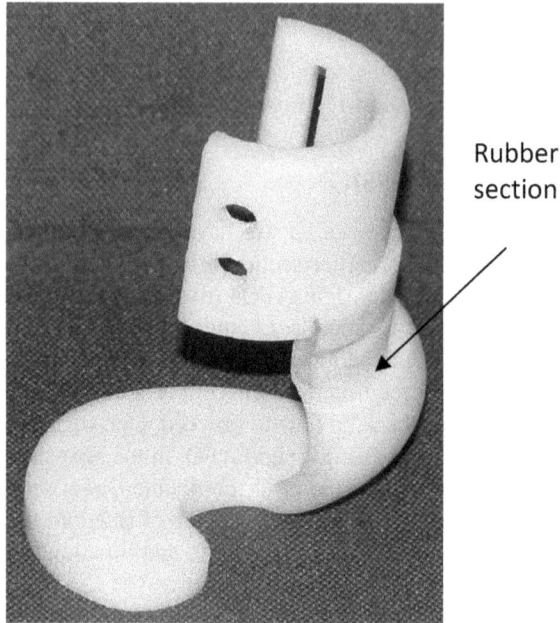

Rubber
section

FIGURE 3.16   Prototype of a flexible AFO [6].

the beneficial correction of a patient's deformed foot. In the future, the design of AFOs will further be modified based on observations from more case studies. This will result in better AFOs, giving success in clubfoot correction, which was never reported earlier. This chapter elaborated an approach for computer-assisted 3D club-foot foot prototype by integrating an MRI modality and a medical image–processing MIMICS tool with an additive manufacturing process. The major outcome of this representation is the geometrical visualization of clubfoot and a fabricated prototype of AFO that assists in better nonsurgical treatment of a historical medical condition of the foot known as clubfoot.

REFERENCES

1. Jacobs, P. F., 1992, *Rapid Prototyping and Manufacturing: Fundamentals of Stereoli-thography*, SME, Dearborn, MI.
2. Gosh, A., 1997, *Rapid Prototyping: A Brief Introduction*, Affiliated East West Press Private Limited, New Delhi, India.
3. Jamieson, R., Holmer, B. and Ashby, A., 1995, How rapid prototyping can assist in the development of new orthopaedic products—a case study, *Rapid Prototyping Journal*, Volume 1, Number 4, pp. 38–41.
4. Kai, C. C. and Fai, L. K., 1997, *Rapid Prototyping: Principles & Applications in Manu-facturing*, John Wiley & Sons, New York.
5. Sanghera, B. Naique, S., Papaharilaous, Y. and Amis, A., 2001, Preliminary study of rapid prototype medical models, *Rapid Prototyping Journal*, Volume 7, Number 5, pp 275–284.

6. Jain Manak L. PhD Thesis, 2004, *Development of a Rapid Prototype Based Ankle Foot Orthosis for Non-Surgical Correction of Clubfoot Deformity in New-Born Babies*, IIT, Kanpur, India.
7. Stratasys Inc., 1998, *FDM System Documentation*, Stratasys Inc., 14940 Martin Drive, Eden Prairie, Minneapolis, pp. 55344–2020.
8. Staats, T. B. and Kriechbaum, C. P. M. P., 1989, Computer aided manufacturing of foot orthosis, *Journal of Prosthetics and Orthotics*, Volume 1, Number 3, pp. 182–186.
9. Athearn, J. N., Case, J. S. and Roberts, J. M., 1995, Impression techniques and model modification of a custom—molded Ankle—Foot orthosis for idiopathic clubfoot, *Journal of Prosthetics and Orthotics (JPO)*, Volume 7, Number 3, pp. 91–95.
10. Mermet, J., 1982, The introduction of CAD in the shoe industry, *Computer in Industry*, Volume 3, pp. 181–186.
11. Swann, S., 1996, Integration of MRI and Stereolithography to build medical models. A case study, *Rapid Prototyping Journal*, Volume 2, Number 4, pp. 41–46.
12. Simon, G. W., 1993, *The Clubfoot—The Present and a View of the Future*, Springer—Verlag, New York.
13. Ponseti, I. V., 1996, *Congenital Clubfoot—Fundamentals of Treatment*, Oxford University Press, Oxford.
14. HEK Germany, 1997, *Operation Manual of MCP Vacuum Casting Machine,* MCP operating manual, MCP Tooling Technologies Limited.

4 The Application of Additive Manufacturing Technology in the Era of COVID-19 Pandemic
A State-of-the-Art Review

Raj Agarwal[1], Jaskaran Singh[2], and Vishal Gupta[3]*

[1,2,3] Mechanical Engineering Department, Thapar Institute of Engineering and Technology Patiala-147004, Punjab, India

CONTENTS

4.1 Introduction 65
4.2 History 66
4.3 AM 66
4.4 COVID-19 and AM Technology 69
4.5 AM of Devices 69
    4.5.1 PPE 70
        4.5.1.1 Face Masks 70
        4.5.1.2 Face Shields 70
    4.5.2 Nasopharyngeal Swabs 72
    4.5.3 Respiratory Valves 73
    4.5.4 Field Respirators 73
    4.5.5 Isolation Chambers and Wards 75
    4.5.6 Antimicrobial Devices 75
    4.5.7 Hands-Free Devices 75
4.6 Prospective Usage of AM Technology for Future Pandemics 75
4.7 Conclusion 76
References 76

4.1 INTRODUCTION

The official name of the currently spreading virus is severe acute respiratory syndrome coronavirus-2 (SARS-COV-2), which causes the disease COVID-19 [1]. The symptoms of a COVID-19 infection seem to start after 5–6 days [2]. This interval may vary depending on a patient's immune system and age. It spreads through droplets when humans sneeze or speak, aerosol, and direct or indirect physical contact

DOI: 10.1201/9781003217961-4

through contaminated surfaces [2]. Once the virus enters the cells of the human body, it starts replicating, potentially invading more and more cells that may prime fever, cough, and fatigue in the human body. It may cause breath shortness, sore throat, a loss of the sense of smell, and a loss of appetite and taste [1–2].

The first patient of COVID-19 was detected in December 2019 in Wuhan, China. After a few months, this virus spread globally very rapidly. At present, COVID-19 is a global health concern and has spread globally as depicted in Figure 4.1a. The worst-affected countries include the United States, India, Brazil, Russia, and many more as presented in Figure 4.1b. The total conformed COVID-19 cases through 14 October 2021 were 239,963,626, and more than 4,889,877 deaths have been reported.

The treatment for patients diagnosed with COVID-19 symptoms includes isolation and quarantine of patients, which caused national lockdowns in various countries. The virus-spreading ratio has led to overloaded health systems around the globe. The sudden increase in the number of patients caused supply chain disruptions and generated a shortage of personal protection equipment (PPE) and medical devices in hospitals for doctors and patients. Additive manufacturing (AM) technology lends itself very well to solving these challenges by being able to quickly prototype and iterate designs for shortages of PPE and medical devices.

This study targets reviewing the use of AM technology during the ongoing COVID-19 pandemic. Moreover, it focuses on various PPE and medical devices. Finally, a perspective for the future of AM during emergencies is presented.

4.2 HISTORY

Viruses were the first living thing on earth, and they hijack other living cells to reproduce and replicate themselves. This is not the first time the world has seen a pandemic. There is a history of pandemics and epidemics in human lives since ancient times. Diseases that transmit from person to person in a particular area very quickly are called epidemics, and diseases that spread from one country to another country are known as pandemics [4]. Table 4.1 provides the information related to disease, time period, prehuman host, countries affected, number of total deaths counted, and type of pandemic or epidemic from ancient times to present day. Most of the deaths were reported due to a lack of medical devices and protective equipment for doctors and patients.

4.3 AM

AM technology is the process of constructing a three-dimensional (3D) object from a computer-aided-design (CAD) model built in a layer-by-layer format [9]. The first AM technique was stereolithography (SLA), invented in 1984. After that milestone, AM technology continued over the years as presented in Figure 4.2. AM has the capability to print any complex structure or detailed 3D construction by creating an accurate physical replica of a model while producing less waste by-product. These unique advantages have allowed this modern technology to be adapted in different domains and diverse applications [10–12]. AM techniques use an extensive range of materials and techniques. Currently, AM technology is utilized in several fields,

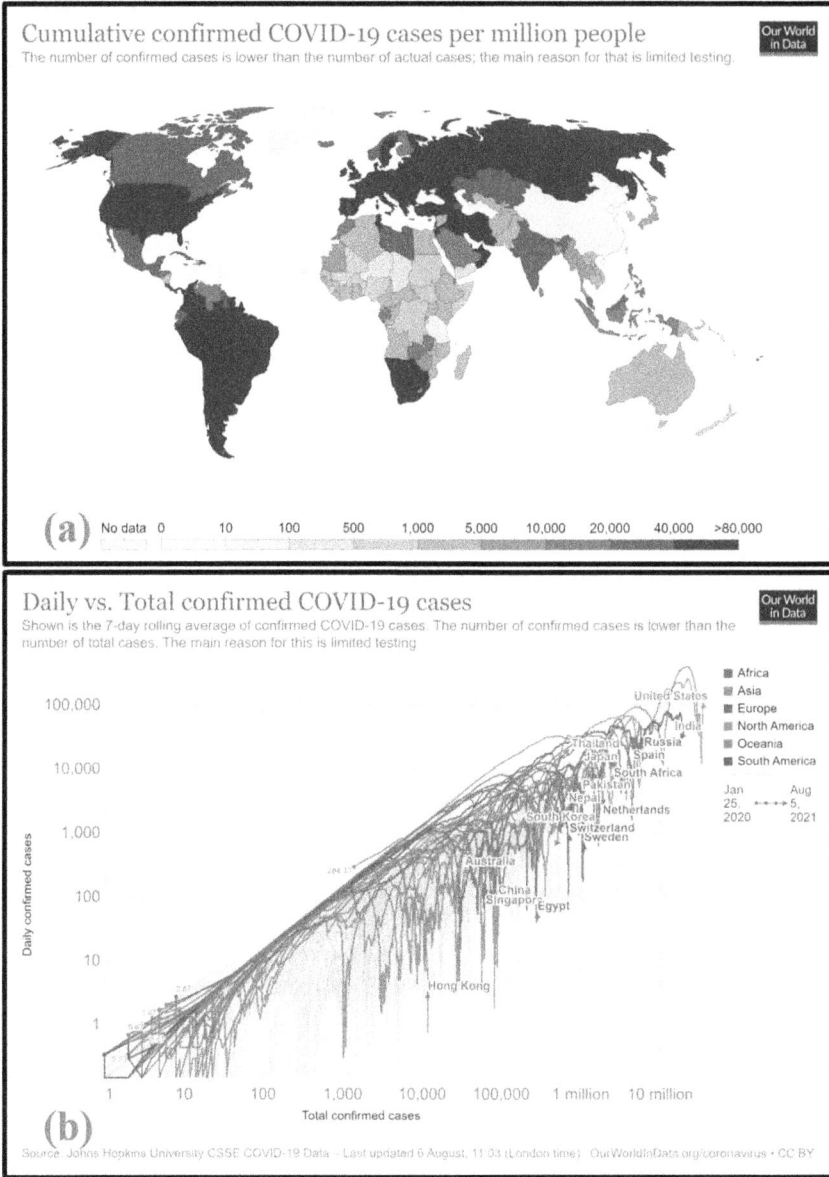

FIGURE 4.1 (a) Globally cumulative confirmed cases of COVID-19 cases; (b) most affected countries with maximum COVID-19 cases [3].

such as the medical, automotive, aerospace, and marine industries [9, 13–14]. AM techniques can be divided into various classifications: material extrusion, material jetting, vat photopolymerization, powder bed fusion, and binder jetting [15–16]. These different AM techniques utilize different materials for part fabrication. The

TABLE 4.1

Epidemics/Pandemics from Ancient Time to Present Day

Disease	Time period	Prehuman host	Country distribution	Total deaths (millions)	Type (WHO)	Reference
Antonina Plague	165–180	Measles or smallpox	Europe, North Africa	5M	Pandemic	[5–6]
Cyprian Plague	250–271	*Yersinia pestis*	Rome	1,90,000	Epidemic	[6–8]
Plague of Justinian	541–542	Bacteria *Yersinia pestis*	Europe, Asia, Africa	50M	Pandemic	[4–6]
Japanese smallpox	735–737	vaccinia virus	Japan	1M	Epidemic	[5–7]
Black death	1347–1351	*Yersinia pestis* bacteria	Europe, Asia, North Africa	200M	Pandemic	[5–6]
Smallpox	1492–onward	Variola virus	All continents	300M	Epidemic	[5–6]
Cocoliztli	1543–1548	Arenavirus	Aztec empire	15M	Epidemic	[5–8]
The Italian Plague	1629–1631	*Yersinia pestis* bacteria	Verona, Bologna and Florence	1M	Epidemic	[5–6]
Great Plague of London	1665–1666	*Yersinia pestis* bacteria	London	1,00,000	Epidemic	[5–6]
Great Plague of Marseilles	1723–1728	*Yersinia pestis* bacteria	Marseilles and Provence	1,00,000	Epidemic	[5–6]
Great North American smallpox	1775–1782	Variola virus	USA, Mexico and Canada	1,30,000	Epidemic	[5–7]
Yellow fever	1793–1889	Arena virus/ Mosquitoes	Philadelphia, Haiti, Louisiana	1,50,000	Epidemic	[5–6]
The Third Plague	1855–1912	*Yersinia pestis* bacteria	All continents	12M	Pandemic	[5–6]
Russian flu	1889–1890	H2N2 virus	Europe and Asia	1M	Pandemic	[5–6]
Spanish flu	1918–1919	H1N1 virus	All continents	50M	Pandemic	[5–6]
Asian flu	1957–1958	H2N2 virus	All continents	1.1M	Pandemic	[5–6]
Hong Kong flu	1968–1970	H3N2 virus	All continents	1M	Pandemic	[5–6]
HIV/AIDS	1981-present	Chimpanzees	All continents	25M	Global epidemic	[5–6]
SARS	2002–2003	Coronavirus/ bats, civets	All continents	774	Epidemic	[4–6]
Swine flu	2009–2010	H1N1 virus	All continents	2,00,000	Pandemic	[4–6]
Ebola	2014–2016	Filo virus		11,000	Pandemic	[4–6]
MERS	2015-present	Bats, camels	Saudi Arabia, Africa, Asia, Europe	858	Pandemic	[4–6]
COVID-19	2019-present	Bats, unknown (possibly pangolins)	All continents	4,889,877 [3] (as of 14 October 2021)	Global pandemic	[6]

Invented SLA	Patented FDM	First biomaterial used for human tissue regeneration	First implantation of bioengineered blood vessels	Bioprinted in vitro liver model	Human scale multimaterial tissue constructs
1984	1989	1996	2001	2014	2016

1986	1993	2000	2002	2015	2019
Development of SLS	3D printing for bone regeneration	First commercial bioprinter	Injected bioprinting	First FDA-approved 3D-printed Spritam drug	First 3D-printed scaffold for spinal cord injury repair

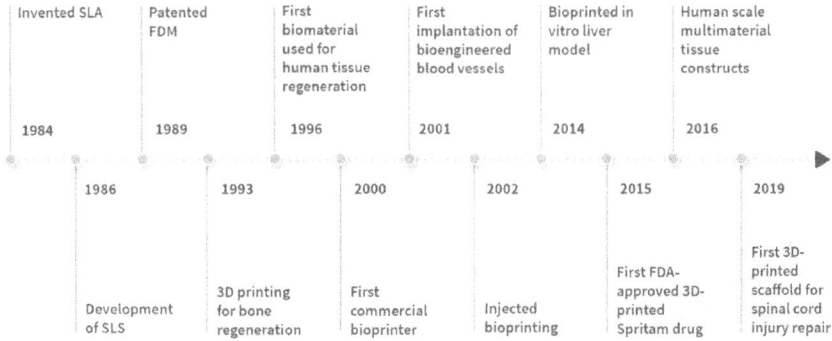

FIGURE 4.2 Milestones in AM technology [19].

materials most often used in different techniques are polymers, metals, and ceramics. These materials have specific mechanical and material properties, chemical and thermal properties, various processing methods, cell–material interactions, and U.S. Food and Drug Administration (FDA) approval [17–18]. Each material is processed with different techniques that have their own limits and applications in producing prototype models.

4.4 COVID-19 AND AM TECHNOLOGY

The COVID-19 pandemic has suddenly amplified the demand for medical devices. It triggered supply chain disruptions and created shortages of PPE and medical devices for doctors and patients [20]. To alleviate the lack of medical devices, various companies and individuals started using AM technology to fabricate different medical equipment to supply to doctors and people facing a shortage of PPE and medical devices [21]. The potential of an AM technique is in helping fabricate various devices and equipment. The major reason for using an AM technique for fabricating these devices is that a higher number of users, many of them are specialized, creative, and innovative [22]. The innovation of fabricating different designs of various devices and equipment is due to ease of using this technology. The other reason of using this technology during COVID-19 pandemic is that people who own 3D printers did not actually have to design a CAD model for fabricating an object. The files used for manufacturing are easily accessed through the internet [15]. The third reason for using this technology is the ease of printing complex parts in less time as compared to traditional subtractive manufacturing. It has an almost negligible lead time for distributing small batches of parts. Therefore, when the demand and need for medical devices and equipment are critical, AM technology can be adjusted and quickly installed to fabricate emergency items.

4.5 AM OF DEVICES

This section presents and discusses the diversified solutions manufactured with the help of AM technology to fight the lack and shortage of PPE and medical devices.

4.5.1 PPE

PPE was the most manufactured device during the COVID-19 pandemic due to its simplicity and low geometrical tolerance requirements. PPE includes face shields, medical protective facemasks, goggles, gloves, surgical hood, outer aprons, and powered air-purifying respirators [23–26]. Of these PPEs, face masks and face shields are considered mandatory for medical workers for protecting themselves from the COVID-19 virus. AM technology is explored in the following for fabricating unique and innovative face masks and face shields.

4.5.1.1 Face Masks

Wearing face masks is important in public as masked breathing in public areas corresponds to a supremely effective way to prevent interhuman transmission [27]. In a critical situation during the COVID-19 pandemic, crucial face masks were provided with the help of AM technology. AM techniques provided the freedom to create customized 3D protective face masks. Customized 3D protective face masks consist of 3D-printed reusable components and a filter membrane support as presented in Figures 4.3a and 4.3b, respectively. Both of these components can be assembled with a changeable, nonwoven particle filter as depicted in Figures 4.3c and 4.3d, respectively. A surgeon wearing such a disposable surgical mask can have reduced exposure with the help of the customized 3D protective face mask shown in Figures 4.3g and 4.3h. Nicholson et al. [28] innovated a snorkel mask with an adaptor with the help of AM technology as depicted in Figures 4.4a, 4.4b, and 4.4c.

4.5.1.2 Face Shields

Face shields are firmly established among the projects of PPE. Face shields are mainly used in the medical, dental, and veterinary domains to provide coverage for the entire face for protection [29–30]. The face shield is a head-worn frame that covers the eyes,

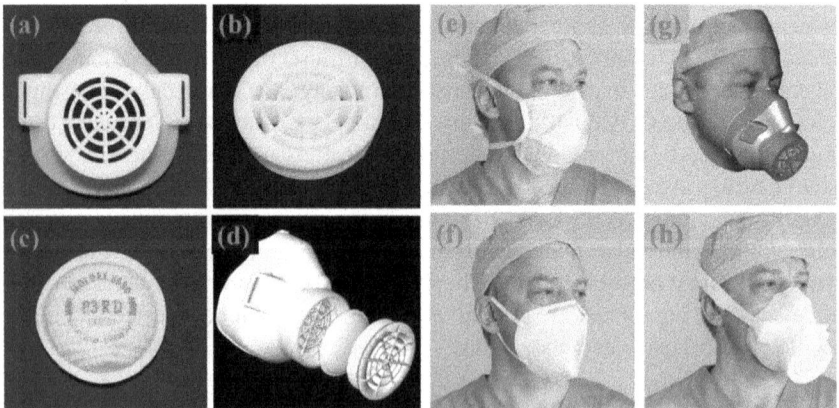

FIGURE 4.3 (a) Reusable 3D-printed face mask; (b) filter support; (c) polypropylene particle filter; (d) face mask prototype 3D image; (e) surgical face mask; (f) filtering face piece 2 (FFP2) face mask; (g) 3D face mask; (h) 3D-printed face mask [27].

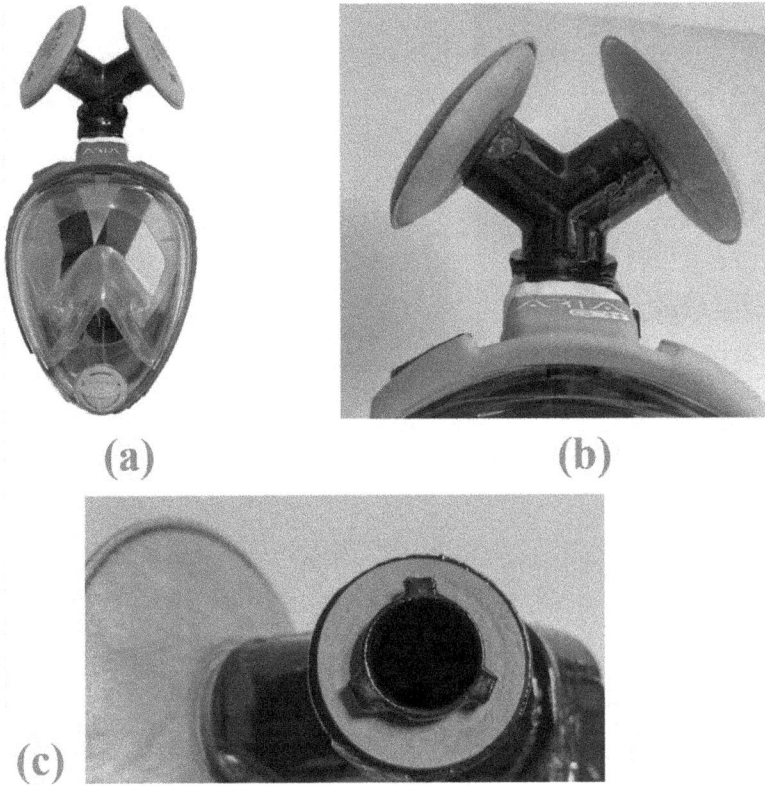

FIGURE 4.4   (a) Snorkel mask; (b) poly-lactic acid adapter with attached filters; (c) inhalation port view [28].

nose, and mouth of an individual to prevent and protect against respiratory droplets and the inhalation of saliva, dust, pollen, and the like. The frame in a face shield is simple geometry that can easily be fabricated with the help of AM technology [30]. Delbarre et al. [31] used AM technology to fabricate shields for slit lamps during the COVID-19 pandemic. Fused deposition modeling (FDM)–based AM technology is used to fabricate face shields as depicted in Figure 4.5a [29]. AM-fabricated face shields contain a 3D-printed headband, a shield, and an elastic strap as presented in Figure 4.5b [29]. Poly-lactic acid (PLA) is used in most FDM-based AM technology [32]. The frame of the face shield is fabricated with the help of AM technology using PLA material as depicted in Figure 4.6a [33]. The transparent film is assembled in the frame of the face shield, and an assembled face-shield prototype is presented in Figure 4.6b [33]. Complete protection is provided to the surgeon with the help of a 3D-printed face shield as shown in Figure 4.6c [33].

To modify the face shields for suitable comfort, they are fabricated with a bottom bracket and foam pads [34]. Along with this, different designs of face shields were compared to monitor fit, comfort, wearing, protection, and overall total comparison

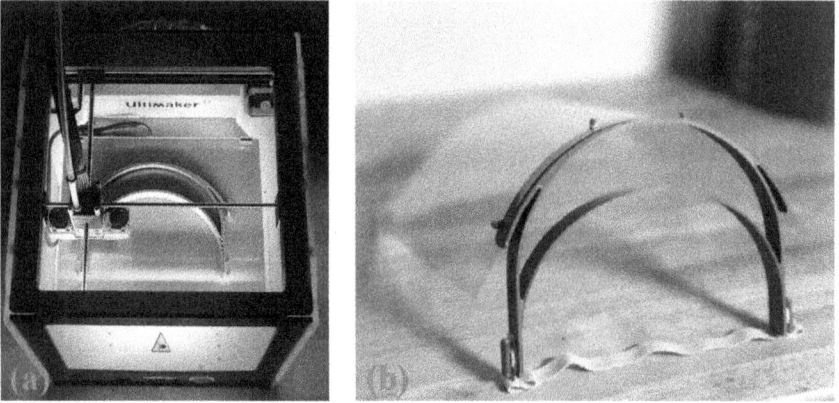

FIGURE 4.5   (a) 3D printing of the headband by FDM; (b) 2-arches 3D-printed headband face shield [29].

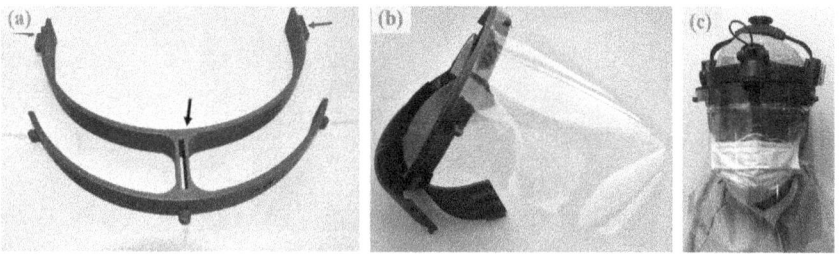

FIGURE 4.6   (a) 3D-printed fame of face shield; (b) assembled face-shield prototype; (c) surgeon wearing 3D-printed face shield [33].

of four different CAD designs of face shields as presented in Figures 4.7a, 4.7b, 4.7c, and 4.7d) [20]. The corresponding fabricated face shields of different designs are depicted in Figure 4.7a1, 4.7 b1, 4.7c1, and 4.7d1 [20]. These face shields were fabricated with a support structure and limited contact area with the printing bed. Based on the weight, printing time, comfort, wearing, fit, protection from respiratory droplets, and large-scale production, the RC2 design is suitable and optimized as presented in Figure 4.7b and Figure 4.7b1.

4.5.2   NASOPHARYNGEAL SWABS

Nasopharyngeal (NP) swabs and nasal swabs are used for the most accurate and safest procedure used to collect samples from patients for a diagnosis of a COVID-19 infection. Callahan et al. [35] validated clinically the use of multiple AM-fabricated nasopharyngeal swabs for collecting samples for high-sensitivity virological testing for the COVID-19 virus. The innovative, cooperative, rapid-response NP swabs were produced with the help of AM technology. Cox and Koepsell [36] used AM

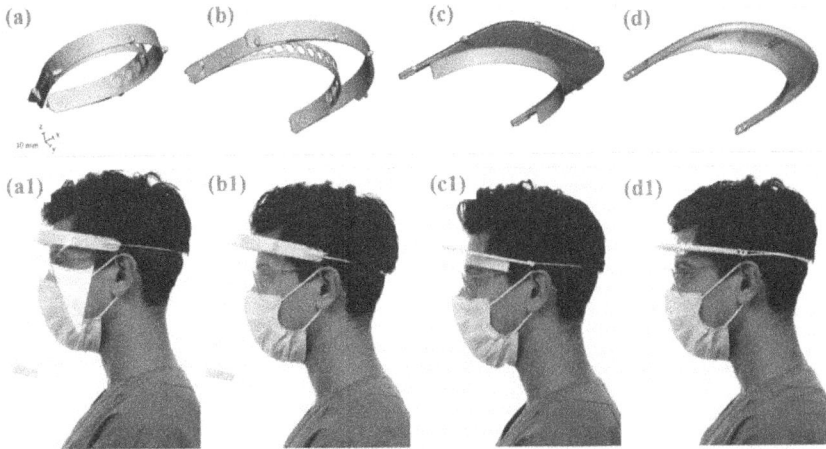

FIGURE 4.7 Four different designs of face shields: (a) RC1; (b) RC2; (c) Budmen V3; (d) easy 3D face shield [20].

technology for fabricating custom-made nasal swabs for the shortage of NP swabs. The 3D-printed NP swabs, along with a photomicrograph of air-dried stained cells collected from the corresponding swab, are represented in Figure 4.8a and Figure 4.8b, respectively.

4.5.3 RESPIRATORY VALVES

Respiratory valves are necessary parts of ventilator breathing machines. Due to the high demand of scale and supply chain disruptions caused due to COVID-19, the fabrication of respiratory valves was innovated with the help of AM technology. The application of the original respiratory valve and the 3D-printed respiratory valve is very similar. Based on the success of 3D-printed respiratory valves, a number of 3D-printed respiratory valves were fabricated in Italy as shown in Figure 4.9c [23].

4.5.4 FIELD RESPIRATORS

Powered air-purifying respirators, or full-face respiratory protective devices, are required in the specific work zones where patients have respiratory symptoms and when handling the bodies of deceased suspected patients (death due to COVID-19). A field respirator is a device used for short-term emergency ventilation. These respirators are designed to guard patients against inhaling hazardous airborne microorganisms. A field respirator helps the wearer breathe easily by letting air out and preventing humidity inside. Petsiuk et al. [37] developed a fully open portable bag-valve mask-based ventilator compression system with the help of AM technology. This automated ventilator can be provided as a temporary emergency ventilator. In this ventilator, various parts are assembled with the help of 3D-printed parts.

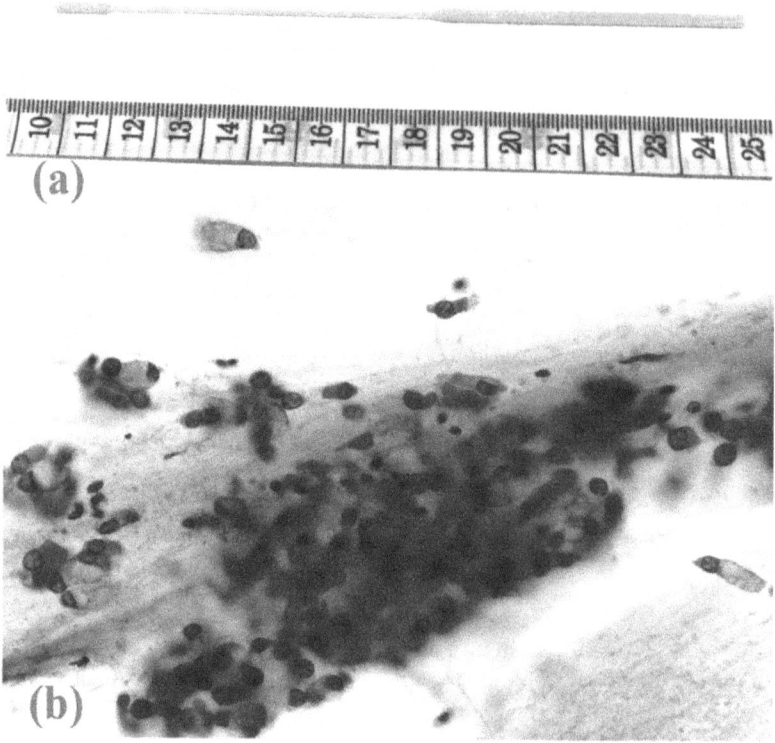

FIGURE 4.8 (a) 3D-printed NP swabs; (b) a photomicrograph of air-dried stained cells collected using a 3D-printed swab [36].

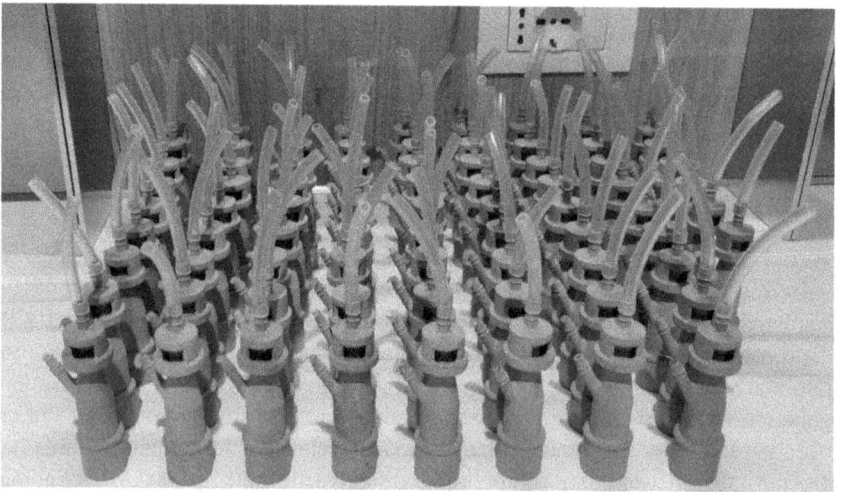

FIGURE 4.9 Respiratory valves developed for Italian hospitals [23].

4.5.5   ISOLATION CHAMBERS AND WARDS

In treating patients having COVID-19 symptoms and for doctors to prevent virus dissemination, quarantine and strict isolation have to be followed. The virus can be spread through aerosols and droplets [15]. AM technology is currently fabricated the isolation chambers and wards for individuals for isolation and self-quarantine. Cubillos et al. [38] innovated a negative airflow isolation chamber. The isolation chamber involves a rigid cubic frame draped with a clear plastic bag. This plastic bag chamber prevents the continuous negative airflow from inside the chamber. AM technology is used for fabricating the ports that allow oxygen delivery.

4.5.6   ANTIMICROBIAL DEVICES

The foremost disadvantage of polymer usage in AM technology during several applications, such as the fabrication of masks and valves, is that the COVID-19 virus might present in the fabricated part. The SARS-CoV-2 virus can stay at surfaces at a high stability (up to 72 hours) [39]. The solution to this problem lies in using several metallic coatings or doping nanoparticles into polymers [15]. The bioactive polymers can be developed with the doping and coating of several metals such as copper and silver, which have antimicrobial characteristics [40]. The process of manufacturing with the usage of antimicrobial polymers for antimicrobial medical devices can be achieved by using copper nanocomposite additives during the mixing of recycled material in pallet's form that might provide an antimicrobial PLA filament. Copper and copper oxide additives have been proved to provide antimicrobial characteristics to the polymer.

4.5.7   HANDS-FREE DEVICES

The SARS-CoV-2 virus might be present on various surfaces up to 72 hours [39, 41–42]. Therefore, in public places, escaping direct contact with surfaces is a significant method for reducing the spread of the virus [43]. The most used objects, such as door handles, switches, buttons, and the like, are possible virus spreaders due to the higher number of human interactions [44].

AM-based technology is used to fabricate door opener with different designs for different door handles [45]. These different sections of door handles help diminish the risk of direct contact between doors and arms of individuals. The application and comparison of various sections (circular, straight, elliptical) of door handles. With the help of AM technology, these 3D-printed contact-free devices are fabricated to help reduce the spread of SARS-CoV-2 virus.

4.6   PROSPECTIVE USAGE OF AM TECHNOLOGY FOR FUTURE PANDEMICS

The current pandemic has indicated that conventional production chain and distribution systems can be tremendously affected due to country lockdowns and the quarantining of patients and doctors. For this, AM technology is proved to be the most innovative, adaptive, and versatile production technology for supporting the supply chain distribution with strong collaboration among countries. The trend of open-source technologies and design data sharing reached a new level as manufacturers, groups, universities, and companies put public welfare over individual interests.

As it is a relatively new technology, 3D printing has not reached its full potential. New materials in polymers, metals, and ceramics are being developed and opening new applications. Furthermore, 4D printing, which uses smart materials as feedstock, will address several issues and leverage a number of solutions in medicine. Bioprinting, a variant technology of 3D printing, promises to produce organs and tissues in the future and can currently create 3D in vitro models that help researchers understand disease spread in tissues and speed up the development of specific drugs. Finally, in AM technology, manufacturing a part in a layer-by-layer format sums to fabricating a complex part with ease, and having freedom in its design correlates to the AM research area, which strongly impacts the products, cost, and productivity of the advanced manufacturing in all areas of industry.

4.7 CONCLUSION

Throughout history, a number of humans have lost their lives because of epidemics and pandemics, and this will occur in future if any infection is not stopped prior to spreading to other populace or nation. Infections can be spread quickly because they are passed on by breathing in the airborne infection. To prevent this ongoing pandemic, vaccination is the major solution, along with making yourself clean and hygienic; not sharing personal things; cleaning your hands appropriately; taking good, healthy, and safe food; and covering your mouth whenever sneeze and cough.

Because of supply chain disruptions and the high demand for protective equipment caused by the COVID-19 pandemic, face masks, face shields, respiratory valves, NP swabs, and hands-free devices were fabricated via AM technology. AM technology is an innovative and game-changing technique known for its ability to construct any complex parts with ease and comfort. This technique is currently used to provide for the demand for necessary medical devices and protective equipment, mostly face masks, face shields, respiratory valves, and NP swabs. AM technology has proved to be a boon during the COVID-19 pandemic for supplying the shortage of medical devices and protective equipment, particularly in the health care industry. Furthermore, AM technology can provide the supply to fulfill the demand for future protective equipment and medical devices necessarily required for forthcoming pandemics.

REFERENCES

1. Zhao X, Ding Y, Du J, Fan Y. 2020 update on human coronaviruses: One health, one world. *Medicine in Novel Technology and Devices*. 2020;8:100043. Elsevier Ltd.
2. Hamid S, Mir MY, Rohela GK. Novel coronavirus disease (COVID-19): A pandemic (epidemiology, pathogenesis and potential therapeutics). *New Microbes and New Infections*. 2020;35:100679. Elsevier Ltd.
3. Singh G, Jain V, Gupta D, Ghai A. Optimization of process parameters for drilled hole quality characteristics during cortical bone drilling using Taguchi method. *Journal of the Mechanical Behavior of Biomedical Materials*. 2016;62:355–65. Elsevier.

4. Kaur H, Garg S, Joshi H, Ayaz S, Sharma S, Bhandari M. A review: Epidemics and pandemics in human history. *International Journal of Pharma Research and Health Sciences*. 2020;8:3139–42.
5. Dasgupta S, Crunkhorn R. A History of pandemics over the ages and the human cost. *The Physician*. 2020;6:1–9.
6. LePan N. Visualizing the history of pandemics. *Visualizing the History of Pandemics*. 2020;2:1–16.
7. Artenstein AW. New generation smallpox vaccines: A review of preclinical and clinical data. *Reviews in Medical Virology*. 2008;18:217–31.
8. Harper K. Pandemics and passages to late antiquity: Rethinking the plague of c.249–270 described by Cyprian. *Journal of Roman Archaeology*. 2015;28:223–60.
9. Salmi M. Additive manufacturing processes in medical applications. *Materials*. 2021;14:1–16.
10. Babbar A, Rai A, Sharma A. Latest trend in building construction: Three-dimensional printing. *Journal of Physics: Conference Series*. 2021;1950:012007.
11. Ahangar P, Cooke ME, Weber MH, Rosenzweig DH. Current biomedical applications of 3D printing and additive manufacturing. *Applied Sciences*. 2019;9:1713.
12. Marinescu R, Popescu D. A review on 3D-printed templates for precontouring fixation plates in orthopedic surgery. *Journal of Clinical Medicine*. 2020;9:2908.
13. Babbar A, Jain V, Gupta D, Prakash C, Singh S, Sharma A. 3D Bioprinting in pharmaceuticals, medicine, and tissue engineering applications. *Advanced Manufacturing and Processing Technology*. 2020:147–161.
14. Majeed A, Ahmed A, Lv J, Peng T, Muzamil M. A state-of-the-art review on energy consumption and quality characteristics in metal additive manufacturing processes. *Journal of the Brazilian Society of Mechanical Sciences and Engineering*. 2020;42:1–25. Springer Berlin Heidelberg.
15. Longhitano GA, Nunes GB, Candido G, da Silva JVL. The role of 3D printing during COVID-19 pandemic: A review. *Progress in Additive Manufacturing*. 2021;6:19–37. Springer International Publishing.
16. Singh D, Babbar A, Jain V, Gupta D, Saxena S, Dwibedi V. Synthesis, characterization, and bioactivity investigation of biomimetic biodegradable PLA scaffold fabricated by fused filament fabrication process. *Journal of the Brazilian Society of Mechanical Sciences and Engineering*. 2019;41:1–13. Springer Berlin Heidelberg.
17. Babbar A, Sharma A, Kumar R, Pundir P, Dhiman V. Functionalized biomaterials for 3D printing: An overview of the literature. *Additive Manufacturing with Functionalized Nanomaterials*. 2021:87–107. Wm. C. Brown Publishers.
18. Babbar A, Jain V, Gupta D, Singh S, Prakash C, Pruncu C. Biomaterials and fabrication methods of scaffolds for tissue engineering applications. *3D Printing in Biomedical Engineering*. 2020:167–86.
19. Pugliese R, Beltrami B, Regondi S, Lunetta C. Polymeric biomaterials for 3D printing in medicine: An overview. *Annals of 3D Printed Medicine*. 2021;2:100011. Elsevier Masson SAS;
20. Wesemann C, Pieralli S, Fretwurst T, Nold J, Nelson K, Schmelzeisen R, et al. 3-D printed protective equipment during COVID-19 pandemic. *Materials*. 2020;13:1–9.
21. Daoulas T, Bizaoui V, Dubrana F, Di Francia R. The role of three-dimensional printing in coronavirus disease-19 medical management: A French nationwide survey. *Annals of 3D Printed Medicine*. 2021;1:100001. Elsevier Masson SAS.
22. Lalièvre L, Adam J, Nataf P, Khonsari RH. 3D-printed suture guide for thoracic and cardiovascular surgery produced during the COVID19 pandemic. *Annals of 3D Printed Medicine*. 2021;1:100005. Elsevier Masson SAS.
23. Singh S, Prakash C, Ramakrishna S. Three-dimensional printing in the fight against novel virus COVID-19: Technology helping society during an infectious disease pandemic. *Technology in Society*. 2020;62:101305. Elsevier Ltd.

24. Vordos N, Gkika DA, Maliaris G, Tilkeridis KE, Antoniou A, Bandekas D V., et al. How 3D printing and social media tackles the PPE shortage during Covid—19 pandemic. *Safety Science*. 2020;130:104870. Elsevier.

25. Agarwal R, Gupta V, Jain V. A novel technique of harvesting cortical bone grafts during orthopaedic surgeries. *Journal of the Brazilian Society of Mechanical Sciences and Engineering*. 2021;8:1–14. Springer Berlin Heidelberg.

26. Rendeki S, Nagy B, Bene M, Pentek A, Toth L, Szanto Z, et al. An overview on personal protective equipment (PPE) fabricated with additive manufacturing technologies in the era of COVID-19 pandemic. *Polymers*. 2020;12:1–18.

27. Swennen GRJ, Pottel L, Haers PE. Custom-made 3D-printed face masks in case of pandemic crisis situations with a lack of commercially available FFP2/3 masks. *International Journal of Oral and Maxillofacial Surgery*. International Association of Oral and Maxillofacial Surgery; 2020;49:673–7.

28. Nicholson K, Henke-Adams A, Henke DM, Kravitz AV, Gay HA. Modified full-face snorkel mask as COVID-19 personal protective equipment: Quantitative results. *HardwareX*. The Authors; 2021;9:e00185.

29. Lemarteleur V, Fouquet V, Le Goff S, Tapie L, Morenton P, Benoit A, et al. 3D-printed protected face shields for health care workers in Covid-19 pandemic. *American Journal of Infection Control*. 2021;49:389–91.

30. Kursat Celik H, Kose O, Ulmeanu ME, Rennie AEW, Abram TN, Akinci I. Design and additive manufacturing of medical face shield for healthcare workers battling coronavirus (COVID-19). *International Journal of Bioprinting*. 2020;6:1–21.

31. Delbarre M, François P-M, Adam J, Caruhel J-B, Froussart-Maille F, Khonsari RH. 3D-printed shields for slit lamps produced during the COVID-19 pandemic. *Annals of 3D Printed Medicine*. 2021;1:100004.

32. Mago J, Kumar R, Agrawal R, Singh A, Srivastava V. Modeling of linear shrinkage in PLA parts fabricated by 3D printing using TOPSIS method. In: Shunmugam MS, Kanthababu M, editor. *Advances in Additive Manufacturing and Joining*. Springer, Singapore, 2020, pp. 267–76.

33. Amin D, Nguyen N. 3D Printing of face shields during COVID-19 pandemic: A technical note. *Journal of Oral Maxillofacial Surgery*. 2020;78:1275–8. Elsevier Inc.

34. Mostaghimi A, Antonini MJ, Plana D, Anderson PD, Beller B, Boyer EW, Fannin A, Freake J, Oakley R, Sinha MS, Smith L. Rapid prototyping and clinical testing of a reusable face shield for health care workers responding to the COVID-19 pandemic. *medRxiv*. Apr 15, 2020.

35. Callahan CJ, Lee R, Zulauf KE, Tamburello L, Smith KP, Previtera J, et al. Open development and clinical validation of multiple 3d-printed nasopharyngeal collection swabs: Rapid resolution of a critical covid-19 testing bottleneck. *Journal of Clinical Microbiology*. 2020;58:1–10.

36. Cox JL, Koepsell SA. 3D-Printing to address COVID-19 testing supply shortages. *Laboratory Medicine*. 2021;51:E45–6.

37. Petsiuk A, Tanikella NG, Dertinger S, Pringle A, Oberloier S, Pearce JM. Partially RepRapable automated open source bag valve mask-based ventilator. *HardwareX*. The Authors; 2020;8:e00131.

38. Cubillos J, Querney J, Rankin A, Moore J, Armstrong K. A multipurpose portable negative air flow isolation chamber for aerosol-generating procedures during the COVID-19 pandemic. *British Journal of Anaesthesia*. 2020;125:e179–81. Elsevier Ltd.

39. Zou L, Ruan F, Huang M, Liang L, Huang H, Hong Z, et al. Aerosol and surface stability of SARS-CoV-2 as compared with SARS-CoV-1. *New England Journal of Medicine*. 2020;382:1177–9.

40. Palza H. Antimicrobial polymers with metal nanoparticles. *International Journal of Molecular Sciences*. 2015;16:2099–116.

41. Agarwal R, Jain V, Gupta V, Saxena S, Dwibedi V. Effect of surface topography on pull-out strength of cortical screw after ultrasonic bone drilling: An in vitro study. *Journal of the Brazilian Society of Mechanical Sciences and Engineering*. 2020;42:1–13. Springer Berlin Heidelberg.
42. Arora PK, Arora R, Haleem A, Kumar H. Application of additive manufacturing in challenges posed by COVID-19. *Materials Today: Proceedings*. 2020;38:466–8. Elsevier Ltd.
43. Tino R, Moore R, Antoline S, Ravi P, Wake N, Ionita CN, et al. COVID-19 and the role of 3D printing in medicine. *3D Printing in Medicine*. 2020;6:1–8.
44. Equbal A, Akhter S, Sood AK, Equbal I. The usefulness of additive manufacturing (AM) in COVID-19. *Annals of 3D Printed Medicine*. 2021;2:100013. Elsevier Masson SAS.
45. François PM, Bonnet X, Kosior J, Adam J, Khonsari RH. 3D-printed contact-free devices designed and dispatched against the COVID-19 pandemic: The 3D COVID initiative. *Journal of Stomatology, Oral and Maxillofacial Surgery*. Sep 1, 2021;122(4):381–5.

5 Relevance of Bio-Inks for 3D Bioprinting

Bhargav Prajwal Pathri[1], Mohd. Shahnawaz Khan[2], and Atul Babbar[3]

[1] Department of Mechanical Engineering,
JK Laksmipat University

[2] Department of Chemical Engineering,
JK Lakshmipat University

[3] Department of Mechanical Engineering,
Shree Guru Gobind Singh Tricentenary
University, Gurugram-122505, India.

CONTENTS

5.1   Introduction.. 81
5.2   Bioprinting Technologies and their Applications 83
5.3   Inkjet Bioprinting... 83
5.4   Bioplotting 87
5.5   Fused Deposition Modeling... 88
5.6   Laser Bioprinting 88
5.7   Extrusion Bioprinting 89
5.8   SLA.. 89
5.9   Bio-Inks and Multicomponent Bio-Inks 90
5.10 Gelatin Methacrylol 91
5.11 Agarose 92
5.12 Alginate.. 92
5.13 Chitosan 92
5.14 Silk Fibroin 93
5.15 Collagen 95
5.16 Hyaluronic Acid... 95
5.17 Conclusion 96
References... 97

5.1   INTRODUCTION

Three-dimensional (3D) bioprinting is the 3D printing of bio-inks in a specific shape of an organ so that the cells grow into the structure that is printed and develop into a fully functional organ. It is an additive manufacturing technology that has gained popularity and interest in the last few decades. Three-dimensional

DOI: 10.1201/9781003217961-5

bioprinting has led to a remarkable advancement in the health sector, especially in regenerative medicine. There is a scarcity of available organs globally that are needed for rehabilitating lost or failed organs and tissues. Regenerative medicine is the branch of medicine that helps regrow and repair cells and organs that are deceased and damaged by either trauma or some congenital issues. Regenerative medicine includes generating tissues and organs by using therapeutic stem cells that facilitate the on-demand printing of tissues, cells, and organs. These technological advancements have led to the foundation of a new scientific field of medicine called "tissue engineering".

Tissue engineering is a new field of medicine in which biologically compatible scaffolds are prepared and implanted in the human body at the place where new tissue is to be formed. Scaffolds are artificial or natural structures that mimic real organs [1]. The tissue grows on these scaffolds to mimic the biological process or structure that can be replaced [2]. Scaffolds are generally created by the cells in the body or can be built from the sources of proteins in the body or naturally man-made plastics. No matter how scaffolds are formed, these scaffolds send signals to the cells that help support and optimize cell functions [3]. Selecting the right stem cells is also a challenge in tissue engineering. Biomolecules in the human body are mostly made up of carbohydrates, lipids, proteins, and nucleic acids. These biomolecules help in forming cell structures and their functions. Proteins help various organs, such as brain, kidney, and heart functions, as well as run the digestive and immune systems. Lipids and proteins help provide necessary antibodies in the body to protect from germs and give structural support and movement. Nucleic acids contain RNA and DNA, giving genetic information cells. There are mainly two types of stem cells available: (1) embryonic stem cells (these cells originates from embryos, usually eggs fertilized outside the body) and (2) adult stem cells (these are found inside each individual human being and multiply, by cell division, to replenish dying cells and tissues) [4]. Many studies have illustrated that when adult stem cells are harvested and then injected at the site of deceased tissue, rehabilitating these tissues is possible under the right conditions. These cells can be collected from blood, bone marrow, fat, dental pulp, skeletal muscle, and the like [5].

Conventional fabrication techniques for manufacturing 3D scaffolds, such as electrospinning, fiber deposition, freeze-drying, gas foaming, and salt leaching, have the least precision regarding internal topology and structure [6–8]. Additive manufacturing is considered a potential solution for creating complex shapes for tissue engineering scaffolds. Three-dimensional bioprinting forms biocompatible complex structures that biological substances can be deposited on the substrate using computer-aided design/manufacturing technology. The working principle of additive manufacturing is that the objects are formed by adding material layer by layer instead of removing material as in conventional manufacturing. Three-dimensional bioprinting is a category of additive manufacturing that focuses on the deposition of biomolecules. It is able to control the shape, size, porosity, and interconnectivity of the scaffold [9]. Some bioprinting technologies are capable of precisely printing biomolecules using fixed-point deposition. This technology has gained immense popularity in the medical field due to its capability in tissue engineering compounds [10].

5.2 BIOPRINTING TECHNOLOGIES AND THEIR APPLICATIONS

Additive manufacturing is revolutionizing product design and on-location manufacturing globally, enabling product design and redesign, which helps in developing new material properties, and the transformation of business capabilities through the production of products in a more sustainable way and at a relatively lower cost [7, 11–12]. Some industrial applications of additive manufacturing and advantages are given in the following Table 5.1.

Any additive manufacturing process will follow a certain sequence for producing its final product. If we take the additive manufacturing process, Figure 5.1 shows the sequence of steps from the CAD model to the final 3D object. The process begins with developing of digital model for prototyping of physical model. A digital model can be produced by reverse engineering using a 3D scanner.

The same principle is applied to the bioprinting process; the most important step in the bioprinting process is the process of imaging. This process involves scanning the injured tissue, organ, or body part. The scanning is done in different ways: 3D scanning of medical imagining is done by computer tomography, commonly called a CT scan. It can be done by magnetic resonance imaging, or MRI, which is widely used in many hospitals. The image obtained by scanning is then converted to a 3D model using software. Once the 3D model is obtained, then the process is the same as that of the additive manufacturing process shown in Figure 5.1. The sequence of operations required for bioprinting is given in Figure 5.2.

In general, bioprinting is the precise positioning of biological constituents—biological living cells—layer by layer by spatial control of the positioning of the functional living cells in the 3D-fabricated structure. Bioprinting methods are classified according to the type of positioning, as given in Figure 5.3

This precise positioning of the cells at respective points is guided by the materials used in the bioprinter. The bioprintable material used in the bioprinting process is known as bio-ink. In regenerative medicine, a wide range of biomaterials are used to repair diseased cells/tissues. But most of these materials are not compatible with bioprinting technologies. For example, biomaterials that need high temperatures in their process of printing are not compatible with living cells. The different bioprinting technologies available for the deposition of bio-inks are depicted in Figure 5.3.

5.3 INKJET BIOPRINTING

Inkjet bioprinting is one of the oldest methods of printing. In this process, the bio-ink is delivered onto the scaffold without contact with the nozzle. These bio-inks can be natural or man-made materials that help support the adhesion, proliferation, and multiplication of the cells. In this process, the bio-ink is forced under pressure through a nozzle and subsequently breaks into a stream of droplets. These printers contain single or multiple print heads. Each print head contains a chamber and a nozzle. The bio-inks are held at the nozzle's orifice by the surface tension of the fluid [14]. Pressure pulses are introduced into the chamber of the print head in three ways. It is given by either piezoelectric inkjet, thermal inkjet, or electrostatic bioprinting, as shown in Figure 5.4.

TABLE 5.1

Industrial Applications and Advantages of Additive Manufacturing [13]

S. No	Industry	Application	Advantages
1	Aerospace and Defense	Landing gears, thrust reverser doors, small surveillance drones, Gimbal eye, grenade launchers, complex brackets, and jet engine components. Repair of turbine blades and high-value components.	• Low-volume production of high-value products with complex geometries • Fuel efficiency through weight reduction of parts • Improved product utility through on-demand production of replacement parts
2	Automotive	Engine bay parts, intake valves, engine components, gearboxes, air inlet, engine control unit, and lower fairing baffle.	• Cost-effective solution for customization of luxury vehicles • Obsolescence management for defective parts • Testing and production of lightweight, high-strength parts
3	Electronics	Wearable devices, soft robots, structural monitoring, building elements, and RFID (radiofrequency identification) devices embedded inside solid substrates.	• High-resolution, multimaterial, large-area fabrication of electronic devices that are free of printed circuit boards (PCBs) • Production of complex, lightweight impact-resistant structures with multiple functionalities • Designing of complex geometry parts with embedded electronics, sensors, and antennas that cannot be produced by conventional manufacturing process • Internal manufacturing of circuits and circuit boards that reduces procurement time and eliminates intellectual property–related issues
4	Healthcare	Surgical models: organs, vasculature, tumor models, and disease models. Surgical instruments: forceps, retractors, medical clamps, and scalpel handles. Implants: limbs, craniofacial implants, casts, and stents. Dental: crown, bridges, and splints	• Production of customized implants, devices, dental crowns, etc. • Reduction in health care costs due to minimal reintervention enabled by accurate diagnosis • Rapid response time during emergencies through rapid scaling of production • Staff training in specific applications, leveraging data sets of patients affected by rare pathologies • Patient-centric health care through personalization of drugs for complex patient-specific release profiles
5	Consumer goods	Consumer electronics, jewelry, shoes, clothing, cosmetics products, toys, figurines, furniture, office accessories, musical instruments, bicycles, and food products	• Fabrication of complex internal and external structures compels innovative product design • Faster time to market and cost-effective customization of customer-centric products. • Decentralized manufacturing, reducing transferred costs to consumers

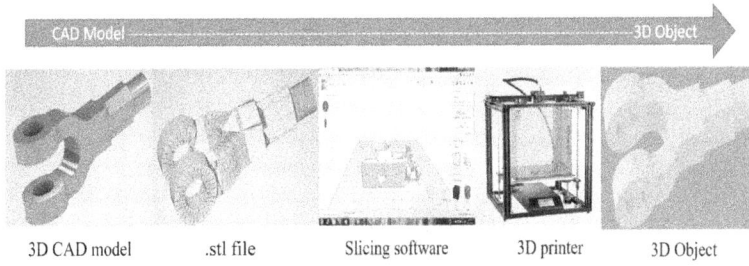

FIGURE 5.1   Basic additive manufacturing process.

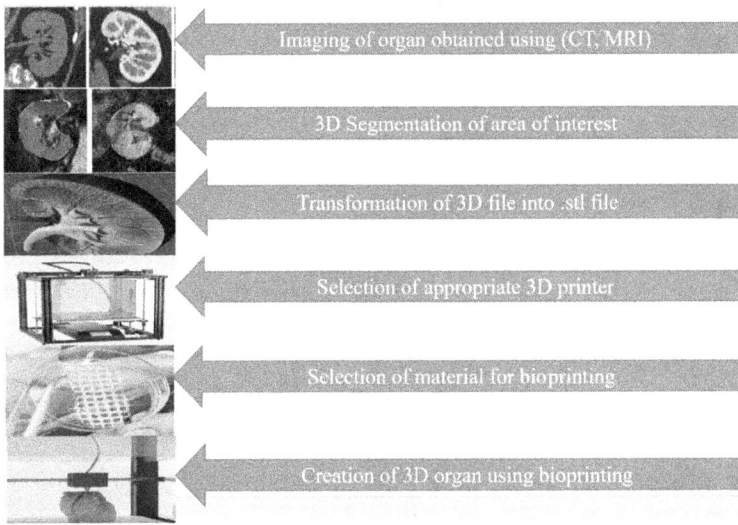

FIGURE 5.2   Sequence of steps for 3D bioprinting.

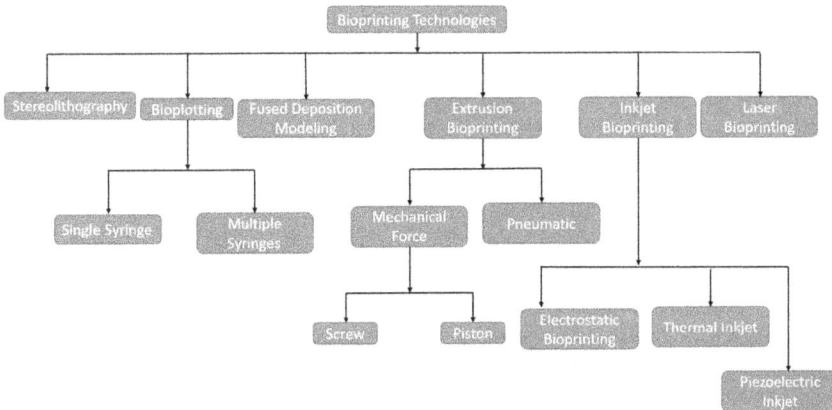

FIGURE 5.3   Bioprinting methods.

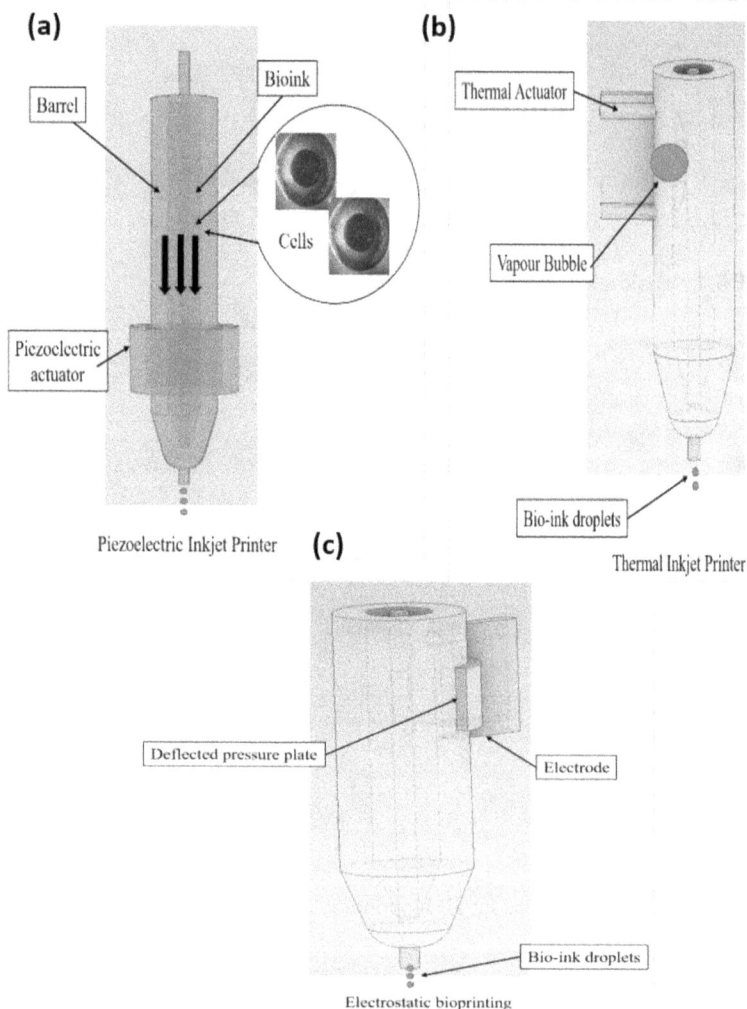

FIGURE 5.4   Various bioprinting technologies: (a) Piezoelectric inkjet printer; (b) thermal inkjet printer; (c) electrostatic bioprinting.

In piezoelectric inkjet printers, the pressure pulses are produced by the actuator in order to deposit the bio-ink; some print heads require backpressure to supplement the pressure pulses in order to generate droplets of the bio-ink. In thermal inkjet printers, the thermal actuator locally heats the bio-ink solution when a voltage pulse is applied to the actuator. Because of local heating, a vapor bubble is formed, as shown in Figure 5.4. This bubble expands rapidly and collapses, which results in a pressure pulse inside the fluid chamber that forces the bio-ink droplets to overcome the surface tension and deposit on the scaffold. Thermal inkjet printers are capable of dispensing various biological elements, such as proteins, mammalian cells, and others. In electrostatic bioprinters, the droplets of bio-ink are delivered by increasing the volume of the fluid chamber, as well as the bio-ink solution attached to the plate. When the voltage is supplied, the pressure plate deflects between the electrode and plate. As the pressure plate regains its position, the fall in voltage creates an ejection of bio-ink [15].

5.4 BIOPLOTTING

Bioplotting is a bioprinting process in which a single or multiple syringes are employed to extrude either cells or spheroids of materials. These types of plotters have several syringes and can extrude different cell materials at a time and at different conditions. Using several syringes enables the production of multiple tissues, which helps in producing bioengineered soft tissues. After the cells have been stacked on one on the other, it is cured with ultraviolet (UV) radiation through a chemical reaction. Besides

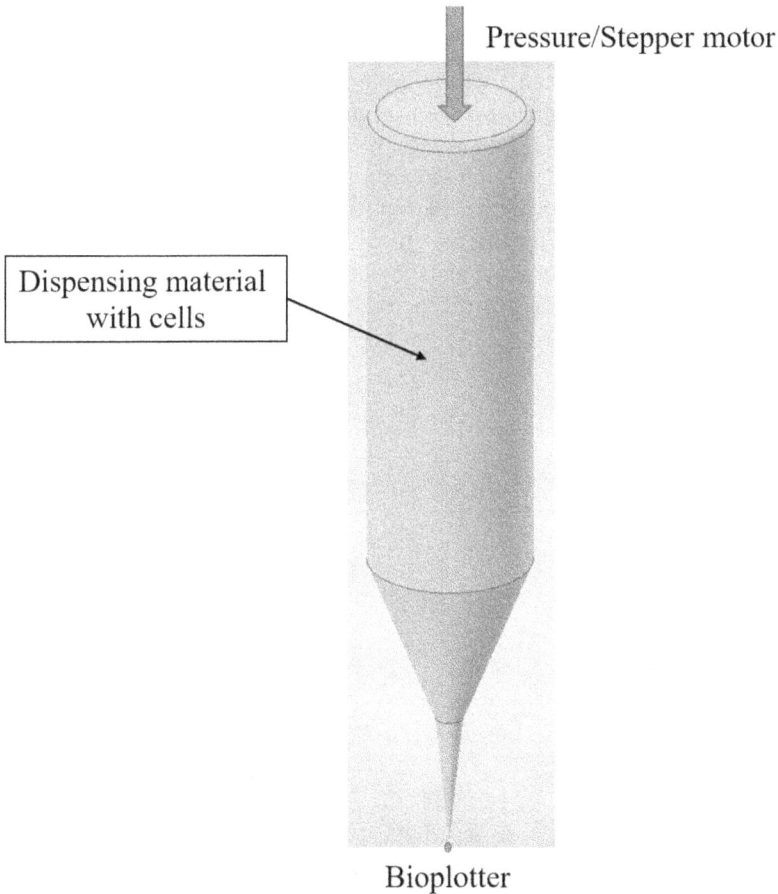

Bioplotter

FIGURE 5.5 Bioplotter.

its advantages, the major challenge is selecting the material for extrusion. The materials that can be extruded in bioplotting should be viscous, provide an environment for cell growth, and support cells. Thermoset resins, polymers, pastes, proteins, and others can be extruded using bioplotting [16].

5.5 FUSED DEPOSITION MODELING

Fused deposition modeling (FDM) is one popular kind of deposition technique in rapid prototyping. This method plays a vital role in improving surface quality, consumes less time, and is considered a cost-effective process. The same technology can be applied in bioprinting, whereby thermoplastic thin layers that can support the hydrogel-inks can be used in FDM. The process of FDM begins with a CAD model being generated; then the thermoplastic material is deposited layer by layer with the help of the nozzle [6]. The temperature of the nozzle is set at the melting point of the thermoplastic material.

5.6 LASER BIOPRINTING

Laser-based bioprinting is also widely used for bioprinting of the living cells onto the substrate. This printing is possible with the help of a high-intensity light source or a long-wavelength light [17–18]. A laser bioprinter mainly contains a pulsed laser, a focusing system to focus the high-intensity light, a laser-absorbing surface/ribbon, a receiving substrate, and material/bio-ink that contains cells. Several parameters influence the resolution of the laser bioprinter, the surface tension of the liquid/bio-ink, the gap between the substrate and the ribbon surface, the absorbance of the substrate, the thickness and viscosity of the organic layer, the laser's light wavelength,

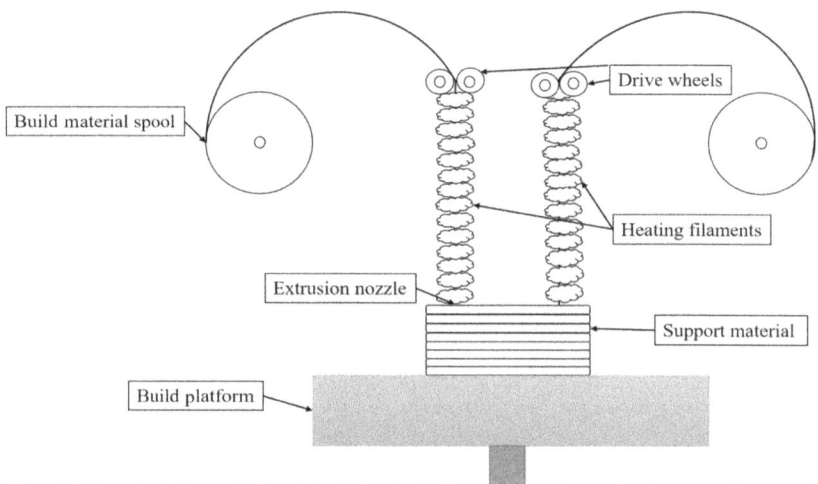

FIGURE 5.6 FDM.

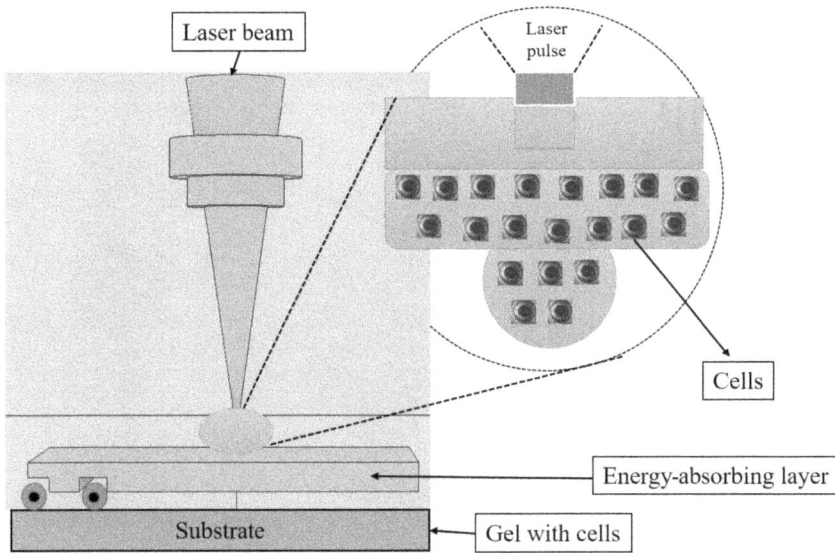

FIGURE 5.7   Laser bioprinting.

and its configuration. Unlike inkjet printers, laser printers are nozzle-free and hence can deposit a high density of bio-ink without clogging, as shown in Figure 5.7.

5.7   EXTRUSION BIOPRINTING

Extrusion-based bioprinting is also widely used in tissue engineering in this type of technology; bio-ink is generally disposed by pneumatic pressure, or a mechanical force (screw or piston) system is used to extrude the bio-ink onto the substrate. The viscosity in these varies from 30 to 6×10^7 mPas [19]. Extrusion bioprinters are controlled by a robotic stage controller. The movement of the head is controlled in the x, y, and z directions. With this method, the bio-ink can be directly dispensed on the substrate placed below it. These printers can dispense high-cell-density bio-inks, special hydrogels with extensive viscosities, and biodegradable thermoplastics, such as polycaprolactone [19]. Extrusion bioprinting will lower the risk of clogging of bio-inks as compared to inkjet printing, but the only drawback with extrusion is we need to ensure that the shear force is not high enough that it compromises the cell viability.

5.8   SLA

It is a free-form technique in which we can deposit light to cross-linked polymer materials. Most SLAs use UV light, which is directed onto the surface of the photo-curable resin. Once the resin is cured, the platform moves upward, and a fresh layer of resin is added. This process repeats until the product is constructed. Despite SLA's advantages, its processing time is slow. Materials are still being developed for its

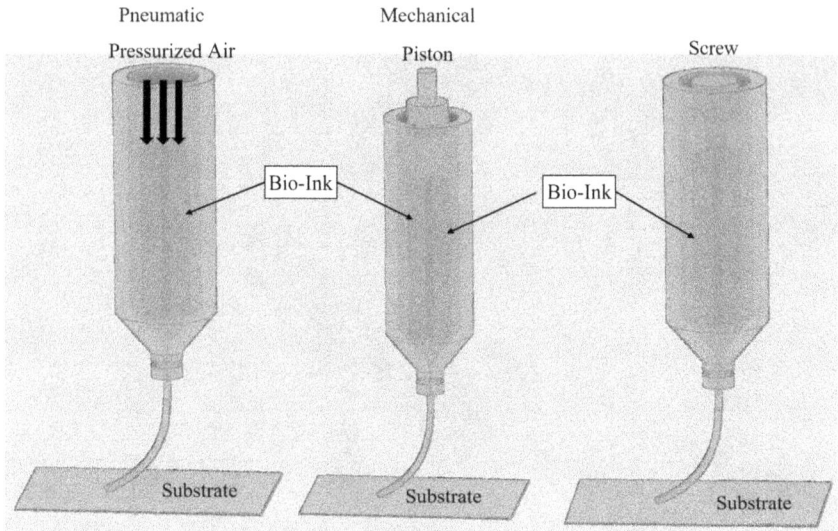

FIGURE 5.8   Extrusion bioprinting.

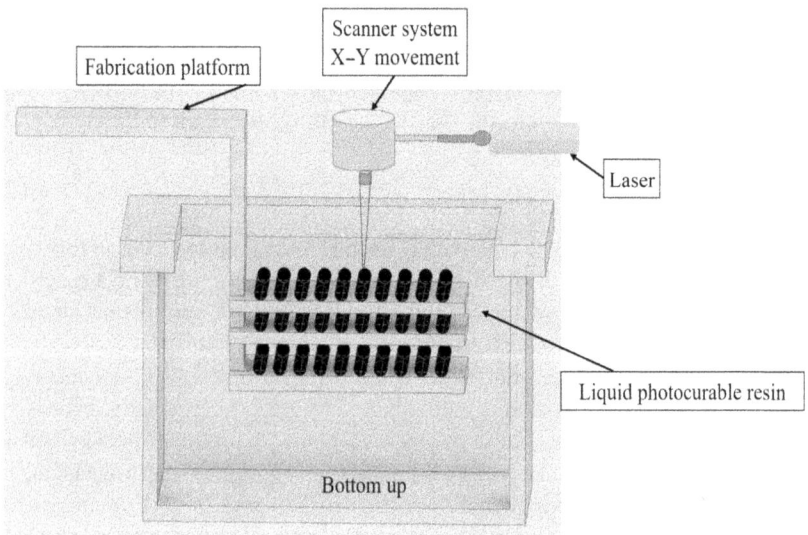

FIGURE 5.9   SLA bioprinting.

appropriate use in tissue engineering. Visible light–based SLA is a popular technology that is been used to dispense bio-inks in difficult applications.

5.9   BIO-INKS AND MULTICOMPONENT BIO-INKS

Bio-inks are those made up of fluid materials that contain three to four matrix components, which are loaded into a bioprinter and deposited onto the scaffold. These scaffolds allow the cells to adhere, support, proliferate, and multiply after printing. This phenomenon of cell growth is important in tissue engineering, which helps in the rehabilitation of diseased tissues and organs. Multicomponent bio-inks are used currently that contain more than one type of biomaterial or biomolecule, one or more cells, and additive materials. These multicomponent bio-inks are used for building different tissue constructs. The reason for using multicomponent bio-inks is that if we go for a general natural polymer, such as gelatin and collagen, which are widely used bio-inks and help in cell attachment and migration, these suffer from low mechanical properties; to avoid these deficiencies, other additives and biomaterials are added to the form multicomponent biomaterial with improved properties. Rheological properties of multicomponent bio-inks play a vital role; it should be precisely controlled in order to achieve proper printability and stability of the structure.

In multicomponent bio-inks, it can have multiple bio-inks in order to produce varying stiffnesses. These bio-inks are made of crosslinked polymers can be solidified just after printing. These bio-inks should be photoreactive in order to form a stiff structure when exposed to UV light. These bio-inks should not solidify too quickly or too slowly. If they solidify too quickly, they may clog inside the nozzle of the printer. If they solidify too slowly, then the construct will collapse. These mutlimaterial combinations of bio-inks should not be toxic in the small and long term [20]. Bio-inks are also classified as shear-thinning and shear-thickening materials [21]. Shear-thinning materials help printers easily dispense with the application of shear force and regains their shape/characteristics once shear force is removed. In shear-thickening materials, gelation occurs under the influence of chemical and physical stimuli. Chemical crosslinking also occurs when exposed to UV rays.

A single-biomaterial bio-ink is not suitable for bioprinting, as this does not meet the mechanical and functional requirements for cells to adhere, proliferate, and spread to form a tissue/organ. The use of biomaterials such as polyethylene glycol (PEG) allows the varying of molecular weight and crosslinking properties, but they lack other properties required to proliferate. If we use natural biomaterials, such as gelatin and fibrin, they are limited by their poor mechanical properties. Therefore, multicomponent bio-inks are composed of more than one bio-ink, improving the properties of the individual materials and supporting the construct with the required environment for the cells to grow. These multicomponent bio-inks are gaining popularity for 3D bioprinting with improved performance. The parameters that influence the viability of the cell are also important characteristics that need to be considered, as given in Figure 5.10.

Some bio-inks may be made by combining natural materials, by combining synthetic materials, or by combining synthetic and natural materials. In Table 5.2, various bio-inks, their advantages, and their properties are described.

5.10 GELATIN METHACRYLOL

Gelatin methacrylol (GelMA) is a hydrogel capable of forming a crosslinking polymer when exposed to UV light. It has great structural fidelity, low stiffness, and high porosity that can well support cell survival and help enhance cell proliferation. GelMA is widely used in endothelial cell morpholisis [22–23], cardiomyocytes, epidermal tissues, tissue constructs, cartilage regeneration, and bone differentiation.

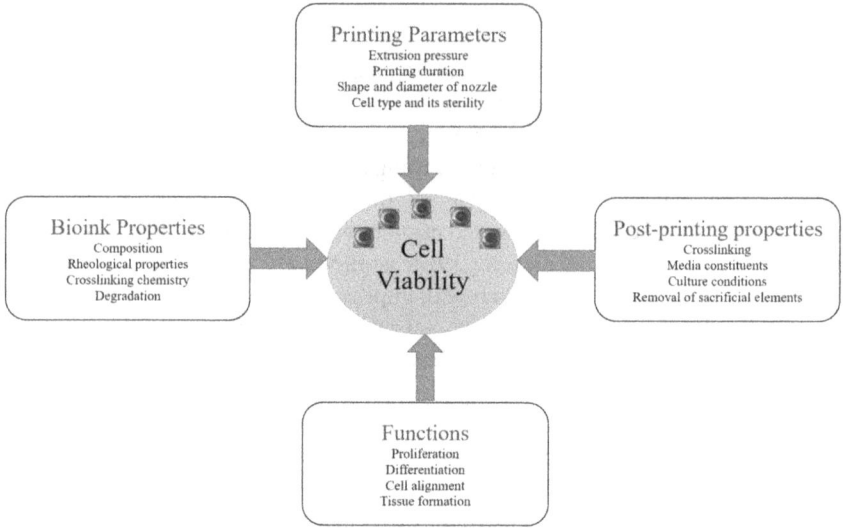

FIGURE 5.10 Parameters influencing the cell viability.

5.11 AGAROSE

Agarose is the most popularly used hydrogel-based bio-ink with other natural polymers for 3D bioprinting. It is made of natural polysaccharide, which has special properties like good crosslinking, biocompatibility, and low-cost availability. It is widely used in tissue engineering for drug and cell delivery, cell encapsulation, and cell adhesion. These bio-inks are printed using inkjet printer, Agarose is mixed with other natural polymers, such as gelatin and fibrinogen, to enhance its cell adhesion [24–25].

5.12 ALGINATE

Alginate is also a natural seaweed-extracted, ion-deficient anionic polysaccharide [26]. It is a rapidly crosslinkable and biocompatible material. This hydrogel solidifies when it is exposed to $CaCl_2$ and leads to the formation of a gel with an ion exchange with sodium-calcium. As alginate is viscous, it provides strong protection for cells when it is been extruded with high pressure onto the scaffold. Alginate can also be combined with polyvinyl alcohol and hydroxyapatite to form a multicomponent bio-ink.

5.13 CHITOSAN

Chitosan is an alkaline polysaccharide biomaterial, which is biocompatible, biodegradable. It has very poor crosslinking properties as well as poor mechanical properties. Chitosan, when compared to alginate, is better for osteogenic cell proliferation and differentiation [27]. Chitosan is a positively charged biomaterial that can be

TABLE 5.2

Natural and Synthetic Bio-Inks and their Characteristics

Molecule Type	Novelty	Overview	Method of Printing	Advantages
Collagen	Polyphenol (tannic acid)/using core shell struts	It can be used as primary structure for skin and other connected tissues	Pressure assisted bioprinting	It has high biological relevance
Elastin	Self-assembling hydrogel	It has excellent hydrophobicity	Pressure assisted bioprinting	It has high biological relevance
Fibrin	Insoluble protein formed during blood clotting	Formed by polymerization of the soluble plasma protein fibrinogen	Extrusion-based bioprinting (mechanical/pneumatic)	Rapid gelation
Gelatin	Hydrogel	Protein substance derived from partial hydrolysis of collagen	Coaxial nozzle extrusion	High biocompatibility High water solubility Thermally reversible gelation
Agarose	Polysaccharide extracted from seaweed	Extracted from seaweed	Pressure-assisted bioprinting	Nontoxic, has good crosslinking and high stability
Alginate	Naturally derived biopolymer from brown algae	Natural bio-ink	Coaxial extrusion printing	Mild cross-linking properties Rapid gelation, high biocompatibility
Chitosan	Polysaccharide obtained from the outer skeleton of shellfish (e.g. shrimp). Non-animal-derived chitosan can be obtained from fungal fermentation.	Natural bio-ink	Coaxial extrusion printing	High biocompatibility Antibacterial Properties
Silk fibroin	Physical and chemical crosslinking	Natural bio-ink	Stereolithography	High biological relevance Rapid gelation

combined with gelatin; it has good printability at room temperature, a high construct strength, and good biocompatibility.

5.14 SILK FIBROIN

There are various kinds of silk fibers that have a wide range of applications in tissue engineering, cartilage regeneration, biosensors, small catalytic motors, and strain

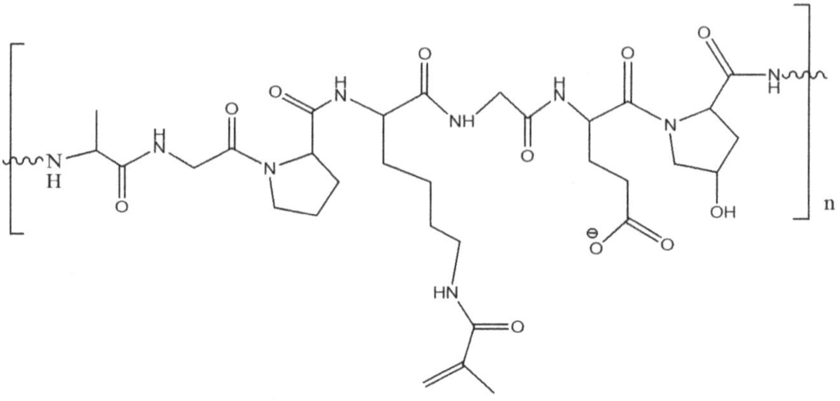

FIGURE 5.11   GelMA.

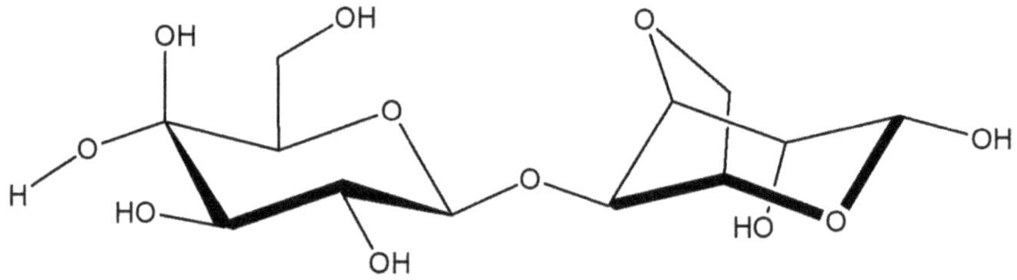

FIGURE 5.12   Agarose structure.

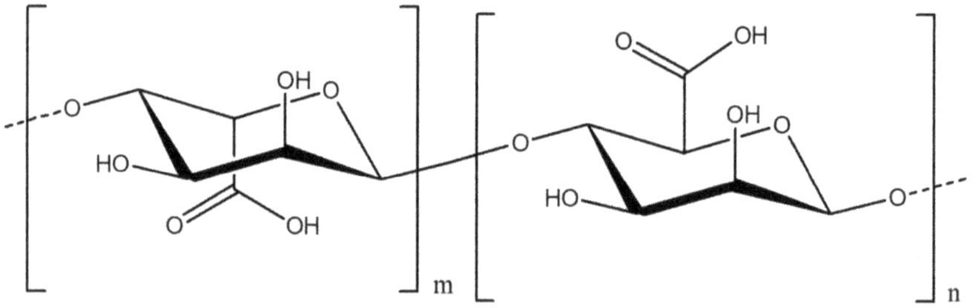

FIGURE 5.13   Alginate structure.

gauges for biological applications. Silk fibroin consists of heavy chains, these chains attached by disulfide bonds. Silk fibroin scaffolds have many advantages compared to other scaffolds, like good mechanical stability, biocompatibility, nontoxicity, and good adhesion properties for the cell to adhere and proliferate. They are printed with inkjet bioprinting process, even some memory shape implants use silk fibroin bio-ink.

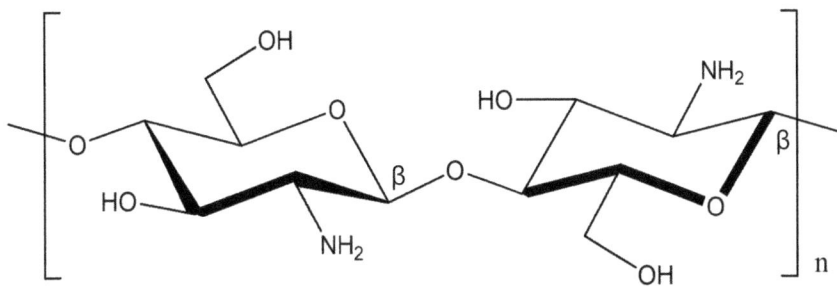

FIGURE 5.14 Chitosan (a linear polysaccharide composed of randomly distributed β-(1→4)-linked D-glucosamine and N-acetyl-D-glucosamine).

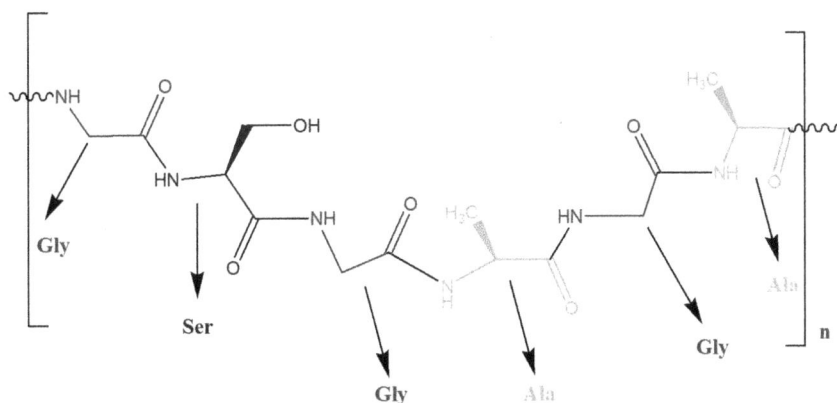

FIGURE 5.15 Silk fibroin a natural polymer bio-ink.

5.15 COLLAGEN

Collagen types I through IV are extracted from the mammalian and marine tissue. Collagen hydrogels alone do not provide the required mechanical stiffness for the scaffold; they even do not have enough of the biological elements essential for cell differential. These collagens, with multicomponent biomaterials, can be used either with laser, inkjet, extrusion, and SLA.

5.16 HYALURONIC ACID

Hyaluronic acid is an extract from the glycosaminoglycan from bovine eyes; it is an anionic biopolymer that is based on D-glucuronic acid and D-N-acetylglucosamine repeating units and behaves similar to the collagen type I bio-ink [28]. This material has good biodegradability, bioresorbability, and biocompatibility and has a potential

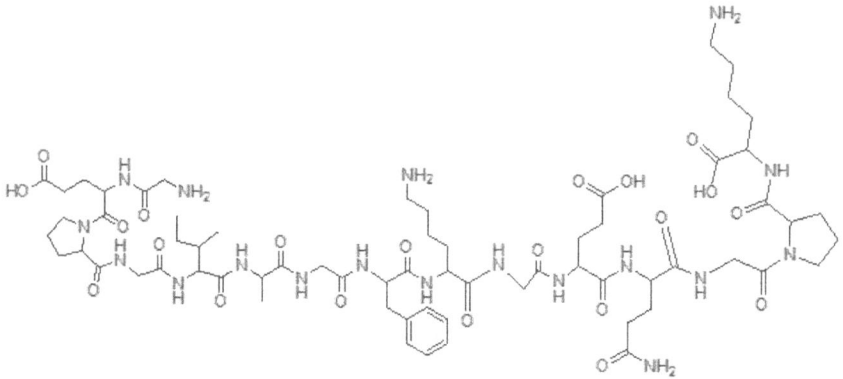

FIGURE 5.16   Collagen type II structure.

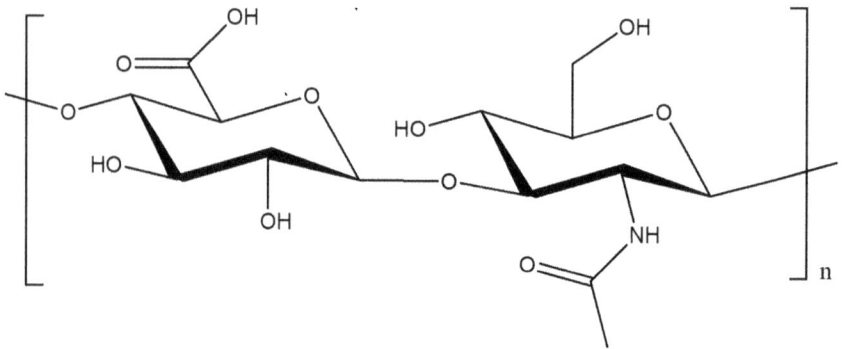

FIGURE 5.17   Hyaluronic acid structure.

to form a flexible hydrogel. This bio-ink is used in extrusion-based 3D-bioprinting applications.

5.17   CONCLUSION

Therefore, 3D bioprinting technology has given us an opportunity to produce hard tissues, organs, 3D models, scaffolds, and more. These bioprinting technologies can be classified into various technologies that can be used according to the application. In tissue engineering, these technologies have been used for patient-specific implants producing porous scaffolds, cell-based constructs, and bioartificial tissues and organs. With these technologies, large tissues and organs could be repaired. Extrusion-based printing technology has played a prominent role in fabricating various scaffolds. The ink- and laser-based 3D printing has been lagging due to its limitations in software capabilities as well as hardware capabilities.

The multicomponent bio-inks have helped many vascular systems for cell growth, proliferation, and differentiation. The gelatin-based natural and synthetic polymers have also provided cells to adhere, grow, proliferate, and differentiate. Although 3D-printing technology has robust features, there are several limitations to it that need to be addressed; more research strategies have to be implemented in order to improve it. In this context, similar to 3D-printing technology, 4D printing is also adding the fourth dimension of time. These 4D-printed structures allow changing their forms or functions with time in response to any stimuli, such as pressure, temperature, air, water, and light. The rapid development and advances in 4D technology will allow us to print more smart materials, which have great applications in vast areas in the near future.

REFERENCES

1. Wang X, Ao Q, Tian X, Fan J, Wei Y, Hou W, et al. 3D bioprinting technologies for hard tissue and organ engineering. *Materials*. 2016;9:1–23.
2. Chang R, Emami K, Wu H, Sun W. Biofabrication of a three-dimensional liver micro-organ as an in vitro drug metabolism model. *Biofabrication*. 2010;2.
3. Matai I, Kaur G, Seyedsalehi A, McClinton A, Laurencin CT. Progress in 3D bioprinting technology for tissue/organ regenerative engineering. *Biomaterials*. 2020;226:119536. Elsevier Ltd.
4. Liu J, Saul D, Böker KO, Ernst J, Lehman W, Schilling AF. Current methods for skeletal muscle tissue repair and regeneration. *BioMed Research International*. 2018;2018.
5. Wong VW, Sorkin M, Gurtner GC. Enabling stem cell therapies for tissue repair: Current and future challenges. *Biotechnology Advances*. 2013;31:744–51. Elsevier B.V.
6. Li J, Chen M, Fan X, Zhou H. Recent advances in bioprinting techniques: Approaches, applications and future prospects. *Journal of Translational Medicine*. BioMed Central; 2016;14:1–15.
7. Singh, D, Babbar, A, Jain V et al. Synthesis, characterization, and bioactivity investigation of biomimetic biodegradable PLA scaffold fabricated by fused filament fabrication process. *Journal of the Brazilian Society of Mechanical Sciences and Engineering*. 2019;41.
8. Bhargav Pathri. Manufacturing of formula one student sports car upright using rapid prototyping. *International Journal of Automotive Technology*. 2011;29:2051–7831.
9. Babbar A, Sharma A, Bansal S, Mago J, Toor V. Potential applications of three-dimensional printing for anatomical simulations and surgical planning. *Materials Today: Proceedings*. 2020 Jan 1;33:1558–61.
10. Babbar A, Jain V, Gupta D., Singh S, Prakash C, Pruncu C. Biomaterials and fabrication methods of scaffolds for tissue engineering applications. *3D Printing in Biomedical Engineering*. 2020:167–86.
11. Babbar A, Jain V, Gupta D, Prakash C, Sunpreet Singh AS. 3D Bioprinting in pharmaceuticals, medicine, and tissue engineering applications. *Advanced Manufacturing and Processing Technology*. 2020:1–15.
12. Atul Babbar AR and AS. Latest trend in building construction: Three-dimensional printing. *International Conference on Mechatronics and Artificial Intelligence*. 2021:1–8.
13. Delhi N. National strategy for additive manufacturing policy. Government of India, 2020.
14. Mobaraki M, Ghaffari M, Yazdanpanah A, Luo Y, Mills DK. Bioinks and bioprinting: A focused review. *Bioprinting*. 2020;18.
15. Tönshoff HK, Hillmann-Apmann H. Diamond tools for wire sawing metal components. *Diamond and Related Materials*. 2002;11:742–8.
16. Pfister A, Landers R, Laib A, Hübner U, Schmelzeisen R, Mülhaupt R. Biofunctional rapid prototyping for tissue-engineering applications: 3D bioplotting versus 3D printing. *Journal of Polymer Science, Part A: Polymer Chemistry*. 2004;42:624–38.

17. Rutz AL, Lewis PL, Shah RN. Toward next-generation bioinks: Tuning material properties pre- and post-printing to optimize cell viability. *MRS Bulletin.* 2017;42:563–70.

18. Sakai S, Kamei H, Mori T, Hotta T, Ohi H, Nakahata M, et al. Visible light-induced hydrogelation of an alginate derivative and application to stereolithographic bioprinting using a visible light projector and acid red. *Biomacromolecules.* 2018;19:672–9.

19. Gurkan UA, El Assal R, Yildiz SE, Sung Y, Trachtenberg AJ, Kuo WP, et al. Engineering anisotropic biomimetic fibrocartilage microenvironment by bioprinting mesenchymal stem cells in nanoliter gel droplets. *Molecular Pharmaceutics.* 2014;11:2151–9.

20. Zhao Y, Li Y, Mao S, Sun W, Yao R. The influence of printing parameters on cell survival rate and printability in microextrusion-based 3D cell printing technology. *Biofabrication.* 2015;7:45002. IOP Publishing.

21. Highley CB, Rodell CB, Burdick JA. Direct 3D printing of shear-thinning hydrogels into self-healing hydrogels. *Advanced Materials.* 2015;27:5075–9.

22. Jose RR, Rodriguez MJ, Dixon TA, Omenetto F, Kaplan DL. Evolution of bioinks and additive manufacturing technologies for 3D bioprinting. *ACS Biomaterials Science and Engineering.* 2016;2:1662–78.

23. Matsiko A, Gleeson JP, O'Brien FJ. Scaffold mean pore size influences mesenchymal stem cell chondrogenic differentiation and matrix deposition. *Tissue Engineering—Part A.* 2015;21:486–97.

24. López-Marcial GR, Zeng AY, Osuna C, Dennis J, García JM, O'Connell GD. Agarose-based hydrogels as suitable bioprinting materials for tissue engineering. *ACS Biomaterials Science and Engineering.* 2018;4:3610–6.

25. Duarte Campos DF, Blaeser A, Buellesbach K, Sen KS, Xun W, Tillmann W, et al. Bioprinting organotypic hydrogels with improved mesenchymal stem cell remodeling and mineralization properties for bone tissue engineering. *Advanced Healthcare Materials.* 2016;5:1336–45.

26. Neufurth M, Wang X, Schröder HC, Feng Q, Diehl-Seifert B, Ziebart T, et al. Engineering a morphogenetically active hydrogel for bioprinting of bioartificial tissue derived from human osteoblast-like SaOS-2 cells. *Biomaterials.* 2014;35:8810–9.

27. Xu C, Lei C, Meng L, Wang C, Song Y. Chitosan as a barrier membrane material in periodontal tissue regeneration. *Journal of Biomedical Materials Research—Part B Applied Biomaterials.* 2012;100 B:1435–43.

28. Coradini D, Pellizzaro C, Miglierini G, Daidone MG, Perbellini A. Hyaluronic acid as drug delivery for sodium butyrate: Improvement of the anti-proliferative activity on a breast-cancer cell line. *International Journal of Cancer.* 1999;81:411–6.

6 Additive Manufacturing of Polymers for Biomedical Applications

Subrata Mondal
Department of Mechanical Engineering, National Institute of Technical Teachers' Training and Research (NITTTR) Kolkata, FC Block, Sector III, Salt Lake City, Kolkata 700106, West Bengal, India

CONTENTS

6.1 Introduction 100
6.2 Various AM Processes for Polymers 100
    6.2.1 Material Extrusion Technique 101
    6.2.2 Material Jetting 103
    6.2.3 Powder Bed Fusion 103
    6.2.4 Sheet Lamination 104
    6.2.5 Binder Jetting 104
    6.2.6 Vat Photopolymerization 104
6.3 Types of Polymers for AM 104
    6.3.1 Thermoplastic Polymers 105
    6.3.2 Thermosetting Polymers 105
    6.3.3 Elastomers 105
6.4 Polymers Composites/Nanocomposites for AM 105
    6.4.1 Fiber Reinforcements 106
    6.4.2 Particle Reinforcements 107
    6.4.3 Nanomaterials Reinforcements 107
6.5 Biomedical Applications of AM for Polymers 107
    6.5.1 Scaffolds 108
    6.5.2 Stents 108
    6.5.3 Prostheses 109
    6.5.4 Dentistry 110
6.6 Conclusion 111
References 112

DOI: 10.1201/9781003217961-6

6.1 INTRODUCTION

Additive manufacturing (AM) is an emerging field and opening up enormous opportunities for several industries and academia [1–4]. AM enables the three-dimensional (3D) printing of lightweight and complex structures that are hardly achievable by other manufacturing technology [5]. This class of manufacturing processes enables the rapid prototyping of complex structures by depositing materials layer by layer via computer-aided design (CAD) [6]. AM has been advanced well beyond prototyping and has been established as a promising technique for transforming traditional manufacturing in the future. The process can build a 3D item from a model created by CAD [7]. Today's additive manufacturing emerged as a versatile technique for customizing parts from metal, ceramic and polymers without the need for complex mold designs or machining that is required for conventional formative fabrication and the subtractive method. AM techniques are basically different from the traditional subtractive manufacturing process, and the structure is constructed into its tailored shape by using a layer-by-layer deposition method, such as extrusion, binding, melting and photopolymerization [8]. In fact, AM permits the construction of 3D structures with high shape complexity [9].

There are several advantages of AM when complex structures are required [10]. The properties of printable materials are specific to the printing method and influence the properties and performance of 3D printed items. Materials used in additive manufacturing are polymers, metals, ceramics, glass and composites. As compared with other materials polymer has advantages, such as low cost, flexibility and tailorable property, which can be engineered prior to the polymer synthesis. Several polymers, such as thermoplastic, thermoset, elastomer, polymer blend, hydrogel, functional polymers and composites, can be used for 3D printing [11]. In comparison to conventional polymer processing, for example, injection molding and subtractive technique, for example, computerized numerical control (CNC) machining, AM allows CAD to drive the manufacturing of multifunctional materials with complex shapes and tailor-made functionalities [9].

An attempt has been made in this chapter to provide an overview of the 3D printing of polymers to manufacture biomedical materials. A brief overview of various AM processes for polymers is provided. Polymer-based 3D-printed parts are weaker compared with metal, ceramic and glass parts. Mechanical properties of polymer 3D-printed parts can be improved by reinforcing them with materials such fibers, particles or even nanoparticles. The various reinforcements of polymers, such as fibers, particles and nanomaterials, for 3D-printed parts are included. The applications of polymer AM parts in various biomedical fields, such as stents, scaffolds, dentistry and others, are described in the chapter. The chapter concludes with the challenges of AM with polymers and the future scope.

6.2 VARIOUS AM PROCESSES FOR POLYMERS

Compared with a subtractive method, such as CNC machining (Figure 6.1a), and formative manufacturing, such as injection molding (Figure 6.1c), the AM process (Figure 6.1b) allows CAD to drive the fabrication of complex shapes with tailor-made

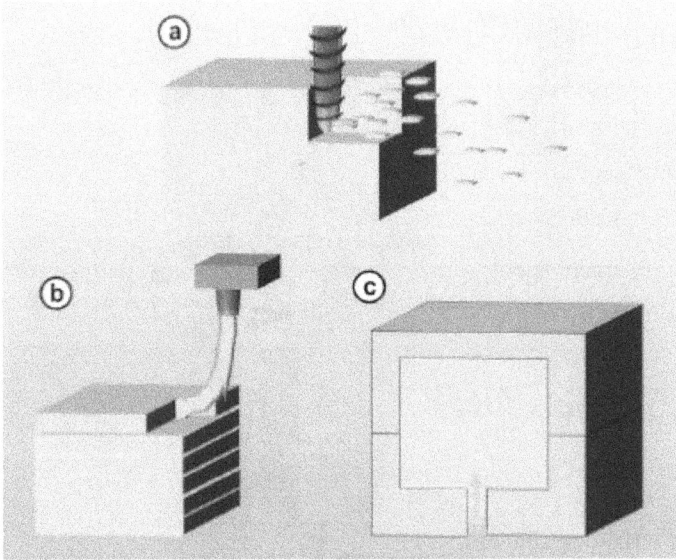

FIGURE 6.1 Schematic showing an example of (a) subtractive manufacturing, (b) additive manufacturing and (c) formative manufacturing techniques [9].

functionalities. As compared with the subtractive method, an additive manufacturing process has several advantages, such as (1) no material loss, (2) passive production (no force required), (3) reproducibility and (4) detail production depends on digitized data [12]. Polymers are widely used as base materials for various additive manufacturing processes. The use of polymers in additive AM includes sheet lamination (e.g., laminated object manufacturing), vat photopolymerization (e.g., stereolithography), powder bed fusion (e.g., selective laser sintering [SLS]), extrusion (such as fused deposition modeling [FDM], 3D dispensing, 3D fiber deposition) and others. Polymer-based AM can be broadly classified as discussed in the following sections [9].

6.2.1 Material Extrusion Technique

In this AM process, a polymer is selectively dispensed through the nozzles. FDM, the fused filament fabrication (FFF) technique and 3D dispensing are typical examples of material extrusion techniques of AM. Among various 3D-printing techniques, FDM is the most popular [13]. A polymer is used as the building material in the FDM process. In order to obtain polymer melt, energy is applied in this process at the pre-deposition stage, and molten polymer is applied through a fine print head or nozzle (Figure 6.2) [10]. FDM is a process of building 3D structures in a layer-by-layer fusion via extrusion of generally nonreactive thermoplastic polymer filaments through heated nozzles. The FDM technique has been widely used by various industries, academia and consumer industries for the fabrication of both prototype and

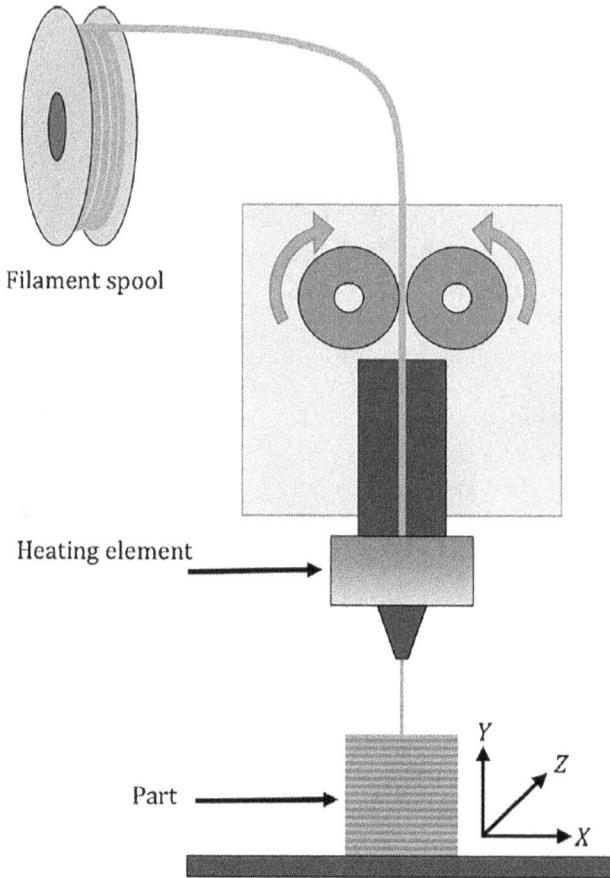

FIGURE 6.2   Schematic showing the FDM technique for layer-by-layer deposition in order to fabricate a 3D part [10].

functional items due to the simplicity, affordability and reliability of the technology. The process required preformed fiber uniform in size and consistency in material properties to be fed through nozzles and roller. FDM printing depends on wide range of parameters that can be broadly categorized into three groups: (1) extruder-, (2) process- and (3) structural-related parameters. For example, nozzle diameter and filament width fall under the category of the first group; printing speed and processing temperature are process-related; and layer thickness, toolpath and infill geometry parameters are grouped under structural parameters [13]. Despite several advantages, FDM has a few intrinsic disadvantages, such as the optimum filament temperature is required for easy flow of the material through nozzle orifice, because the viscosity of the molten filament material depends on the filament's temperature. Furthermore, the deposited filament should provide sufficient structural support for the subsequent layers. Other disadvantages are weak mechanical properties and the cost of printed parts [13].

6.2.2 MATERIAL JETTING

Droplets of photopolymers and thermoplastic polymers are selectively deposited by this technique to fabricate the complex structure. Materials used in this technique are liquid thermoset photopolymers. The inkjet printing technique is an example of this kind of AM technique. Material jetting can be used for photosensitive resin, wax, thermoplastic and reactive materials [14]. The polymer jet printing process involves curing the deposited polymer with ultraviolet (UV) light. The main advantage of this process is the elimination of postprocessing. However, one drawback of this process is the high printing cost with single material [6].

6.2.3 POWDER BED FUSION

Selective regions of powder bed are fused in this technique by using thermal energy provided by laser or electron beam. SLS, selective laser melting and electron beam machining are examples of the powder bed fusion technique of AM. Laser sintering of polymer powder is schematically depicted in Figure 6.3 [15]. When a laser beam hits the polymer bed (Figure 6.3a), principally, three effects can occur, namely, reflection, energy absorption and transmission. A polymer consisting of an aliphatic linkage (C-H) should have the capability of absorbing the relevant portion of 10.6-μm CO_2 laser energy. Reflection and transmission become relevant as well during the laser sintering process. The transmission part can provide sufficient energy in the form of radiation into the deeper portion of the powder bed for adequate layer adhesion so that the sintered layers are well connected (Figure 6.3b). Furthermore, poor absorption and transmission due to the loss of energy by a certain amount of reflection can be compensated by increasing laser power. However, too high laser energy can destroy the polymer. Therefore, the shape of the polymer powder will play a significant role in powder flowability. Milled powder is unfavorable, while a spherical-shaped polymer particle can provide good flowability [15].

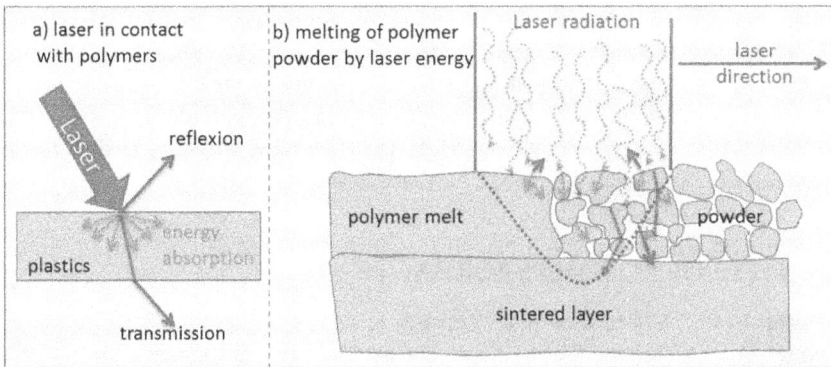

FIGURE 6.3 Schematic showing laser sintering of polymer bed: (a) Energy distribution in the polymer bed; (b) melting of polymer powder in presence of laser energy and formation of a structure layer by layer [15].

6.2.4 Sheet Lamination

As its name implies, in this AM technique, sheets of polymeric materials are stacked and bonded together to produce a 3D structure. Prior to lamination, the sheets are cut as per the required shapes, or the sheets are laminated together and afterward are cut as per the required shape [5]. Therefore, this process of AM is a combination of subtractive and additive manufacturing [8]. The subtractive part involves the cutting and lamination of bulk material sheets in order to form a 2D pattern, while the additive portion of the process involves adhesion bulk material sheets layer by layer to fabricate the 3D structure [8].

6.2.5 Binder Jetting

This technique of AM creates 3D parts by a process in which liquid bonding materials are selectively deposited to fuse powder material while a roller spread powder is used over a build stage to form the subsequent layers. The printer jet is specifically designed for dropping the bonding liquid onto the powder particles that are kept on the platform. This technique can incorporate a wide range of materials together with polymers, such as metals, ceramics, various colors and the like. The process is capable of cost-effectively building large and complex high-value structurally robust components as compared with others using a direct 3D-printing process. Various factors affect jet ability and printability including powder characteristics, print head design, binder material, binder solvent and others [16–17].

6.2.6 Vat Photopolymerization

Vat photopolymerization process can create high-resolution complex structures with excellent accuracy to customize 3D parts for patient-specific requirements [18–19]. In this AM process, light-activated photopolymerization process selectively cured liquid photopolymer in a vat. The technique used a vat of liquid photocurable resin [14, 19–20]. Solid 3D items are built layer by layer using a suitable laser that selectively hardens the photosensitive liquid resin. Stereolithography, digital light processing and two-photon polymerization fall under this category. Vat polymerization is an emerging AM process for fabricating various shapes and items for tissue engineering applications because of the high accuracy in printing. Vat polymerization 3D printing depends on various parameters, namely, laser scanning speed, layer thickness, Z compensation for material thickness, part orientation and others. [21].

6.3 TYPES OF POLYMERS FOR AM

The properties of 3D-printed parts depend on both the material structure and the printing process. Polymers are extensively used as the feed material in 3D printing due to their ease of processability and their printing cost-effective, functional items with tailor-made properties and capabilities. Selecting polymers for biomedical applications depends on a wide range of mechanical properties, including tensile strength, compressive strength, toughness and flexibility, as well as biocompatibility, biostability/biodegradability and others. [22]. Thermoplastic, thermoset, elastomer, hydrogel, functional polymers, polymer-blend and polymer matrix composites can be used in AM for biomedical parts fabrication [9, 11].

6.3.1 THERMOPLASTIC POLYMERS

These materials are softened by heating so they can be moldable, and on cooling, they solidify to provide the given shape. The process can be repeated since the long-chain polymers are held by a weak Van der Waals force. Examples of thermoplastic polymers are polyethylene, polystyrene, nylons, polycarbonate, polyether imide and others. Traditional processes, such as injection molding and material extrusion, are used to produce thermoplastic parts. Three-dimensional printing technology, such as FDM and SLS, can create complex parts by using thermoplastic polymer. Commonly used thermoplastic polymers in FDM are acrylonitrile butadiene styrene, polylactide, polyamide, polycarbonate, glass-filled nylon, polyether ester ketone (PEEK) and polyetherimide [7]. In SLS and multijet techniques, polyamides and thermoplastic polyurethane are most commonly used [15].

6.3.2 THERMOSETTING POLYMERS

Thermosetting plastic, once molded, cannot be remolded because during the curing process, crosslinking bonds are formed between the polymer chains that prevent the polymer chain from undergoing a reversible change. Examples of thermosetting polymers are epoxides, polyesters resin, phenolics resin, silicone resin and others. Thermosetting polymers are widely used for various high-tech applications due to their excellent mechanical, chemical and thermal resistance properties. AM processes, such as stereolithography, direct ink writing and others, use thermosetting polymer in their liquid state and the polymers are solidified after curing. In fact, thermosetting acrylate, crosslinked polyester, polyurethane, epoxy resin and photosensitive polymer resins are widely used in AM [23–24].

6.3.3 ELASTOMERS

Elastomers are polymeric materials with high stretchability due to the low intermolecular forces that enable them to have high stretchability [25]. Examples of elastomers are natural rubber, synthetic polyisoprene, butyl rubber, epichlorohydrin rubber, silicone rubber, thermoplastic elastomers and others. Some of the elastomers used in 3D printing are silicon elastomer, thermoplastic elastomer, hydrogel elastomer, liquid crystal elastomer, polydimethyl siloxane elastomer and the like [26–31].

6.4   POLYMERS COMPOSITES/NANOCOMPOSITES FOR AM

Three-dimensionally printed structures with improved mechanical properties are required for various load-bearing components. However, 3D-printed polymer items are weaker compared with conventionally fabricated parts. This problem can be overcome by fabricating 3D-printed polymer composite or nanocomposite parts [32].

TABLE 6.1
Properties Enhancement in AM Parts by Reinforcing Appropriate Material in the Polymer Matrix

Matrix Material	Reinforcement Material	Properties Enhancement	Reference
Nylon blend	Chopped carbon fiber	Tensile strength, fracture resistance	[34]
Epoxy resin	Fiber glass	Tensile strength, fatigue life	[35]
Nylon 11	Silica	Tensile and compressive properties	[36]
Epoxy	Multiwalled carbon nanotube	Tensile strength, fracture resistance	[37]
ABS	Graphene	Thermal properties	[38]
Epoxy acrylate	TiO_2	Tensile properties, flexural and hardness	[39]
ABS	Carbon fiber	Tensile properties	[40]
Nylon	Carbon, glass and Kevlar	Interlaminar shear strength	[41]
ABS	Carbon fiber	Thermal property	[42]

ABS, acrylonitrile butadiene styrene.

Composites materials consist of at least two different phases separated by a distinct interface. Different phases are combined appropriately to achieve a material system with improved structural or functional properties not attainable by individual materials. Different types of reinforcing materials can be selected for printing 3D-printed polymer composite parts in order to enhance their properties (Table 6.1). In polymer matrix composites, the polymer is a continuous phase, and reinforcements serve as a discontinuous phase. Reinforcements are bonded with a matrix phase by physical and chemical bonding to retain their identities. The mechanical properties of composite materials depend on the properties of the matrix polymer, reinforcing materials, their concentration and the interfacial interaction between two dissimilar phases. Particle-reinforced polymer composites composed of particle reinforcement in the polymer matrix. The particles vary in shape, size and morphology. Selecting the reinforcing materials depends on expected properties of the composite [5]. In polymer nanocomposites, polymer is a matrix material, while nanoparticles are used as the reinforcing material. The combination of nanotechnology and AM allows material scientists to construct 3D-printed parts with tailor-made properties and multifunctionality [33].

6.4.1 FIBER REINFORCEMENTS

Fibrous polymer composite reinforced with either continuous or chopped (whiskers) fibers in a matrix material. Whiskers are short, stubby fibers whereas continuous fibers are long fibers. Two categories of fibers can be used for the AM of fiber-reinforced polymer composites, namely, natural fiber and synthetic fiber [43]. Various synthetic fibers, namely, carbon fiber, glass fiber and Kevlar, can improve the mechanical properties of final 3D-printed polymer parts. Natural fibers are derived from plants or animals. Cellulose fibers are widely used as reinforcement in the polymer matrix [43]. Natural fiber reinforcement does not decline the biodegradability of various biodegradable polymers used for the fabrication of biomedical parts. Therefore, natural fiber reinforcement can be used for the biodegradable biomaterials items to improve the mechanical properties without affecting the biodegradability of polymers much [6]. Fiber-reinforced AM item exhibits significantly improved mechanical properties as compared with unreinforced polymers [34–35, 44–47].

6.4.2 PARTICLE REINFORCEMENTS

A particulate composite consists of particles suspended in a matrix. Particulates can be subclassed into two groups, namely, flake and filled/skeletal. Particle reinforcements are widely used for the fabrication of 3D-printed parts due to their low cost and easy processability with polymeric materials. For example, ceramic particle–like alumina (Al_2O_3) can be selected for various polymer matrices in the 3D printing of polymer composites [6].

6.4.3 NANOMATERIALS REINFORCEMENTS

Nanocomposites are materials that are created by introducing nano-particulates (often referred to as *nano-reinforcements*) into a macroscopic sample material (often referred to as the *matrix*). Various nanoparticles as reinforcing materials opened up opportunities to enhance properties, such as mechanical, electrical, thermal, chemical properties and so on, for the 3D-printed parts [6]. Some of the nano-reinforcing materials can be used in 3D printing are carbon nanotubes, graphene, nanoclays, SiC, nano-cellulose and others. [8]. Homogeneous dispersion, the distribution of nanoparticles in the polymer matrix and their strong interfacial interaction are key factors for the uniform properties of composite materials. The advantages of using nano-reinforcing materials for biomedical applications include enhancing biocompatibility, improving physical or chemical characteristics of the scaffold and enhancing tissue growth around the implant.

6.5 BIOMEDICAL APPLICATIONS OF AM FOR POLYMERS

AM is a rapidly growing technique that has enormous opportunities in various industries such as aerospace, engineering, art, academia, medicine and others. This is flexible technology that has the ability to print a range of dimensions by using multiple materials in order to fabricate multifunctional 3D structure systems [11]. Three-dimensionally printed items are widely used in various biomedical applications, because of its ability to customize medical items, its cost-effectiveness, its design flexibility and the like [31]. Two key properties required of the materials for biomedical applications are biocompatibility and biodegradability/bio-stability. Both biodegradable and bio-stable polymers are used for the 3D printing of biomaterial parts. Biodegradable polymers are used for soft tissue engineering, in which the tissue grows at the same rate the scaffolds are degraded. However, bio-stable polymers are used for structural implants.

Biomedical applications of AM are promising [48–50]. Tailor-designed polymeric biomaterials items from tomographic images can be used to 3D-print objects contoured for patients when customized therapies, medicines, tools and organ replacements are required. Polymeric materials can be used in the biomedical field for hard and soft tissue engineering and implant biomaterials. Improved mechanical properties are required for few key biomedical applications, such as load-bearing soft tissue replacement, artificial muscles, medical devices and others [11, 33, 51].

6.5.1 SCAFFOLDS

There is significant research interest in fabricating soft tissue scaffolds due to musculoskeletal, cardiovascular and connective tissue injuries and their subsequent replacement requirement. Accurately replacing these damaged tissues is quite challenging due to the variation in shape, size and strength of various tissues. Tailoring the biological, mechanical and chemical properties is required for tissue engineering scaffold [52]. Three-dimensional polymer printing is gaining interest in tissue engineering scaffolds, for which material properties, design strategies and processes play vital roles in tailoring the scaffold structure. Targeted tissues for 3D-printed materials can be bone, skin, ligament, neurons and skeletal muscles, among others [22]. For soft tissue replacement applications, the scaffold must degrade at a similar rate as the new tissue regenerates. Jackson et al. presented an SLS 3D-printed nylon-12 scaffold for cell differentiation, growth and biomineral formation. Nylon-12 possesses biocompatibility while SLS printing can provide a highly porous structure with a high surface area for surface modification and cell growth. Various SLS 3D-printed shapes in nylon-12 are depicted in Figure 6.4. These 3D-printed matrices presented enormous potential in bone grafting, implants, skeletal repairs and so on [53].

6.5.2 STENTS

Stents have been generally used in percutaneous coronary intervention and following nephrological procedures. Prior to being inserted into the blood vessel, the large stent is first folded to fit into a catheter. In the case of polymer-based stents, shape memory polymers are used to fabricate the stents. Inside the blood vessel, the stent deploys under body temperature utilizing the shape memory effect of polymer. The superelasticity of the shape memory material has been utilized to provide a force that can keep the vessel open. Yeazel and Becker reported bioresorbable and shape memory material–based 3D-printed stents that could eliminate the need for balloon expansion and limit stent migration [54]. Esophageal stents' palliation therapy is a current treatment for a patient with inoperable esophageal malignancies. Commonly used plastic stents for these purposes can create complications, such as tumor ingrowth as well as stent migration into the stomach. In order to overcome these issues, Lin et al. reported a specially designed 3D-printed stent made with two polymers, such as flexible thermoplastic polyurethane, which provided flexibility for the ease of deployment and self-expansion force. They have selected poly(lactic acid) to improve the mechanical properties so that it can open the blocked esophagus at the beginning. Poly(lactic acid) component can impart slow degradation of the inserted stent, and this eliminates the need for reintervention [55]. Wang et al. reported a screw extrusion–based 3D-printed cardiovascular stent with a zero Poisson's ratio in

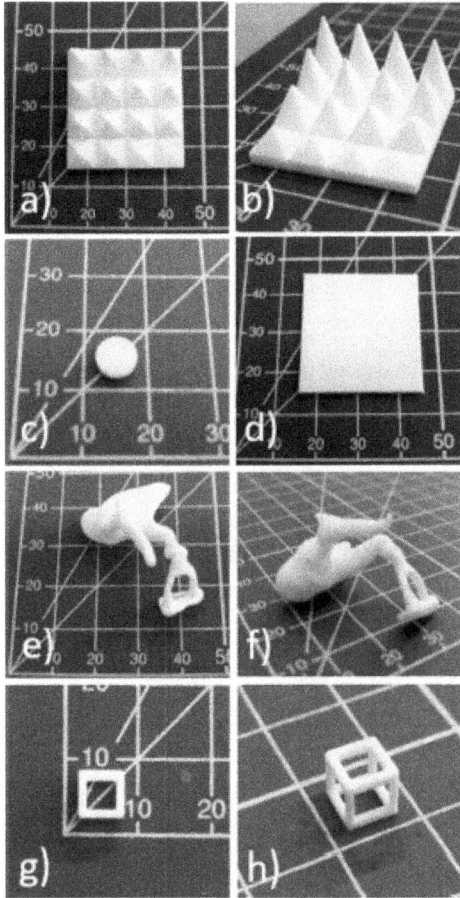

FIGURE 6.4 Images showing selective laser sintering printed various 3D items: (a, b) Spike arrays; (c, d) plates; (e, f) human ear bones; (g, h) hollow cubes. Grid scale in millimeters [53].

longitudinal deformation (Figure 6.5). Polycaprolactone (PCL)- and poly(l-lactide) acid–based customized stents with different shapes and geometric configurations have been fabricated using the overlapping printing approach. Poly(l-lactide) acid, with improved strength and a lower elongation rate, could be a good candidate for customizing stents [56].

6.5.3 PROSTHESES

The 3D printing of polymers can offer a wide variety of prosthetics customized for a person's needs [22, 57]. He et al. reported soft tissue prostheses, for example, artificial noses, ears and eyes for maxillofacial rehabilitation, using an AM method, namely, scanning, printing, polishing and casting. The process of fabricating a silicon prosthesis is simple and cheap [58]. Arjun et al. reported 3D-printable hand prostheses based

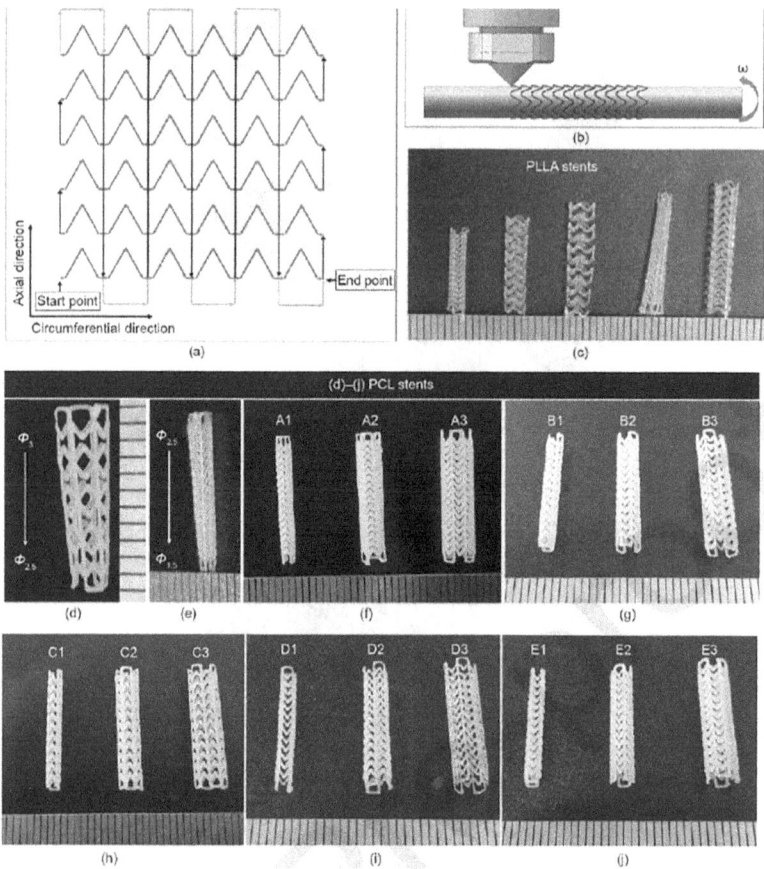

FIGURE 6.5 3D printing of cardiovascular stents: (a) Printing trajectory of stents; (b) schematic of stent fabrication; (c) stents with different geometrical structures; (d, e) tapered stents; (f–j) stents with different diameters and heights [56].

on an electro-thermal actuator on nylon 6,6–based muscles. A 3D-printed fabricated prosthetic hand has the ability to move all fingers, individually, and grasp a variety of objects [59]. Zuniga reported polylactic acid–based 3D-printed finger prostheses with antibacterial properties. Three-dimensional printing antibacterial filament has the potential to revolutionize fabricating medical devices [60]. Stenvall et al. reported a custom-made prosthetic product using microfibrilated cellulose (MFC)–reinforced polypropylene composite. The FDM technique of AM has been employed to fabricate the prostheses and orthosis solution. They have reported the clinical trial in terms of wearing experience, appearance and acceptance of material and technique [21].

6.5.4 Dentistry

AM parts are increasingly being used in the field of dentistry [61]. Five AM processes are commonly used for 3D printing dental items, and these are vat polymerization

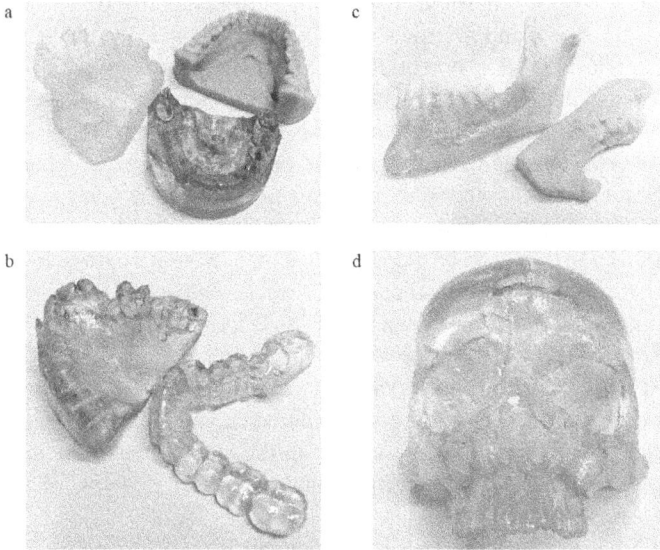

FIGURE 6.6 Images showing dental items produced by AM of polymers: (a) Cast; (b) implant drilling guides; (c, d) simulation models in surgery [12].

technique, digital light processing, polymer jetting, laser stereolithography and FDM [12]. The vat polymerization technique can be utilized in implant dentistry [6]. Vinyl polymers are widely used for dentistry because of their tunable properties. Many of them are biocompatible and nondegradable, which are prerequisites for dental implants. In the 3D printing of dental implants, vinyl polymers are widely used in sintering (e.g., SLS) or photopolymerization (e.g., stereolithography). Photopolymers are composed of a monomer, an oligomer and a photo-initiator. The curing effect of the photopolymer depends on wavelength, the power of light and radiation time [62]. Other polymers used in dental 3D printing are polyesters (such as polycaprolactone, polycarbonate, polylactic acid) and polystyrene (such as polystyrene and acrylonitrile butadiene styrene). The AM of polymers in dental applications can be completed in different ways. Some of the application has been depicted in Figure 6.6. The material selection for AM dental application is crucial. The materials should be biocompatible and mechanically stable with optimum postprocessing requirements [12]. Other applications of 3D-printed polymers in dental fields include the healing of periodontal defects using guided tissue regeneration, prosthodontics crowns and bridges for provisional and fixed dental restoration and the fabrication of removable prostheses, orthodontic mini screws and others [22, 31, 61].

6.6 CONCLUSION

AM technology is a rapidly growing field in medicine due to its inherent advantages, which include ease of use and a wide range of applications in the biomedical field. AM techniques allow design flexibility, customization and rapid prototyping.

Furthermore, AM offers enormous opportunities to design complex structures. This chapter presents review and overview of advances in the field of AM of polymers for biomedical applications. The potential of AM still needs more research in the areas of fabrication and design development from rapid prototyping to large-scale manufacturing. First and foremost, more research is required to improve the slow production speed of AM. Furthermore, research on developing novel functional polymers for biomedical application and new processes to sustain AM process are required. The poor strength of 3D printed parts is an important issue. Incorporating reinforcing materials as a strategy can be employed to enhance the strength of the 3D-printed items. However, some of the challenges for fiber-reinforced 3D-printed items are surface roughness, void formation and poor bond formation between reinforcement and polymer matrix. It will be interesting to perform more research on the development of AM parts based on smart polymers that are biocompatible and display the stimuli-responsive properties required for biomedical applications. Finally, it can be concluded that AM will continue to develop in the biomedical fields, improving the properties of biomaterials and novel functionality.

REFERENCES

1. A. A. Shapiro *et al.*, "Additive manufacturing for aerospace flight applications," *Journal of Spacecraft and Rockets*, vol. 53, no. 5, pp. 952–959, Sep 2016.
2. P. Ahangar, M. E. Cooke, M. H. Weber, and D. H. Rosenzweig, "Current biomedical applications of 3D printing and additive manufacturing," *Applied Sciences-Basel*, vol. 9, no. 8, Apr 2019, Art. no. 1713.
3. B. Aslan and A. R. Yildiz, "Optimum design of automobile components using lattice structures for additive manufacturing," *Materials Testing*, vol. 62, no. 6, pp. 633–639, Jun 2020.
4. J. Li *et al.*, "Micro electronic systems via multifunctional additive manufacturing," *Rapid Prototyping Journal*, vol. 24, no. 4, pp. 752–763, 2018.
5. S. Wickramasinghe, T. Do, and P. Tran, "FDM-based 3D printing of polymer and associated composite: A review on mechanical properties, defects and treatments," *Polymers*, vol. 12, no. 7, Jul 2020, Art. no. 1529.
6. S. D. Nath and S. Nilufar, "An overview of additive manufacturing of polymers and associated composites," *Polymers*, vol. 12, no. 11, Nov 2020, Art. no. 2719.
7. S. Saleh Alghamdi, S. John, N. Roy Choudhury, and N. K. Dutta, "Additive manufacturing of polymer materials: Progress, promise and challenges," (in eng), *Polymers*, vol. 13, no. 5, p. 753, 2021.
8. A. C. de Leon, Q. Chen, N. B. Palaganas, J. O. Palaganas, J. Manapat, and R. C. Advincula, "High performance polymer nanocomposites for additive manufacturing applications," *Reactive and Functional Polymers*, vol. 103, pp. 141–155, Jun 1, 2016.
9. S. C. Ligon, R. Liska, J. Stampfl, M. Gurr, and R. Mulhaupt, "Polymers for 3D printing and customized additive manufacturing," *Chemical Reviews*, vol. 117, no. 15, pp. 10212–10290, Aug 2017.
10. J. W. Stansbury and M. J. Idacavage, "3D printing with polymers: Challenges among expanding options and opportunities," *Dental Materials*, vol. 32, no. 1, pp. 54–64, Jan 2016.
11. Z. Jiang, B. Diggle, M. L. Tan, J. Viktorova, C. W. Bennett, and L. A. Connal, "Extrusion 3D printing of polymeric materials with advanced properties," *Advanced Science*, vol. 7, no. 17, Sep 2020, Art. no. 2001379.

12. J. Jockusch and M. Ozcan, "Additive manufacturing of dental polymers: An overview on processes, materials and applications," *Dental Materials Journal*, vol. 39, no. 3, pp. 345–354, Jun 2020.

13. V. Mazzanti, L. Malagutti, and F. Mollica, "FDM 3D printing of polymers containing natural fillers: A review of their mechanical properties," *Polymers*, vol. 11, no. 7, Jul 2019, Art. no. 1094.

14. L. J. Y. Tan, W. Zhu, and K. Zhou, "Recent progress on polymer materials for additive manufacturing," *Advanced Functional Materials*, vol. 30, no. 43, Oct 2020, Art. no. 2003062.

15. M. Schmid and K. Wegener, "Additive manufacturing: Polymers applicable for laser sintering (LS)," *Procedia Engineering*, vol. 149, pp. 457–464, Jun 1, 2016.

16. E. M. Wilts and T. E. Long, "Sustainable additive manufacturing: Predicting binder jettability of water-soluble, biodegradable and recyclable polymers," *Polymer International*, vol. 70, no. 7, pp. 958–963, Jul 2021.

17. D. H. Kim *et al.*, "Mechanical analysis of ceramic/polymer composite with mesh-type lightweight design using binder-jet 3D printing," *Materials*, vol. 11, no. 10, Oct 2018, Art. no. 1941.

18. D. C. Aduba *et al.*, "Vat photopolymerization 3D printing of acid-cleavable PEG-methacrylate networks for biomaterial applications," *Materials Today Communications*, vol. 19, pp. 204–211, Jun 2019.

19. W. L. Li, L. S. Mille, J. A. Robledo, T. Uribe, V. Huerta, and Y. S. Zhang, "Recent advances in formulating and processing biomaterial inks for vat polymerization-based 3D printing," *Advanced Healthcare Materials*, vol. 9, no. 15, Aug 2020, Art. no. 2000156.

20. G. Gonzalez *et al.*, "Materials testing for the development of biocompatible devices through vat-polymerization 3D printing," *Nanomaterials*, vol. 10, no. 9, Sep 2020, Art. no. 1788.

21. E. Stenvall *et al.*, "Additive manufacturing of prostheses using forest-based composites," (in eng), *Bioengineering (Basel, Switzerland)*, vol. 7, no. 3, p. 103, 2020.

22. A. M. E. Arefin, N. R. Khatri, N. Kulkarni, and P. F. Egan, "Polymer 3D printing review: Materials, process, and design strategies for medical applications," *Polymers*, vol. 13, no. 9, May 2021, Art. no. 1499.

23. D. Lei *et al.*, "A general strategy of 3D printing thermosets for diverse applications," *Materials Horizons*, 10.1039/C8MH00937F vol. 6, no. 2, pp. 394–404, 2019.

24. E. S. Bud *et al.*, "Accuracy of three-dimensional (3D) printed dental digital models generated with three types of resin polymers by extra-oral optical scanning," *Journal of Clinical Medicine*, vol. 10, no. 9, May 2021, Art. no. 1908.

25. T. Özdemir, "Chapter 5 — Elastomeric micro- and nanocomposites for neutron shielding," in *Micro and Nanostructured Composite Materials for Neutron Shielding Applications*, S. T. Abdulrahman, S. Thomas, and Z. Ahmad, Eds. Woodhead Publishing, 2020, pp. 125–137.

26. L. Y. Zhou *et al.*, "Multimaterial 3D printing of highly stretchable silicone elastomers," *Acs Applied Materials & Interfaces*, vol. 11, no. 26, pp. 23573–23583, Jul 2019.

27. D. McCoul, S. Rosset, S. Schlatter, and H. Shea, "Inkjet 3D printing of UV and thermal cure silicone elastomers for dielectric elastomer actuators," *Smart Materials and Structures*, vol. 26, no. 12, Dec 2017, Art. no. 125022.

28. K. Tian *et al.*, "3D printing of transparent and conductive heterogeneous hydrogel-elastomer systems," *Advanced Materials*, vol. 29, no. 10, Mar 2017, Art. no. 1604827.

29. S. Woska *et al.*, "Tunable photonic devices by 3D laser printing of liquid crystal elastomers," *Optical Materials Express*, vol. 10, no. 11, pp. 2920–2935, Nov 2020.

30. S. J. Sun *et al.*, "Covalent adaptable networks of polydimethylsiloxane elastomer for selective laser sintering 3D printing," *Chemical Engineering Journal*, vol. 412, May 2021.

31. Y. T. Wang, J. H. Yu, L. J. Lo, P. H. Hsu, and C. L. Lin, "Developing customized dental miniscrew surgical template from thermoplastic polymer material using image super-imposition, CAD system, and 3D printing," *Biomed Research International*, vol. 2017, 2017, Art. no. 1906197.

32. N. S. Hmeidat, R. C. Pack, S. J. Talley, R. B. Moore, and B. G. Compton, "Mechanical anisotropy in polymer composites produced by material extrusion additive manufacturing," *Additive Manufacturing*, vol. 34, Aug 2020, Art. no. 101385.

33. H. Wu *et al.*, "Recent developments in polymers/polymer nanocomposites for additive manufacturing," *Progress in Materials Science*, vol. 111, Jun 2020, Art. no. 100638.

34. F. Akasheh and H. Aglan, "Fracture toughness enhancement of carbon fiber-reinforced polymer composites utilizing additive manufacturing fabrication," *Journal of Elastomers and Plastics*, vol. 51, no. 7–8, pp. 698–711, Nov 2019.

35. K. Agarwal, S. K. Kuchipudi, B. Girard, and M. Houser, "Mechanical properties of fiber reinforced polymer composites: A comparative study of conventional and additive manufacturing methods," *Journal of Composite Materials*, vol. 52, no. 23, pp. 3173–3181, Sep 2018.

36. H. Chung and S. Das, "Functionally graded Nylon-11/silica nanocomposites produced by selective laser sintering," *Materials Science and Engineering a-Structural Materials Properties Microstructure and Processing*, vol. 487, no. 1–2, pp. 251–257, Jul 2008.

37. J. H. Sandoval and R. B. Wicker, "Functionalizing stereolithography resins: Effects of dispersed multi-walled carbon nanotubes on physical properties," *Rapid Prototyping Journal*, vol. 12, no. 5, pp. 292–303, 2006.

38. X. J. Wei *et al.*, "3D printable graphene composite," *Scientific Reports*, vol. 5, Jul 2015, Art. no. 11181.

39. Y. G. Duan, Y. Zhou, Y. P. Tang, and D. C. Li, "Nano-TiO2-modified photosensitive resin for RP," *Rapid Prototyping Journal*, vol. 17, no. 4, pp. 247–252, 2011.

40. H. L. Tekinalp *et al.*, "Highly oriented carbon fiber-polymer composites via additive manufacturing," *Composites Science and Technology*, vol. 105, pp. 144–150, Dec 2014.

41. H. J. O'Connor and D. P. Dowling, "Low-pressure additive manufacturing of continuous fiber-reinforced polymer composites," *Polymer Composites*, vol. 40, no. 11, pp. 4329–4339, Nov 2019.

42. B. G. Compton, B. K. Post, C. E. Duty, L. Love, and V. Kunc, "Thermal analysis of additive manufacturing of large-scale thermoplastic polymer composites," *Additive Manufacturing*, vol. 17, pp. 77–86, Oct 2017.

43. T. Hofstatter, D. B. Pedersen, G. Tosello, and H. N. Hansen, "State-of-the-art of fiber-reinforced polymers in additive manufacturing technologies," *Journal of Reinforced Plastics and Composites*, vol. 36, no. 15, pp. 1061–1073, Aug 2017.

44. P. Parandoush and D. Lin, "A review on additive manufacturing of polymer-fiber composites," *Composite Structures*, vol. 182, pp. 36–53, Dec 2017.

45. A. El Moumen, M. Tarfaoui, and K. Lafdi, "Additive manufacturing of polymer composites: Processing and modeling approaches," *Composites Part B-Engineering*, vol. 171, pp. 166–182, Aug 2019.

46. V. K. Balla, K. H. Kate, J. Satyavolu, P. Singh, and J. G. D. Tadimeti, "Additive manufacturing of natural fiber reinforced polymer composites: Processing and prospects," *Composites Part B-Engineering*, vol. 174, Oct 2019, Art. no. 106956.

47. M. E. Gebel and M. Ermurat, "Investigation of polymer matrix continuous fiber reinforced composite part manufacturability for composite additive manufacturing," *Journal of the Faculty of Engineering and Architecture of Gazi University*, vol. 36, no. 1, pp. 57–67, 2021.

48. C. M. Gonzalez-Henriquez, M. A. Sarabia-Vallejos, and J. R. Hernandez, "Antimicrobial polymers for additive manufacturing," *International Journal of Molecular Sciences*, vol. 20, no. 5, Mar 2019, Art. no. 1210.

49. A. E. Jakus, A. L. Rutz, and R. N. Shah, "Advancing the field of 3D biomaterial printing," *Biomedical Materials*, vol. 11, no. 1, Feb 2016, Art. no. 014102.

50. J. G. Ma *et al.*, "3D printing of strontium silicate microcylinder-containing multicellular biomaterial inks for vascularized skin regeneration," *Advanced Healthcare Materials*, 2021, Art. no. 2100523.

51. C. M. Cristache, A. R. Grosu, G. Cristache, A. C. Didilescu, and E. E. Totu, "Additive manufacturing and synthetic polymers for bone reconstruction in the maxillofacial region," *Materiale Plastice*, vol. 55, no. 4, pp. 555–562, Dec 2018.

52. R. J. Mondschein, A. Kanitkar, C. B. Williams, S. S. Verbridge, and T. E. Long, "Polymer structure-property requirements for stereolithographic 3D printing of soft tissue engineering scaffolds," *Biomaterials*, vol. 140, pp. 170–188, Sep 2017.

53. R. J. Jackson *et al.*, "Chemically treated 3D printed polymer scaffolds for biomineral formation," *Acs Omega*, vol. 3, no. 4, pp. 4342–4351, Apr 2018.

54. T. R. Yeazel and M. L. Becker, "Advancing toward 3D printing of oresorbable shape memory polymer stents," *Biomacromolecules*, vol. 21, no. 10, pp. 3957–3965, Oct 2020.

55. M. H. Lin, N. Firoozi, C. T. Tsai, M. B. Wallace, and Y. Q. Kang, "3D-printed flexible polymer stents for potential applications in inoperable esophageal malignancies," *Acta Biomaterialia*, vol. 83, pp. 119–129, Jan 2019.

56. C. Wang, L. Zhang, Y. Fang, and W. Sun, "Design, characterization, and 3D printing of cardiovascular stents with zero Poisson's ratio in longitudinal deformation," *Engineering*, vol. 7, Jul 24, 2020.

57. P. Honigmann, N. Sharma, R. Schumacher, J. Rueegg, M. Haefeli, and F. Thieringer, "In-hospital 3D printed scaphoid prosthesis using medical-grade polyetheretherketone (PEEK) biomaterial," *Biomed Research International*, vol. 2021, Jan 2021, Art. no. 1301028.

58. Y. He, G. H. Xue, and J. Z. Fu, "Fabrication of low cost soft tissue prostheses with the desktop 3D printer," *Scientific Reports*, vol. 4, Nov 2014, Art. no. 6973.

59. A. Arjun, L. Saharan, and Y. Tadesse, "Design of a 3D printed hand prosthesis actuated by nylon 6–6 polymer based artificial muscles," in *2016 IEEE International Conference on Automation Science and Engineering (CASE)*, IEEE Explore, 2016, pp. 910–915.

60. J. M. Zuniga, "3D printed antibacterial prostheses," *Applied Sciences-Basel*, vol. 8, no. 9, Sep 2018, Art. no. 1651.

61. S. Pillai *et al.*, "Dental 3D-printing: Transferring art from the laboratories to the clinics," *Polymers*, vol. 13, no. 1, Jan 2021, Art. no. 157.

62. J. Kim and D. H. Lee, "Influence of the postcuring process on dimensional accuracy and seating of 3D-printed polymeric fixed prostheses," *Biomed Research International*, vol. 2020, Nov 2020, Art. no. 2150182.

7 Additive Manufacturing for Presurgical and Postsurgical Planning
A State-of-the-Art Review

Satadru Kashyap
Department of Mechanical Engineering, Tezpur
University, Napam, Sonitpur, Assam (India)

CONTENTS

7.1 Introduction 118
7.2 Role of AM in Presurgical Planning 120
    7.2.1 Presurgical Planning in Cardiology 120
    7.2.2 Presurgical Planning in Orthopedics 122
        7.2.2.1 3D Models 122
        7.2.2.2 Surgical Devices and Guides 123
        7.2.2.3 Abnormalities in Bone 123
        7.2.2.4 Designing Patient-Specific Implants 123
        7.2.2.5 Better Care of Patients and Surgical Precision 123
        7.2.2.6 Teaching and Learning 124
    7.2.3 Presurgical Planning in Dentistry 124
        7.2.3.1 3D Dental Models/Implants 124
        7.2.3.2 Designing Orthodontic Models and Replacement of
                 Damaged Teeth 124
        7.2.3.3 Surgical Devices and Guides 125
        7.2.3.4 Design of Dentistry Tools 125
        7.2.3.5 Teaching and Education 125
    7.2.4 Presurgical Planning in Drug Delivery 125
        7.2.4.1 Oral Medications 126
        7.2.4.2 Vaginal and Rectal Medicine 126
        7.2.4.3 Intravenous Catheters 127
        7.2.4.4 Transdermal Medicine 127
        7.2.4.5 Implants and Scaffolds 127
7.3 Role of AM in Postsurgical Planning 127
    7.3.1 Postsurgical Planning in Orthoses and Prostheses 128
        7.3.1.1 FOs 128
        7.3.1.2 AFOs 129

DOI: 10.1201/9781003217961-7

       7.3.1.3   Prosthetic Sockets of the Lower Limb 130
       7.3.1.4   Miscellaneous Applications 131
7.4   Major Findings through the Study 131
7.5   Challenges in Using AM for Pre- and Postsurgical Planning 132
7.6   Conclusion 133
References 134

7.1   INTRODUCTION

Additive manufacturing (AM) today is an emerging technology that has numerous different applications in medical, military, automotive aerospace and a host of other industries [1]. It provides the advantages of extensively duplicating body parts and organs, prosthetics, surgical instruments and others through customized printing of these products. AM guarantees novelty by manufacturing exceptionally multifarious components by developing them in a layer-by-layer fashion. This provides flexibility in fabricating complex parts that in other cases may not be produced by conventional subtractive machining techniques. Three-dimensional (3D) patient data of soft tissues, bones, organs and vascular structures are collected through techniques such as computerized tomography (CT), magnetic resonance imaging (MRI), laser scanning, ultrasound and others [2]. The patient-specific components can be tailored, designed and manufactured with the assistance of AM technology. The models are developed with a 3D computer-aided-design (CAD) software in order to fine-tune the component and incorporate any modifications/implants and additive pieces. Once the model is complete, it is further converted into a standard triangulate (STL) format, used for rapid prototyping (RP) of the final product through 3D printers [3]. Presently, AM is extensively used in the manufacturing of medical models and prosthetics, which offers advantages such as shorter manufacturing time and low cost [4]. Tuomi has earlier categorized the application of AM in medical fields into five main domains: (a) surgical implants, (b) medical models, (c) surgical guides, (d) external aids or prosthesis and (e) biomanufacturing [5]. Additionally, rapid prototyping is also used in the fabrication of tailor-made maxillofacial prostheses, dentistry and various orthopedic components [6].

Numerous surgical tools required for presurgery, during surgery and postsurgery have been designed and innovated through AM. With the considerable development of rapid prototyping techniques, such as stereolithography (SLA), fused deposition modeling (FDM), 3D inkjet printing and others, AM has slowly replaced the wax pattern of model development. The addition of upcoming technology in the form of techniques like selective laser melting (SLM), selective laser sintering (SLS) and electron beam melting (EBM) has enabled the construction of medical components in dense metallic form. Thus, rapid prototyping in the medical field has slowly overtaken the conventional methods of product development through casting and machining [7–8]. AM in the field of medicine is today employed in tailored masks, organ development, implant design, teaching and learning, presurgical requirements, during operation and during postsurgical rehabilitation.

Presurgical assessment of complex surgeries currently is paramount for the development of surgical protocols. The success of such complex surgeries heavily depends on a meticulous preoperative assessment, planning and preparation of surgical protocols, efficient restoration of the problem and effective postsurgical rehabilitation procedure. Originally, conventional techniques such as X-ray, 2D CT and cephalometry were employed to understand anatomical geometry. However, preoperative assessment becomes limited due to the restrictions in visualizing the defects or problems as a result of the 2D features [9]. However, with the advent of MRI and CT scans, 3D modeling of the anatomical structures has been made possible, which has made interpretation of the patient data much easier. Three-dimensional reconstructions developed through MRI or CT scans can help surgeons effectively plan the complicated surgical procedure, predetermine the safe pathway for removal of any tumor or foreign body and use the model as an educative instrument for the patient and medical students. Thus, through presurgical planning or simulation, a complicated surgery can be effectively optimized for the patients' benefit. Presurgical planning also involves custom-designing implants that can be fabricated through RP with precision as per individual's requirement with a shorter delivery period and reduced operation times. The categorization of the various applications of AM domain-wise based on presurgical and postsurgical planning is shown in Figure 7.1.

The accurateness between the virtually designed implant model and the required fit in the patient can be assessed using a physical model developed through RP. This

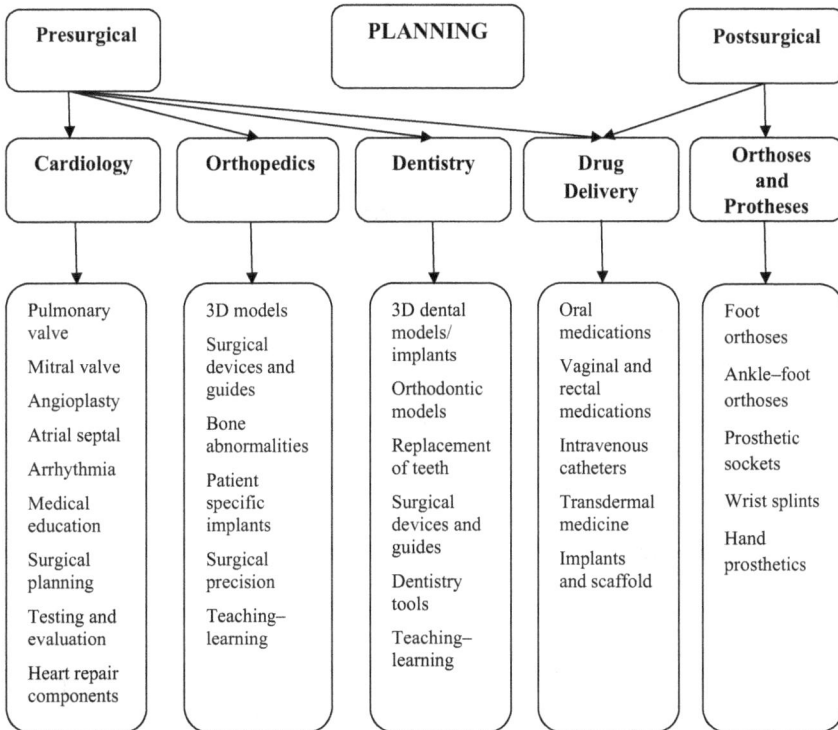

FIGURE 7.1   AM applications in presurgical and postsurgical planning.

will facilitate correcting all errors in the shape of the implant before surgery, thus reducing the risk of a subsequent intervention, a loss of money and time and stress on the patient [10]. In a similar manner, AM has been a significant contributor toward facilitating postsurgical rehabilitation as well. Postsurgical interventions, such as AM-fabricated customized devices, assist poststroke individuals, in limb and ana-tomical prosthesis posttrauma surgeries, in customized elbow orthosis that simulate the action of physiotherapists for postsurgical rehabilitation and others [11–12]. AM has been instrumental in creating a revolution in the field of medical science, which has led to increased efficiency in preoperative planning and increased accuracy in surgical procedures and postsurgical rehabilitation. This chapter reviews the contri-bution of AM in the various aspects of the pre- and postsurgical planning process.

7.2   ROLE OF AM IN PRESURGICAL PLANNING

Presurgical or preoperative planning is basically the blueprint of the surgical pro-tocol that is to be laid down before the actual surgery. Preoperative planning can be categorized into visualization—imagining the actual organs of interest, origi-nal images, implants and structure; modeling—3D representations of the points of interest through mapping software; investigation—an examination of the modeled structure and optimization; and, finally, the generation of a protocol based on the investigation the best intervention procedure is chosen. AM has been significant in the presurgical planning by providing surgeons with various models, guides, implants and drug delivery platforms for planning the presurgical protocols before actual intervention. Works conducted by various researchers employing AM in pre-surgical planning on various domains of the health industry are studied under the following heads.

7.2.1   PRESURGICAL PLANNING IN CARDIOLOGY

AM has been instrumental in the treatment of cardiovascular diseases, which has paved a road toward greatly improving the efficacy of a heart surgeon. Through AM, it is possible to generate an exact an *in vitro* physical model of the heart muscle that enhances operational safety, reduces the complexity of the surgery, reduces operation time and creates collaboration between the surgery and the surgeon. Additionally, bioprinting customized cardiac valves through AM using biocompatible materials can facilitate valve replacement in patients [13]. Cardiac surgeries, for example, for congenital heart conditions, are mostly complex in nature, and a great variation occurs in terms of preoperative planning from patient to patient. Models generated by AM assist the surgical team in practicing and teaching surgery, operative demon-stration, patient-specific surgical preparation, explanations to patients, improved operative accuracy and reduced time. Thus, AM is paramount in planning and con-ducting complex cardiac, which assist surgeons in swiftly assessing the health of the heart [14–16]. Earlier, research was conducted in which 3D printing was incorporated during congenital heart disease simulation and while training doctors [17–18]. AM has also been used in deciding the placement of stents in customized patient-specific cases. Additionally, 3D printing these components with specific components is also developing at a rapid pace [19–20]. Emerging AM technology has also facilitated the development of an artificial silicone heart whose beating resembles the normal human heart but has a limited life. Such innovations are minute steps taken toward entirely replacing a diseased human heart [19]. AM also facilitates the correct prediction of the efficacy of the four heart valves responsible for sustaining a unidirectional blood flow during heart pumping, thus communicating the status of the heart and its valves [21–22]. AM fabricated heart models and valves facilitate the surgeon to test and determine whether the customized patient-specific valves fit the patient. This would prevent any complication during actual surgery or prevent any further surgeries after the valves are fitted in the patient.

The major advantages of using AM in cardiology include the following [23]:

1. *Visualization:* Fabrication of a heat model through 3D printing to visualize the heart anatomy and its defects
2. *Different insights:* 3D-printed model that can be used to provide specific insights from different angles in complicated cases
3. *Surgical planning:* Surgeons preparing and predicting the consequences during actual surgery based on the evaluation of the model
4. *Education:* 3D-printed model that can be used as a tool to demonstrate and teach surgeons, medical students and even patients about heart-related complications

The role of AM in the presurgical planning in the cardiology domain has been reviewed at length under the following headings:

- **Pulmonary valve:** The design of pulmonary valves has been successfully conducted subsequent using AM, whereby 3D models depicting the proper ventricular outflow and arterial tract have been constructed. The future looks bright for their extensive implementation in heart surgeries [24–25].
- **Mitral valve:** AM has been used in the mitral valve annuloplasty for the repair of the mitral valve and mitral regurgitation. A 3D model printed via AM has been successfully used in treating mitral valve and aortic valves complications in heart disease patients [26–27].
- **Angioplasty:** AM-printed models are hugely helpful in determining stent length, stent positioning and balloon size before angioplasty (endovascular stenting). Additionally, AM has the ability to deliver stents in the treatment of heart blockage and conditions that cause aortic enlargement and localized weakness [28–30].
- **Atrial septal:** Researchers have shown that AM has the potential to fabricate medical components that would seal the hole in the valve wall (atrial septal defect) in the upper compartments of the heart, causing oxygen-rich blood to leak from the left to the right [31–32].
- **Treating arrhythmia:** AM techniques can absorb data from CT scans and MRIs and print 3D models that can assist doctors and health professionals in assessing the damage caused by arrhythmias and plan the future course of action in treating the patients [33–34].

- **Medical Education:** AM assists in creating 3D heart and its accessory models out of different materials for doctors, medical students and professionals to visualize the anatomy and patient-specific complications so that they can determine the differences between a regular and irregular structure [35–36].
- **Surgical planning:** AM facilitates presurgical planning, fixing operative protocols and simulation as the 3D-printed heart model provides inclusive knowledge on a variety of patient-specific heart conditions. Three-dimensional models of stents act as pathways to clear blocked or narrowing blood vessels/arteries/veins that carry blood to and from the heart. AM models are also used for interventional, critical care training and integrative treatment of heart ailments [37–39].
- **Functional models for testing and evaluation:** AM can manufacture rapidly patient-specific functional models of heart, valves and other heart components that would assist surgeons in evaluating the status of effective blood flow, valve and heart health *in vitro* in patients. Additionally, these functional models are also effective in facilitating a controlled test bed for evaluation of the flow status in patient-specific circumstances [40–41].
- **Creating heart repair components:** AM can design and redesign innovative medical components for heart ailments rapidly. Many researchers have put forward their ideas related to product innovation, novel material selection, design legalization, surgical planning and clinical trials [42–44].

7.2.2　PRESURGICAL PLANNING IN ORTHOPEDICS

AM has the ability to construct a 3D bone image from the data obtained from MRI or CT scans. Subsequently, it can generate the bone prototype through the layer-by-layer deposition of the specific material chosen. Additionally, it can also generate a missing bone image and construct the part through reverse engineering. This AM methodology is significant in its role as a teaching tool, surgical design procedures and visualization of complex surgeries, all of which form important domains of preoperative planning procedures. This process is rapid with reduced processing times and low cost as compared to traditional methods of manufacturing. AM has significant benefits in creating complex bone models and parts of various shapes and sizes, which helps the surgeons in better understanding as well as creates accurate orthopedic implants. The role of AM in presurgical planning can be categorized as discussed in the following sections.

7.2.2.1　3D Models

It is known that conventional methodology employed 2D CT scans, X-ray reports for assessing the anatomy and the extent of patient-specific defects in the bone. However, with advanced technological software, the conversion from CT scans and MRI reports to 3D models has become much easier and faster. Acquiring of images digitally from a data acquisition device such as multidetector computed tomography scan and generating images in Digital Imaging and Communications in Medicine (DICOM), along with high-contrast postprocessing of images employing segmenting technique (labeling the structures of interest) in software such as ITK-SNAP has come a long way in generating 3D high-resolution and -contrast 3D images or nonaxial reformatted images. DICOM is significant in investigating skeletal construction and thorough information about joint placements and fractures. CAD software converts the 3D images into a series of polygons and changes the data into standard STL format, which is used for 3D printing. These 3D models assist surgeons in visualizing, tactile understanding and finalizing the plan of action before actual surgery [45–48]. Three-dimensional models based on these images can be printed with the chosen materials which are subsequently used in understanding anatomical defects and bone fractures, in planning implant location/sizes/shapes and in teaching.

7.2.2.2 Surgical Devices and Guides

Presurgical planning also involves designing and fabricating surgical devices that would be required for a patient-specific surgery. For this purpose, AM can custom print innovative 3D devices and guides based on the surgery and the surgeon's requirement. Surgeons can design cutting tools and guides along with other surgical instruments that would accurately fit the anatomy of the patient. Additionally, based on the testing and evaluation of 3D models, the surgical guides and tools can be redesigned and refabricated without a second operative intervention on the patient. Custom-designed surgical devices have been used before in the treatment/surgery for joint arthroplasty, tumors and adjustment of deformities. Moreover, AM can also be used to custom print synthetic devices and implants used for complicated surgeries on even bone tissue and tumors (spinal, pelvic, etc.) [49–51].

7.2.2.3 Abnormalities in Bone

AM can generate 3D images of bone abnormalities that can be converted into 3D physical models—for correct surgical visualization, teaching–learning, presurgical planning and rehabilitation planning. Doctors can easily detect the extent of damage or deformation in the bone, plan corrective action and conduct the surgery precisely without the need for a second intervention [52]. Earlier, researchers and surgeons 3D-printed wrist arthroplasty in order to treat complex and severe wrist bone defects [53]

7.2.2.4 Designing Patient-Specific Implants

Developments in AM have provided the leeway for doctors and health professionals today to custom design and fabricate implants with exact fit, shape and size for each individual patient. This has significantly removed the requirements of conventional implant fabrication techniques as they came in standard sizes that do not fit all patients accurately. This led to complications in the functional aspects of the implants and distress in patients [54–55].

7.2.2.5 Better Care of Patients and Surgical Precision

Proper surgical planning and fabrication of 3D models and implants have lowered the risk of any operative mishaps during intervention. The need for a second intervention has reduced to a bare minimum as surgeons can efficiently practice on preprinted models, learn and visualize the patient-specific defects, custom print surgical guides beforehand for a specific surgery and ably perform surgeries with minimal invasion, which lowers the overall risk and stress on the patient [56–57].

7.2.2.6 Teaching and Learning

AM-fabricated 3D models have been thoroughly used not only in the orthopedics domains but through all the domains of medicine as well. Three-dimensionally printed models have been used in order to teach and understand different bone-related diseases—Perthe's disease, Blount disease, bone coalitions and others. These 3D models provide a better knowledge of the human anatomy, specifically the musculoskeletal system. The knowledge obtained regarding the bone defects or diseases can be also extended to medical students and the families of the patient for training, patient well-being and satisfaction. Additionally, surgeons can also practice their procedures on the 3D models to enhance their surgical capabilities on the patient-specific defects/cases [25, 58–59].

7.2.3 PRESURGICAL PLANNING IN DENTISTRY

Before a dental surgery, surgeons usually examine the patient's jaw and take an image of it. Based on the image, the surgeon decides on the location of dental surgery (drilling, root canal, etc.). However, this technique is entirely based on the visualization and assessment of the surgeon. With the advent of AM technology, it is now possible to exactly pinpoint the location of surgery or drilling, which, in turn, increases the accuracy of drilling location. Additionally, dental implants and artificial teeth sets (dentures) can also be custom designed based on the data received through AM so that they comfortably fit the mouth [60–62]. AM technology can also be useful in performing complex dental procedures. Presurgical planning under the dentistry domain can be categorized under the following domains.

7.2.3.1 3D Dental Models/Implants

Three-dimensional models of dental implants can be created through AM technology that will assist dental surgeons in creating the most accurate implants/dentures for the damaged tooth/teeth. It is a much more precise and accurate method when compared to the traditional "scan and create" methodology. Three-dimensionally printed implants have an excellent surface finish, which creates a comfortable fit in the patient's teeth. Additionally, the AM techniques are faster and more cost-effective than conventional methods of implant fabrication [63–66].

7.2.3.2 Designing Orthodontic Models and Replacement of Damaged Teeth

AM can also be used in the creation of models that are used for teaching and treating irregularities in jaws and teeth (orthodontic models). This assists in presurgical planning during patient-specific treatment of the deformities in the teeth or jaws. The defective teeth or jaws are scanned first, converted into a 3D image and finally 3D-printed. CAD software assists in digital customization of 3D models of damaged teeth, crowns, braces, dental molds and dentures as a part of presurgery requirements so that dentists can evaluate and test the fit and alignment of these components before actual operation [67–69].

7.2.3.3 Surgical Devices and Guides

AM technology helps in scanning the teeth and jaws of patients, which, in turn, can be easily converted into 3D form. These 3D models can assist dental surgeons in designing custom-made surgical guides and devices as a part of preoperative surgical planning. These guides make complicated surgical procedures much easier and more accurate, thus preventing the need for a second intervention [70–73].

7.2.3.4 Design of Dentistry Tools

AM facilitates innovative designs of dentistry tools and instruments as per surgeons' ergonomic requirements. Preplanning the design of these tools before surgery, and subsequently their 3D printing, would facilitate surgeons to conduct complex dental procedures with more ease and accuracy. Tools can also be 3D-printed based on the patient's teeth anatomy. Three-dimensional scanning and designing through AM also enable design, innovation and the development of newer and more sophisticated tools (e.g., drill guides) in the field of dentistry [74–77].

7.2.3.5 Teaching and Education

The training of medical students and health professionals is paramount for their proficiency in the field of dentistry. Three-dimensionally printed teeth, jaws and implants can serve the purpose of teaching-learning tools through visualization, trials and practice before the actual surgery. Three-dimensional models of damaged teeth, implants, crowns, braces, dental molds and dentures are used as a part of pre-surgery planning requirements so that prospective dentists can evaluate and test their proficiency on the models before actual intervention [78–80].

7.2.4 Presurgical Planning in Drug Delivery

Drug delivery is a complex process as many issues come up during administering drugs due to the disparity in the nature of patients varying in terms of age, gender, race, levels of fitness, health conditions, diseases, pharmacodynamics and pharmacokinetics. Due to this, administering medicines requires patient-specific customized drug delivery systems that have the ability to release a specific amount of drugs depending on the patient. However, traditional methods of drug delivery are very standard and not patient-specific. In this regard, AM facilitates innovative design specifications, complete customization and tailor-made drug delivery platforms with rapid fabrication times. As such, with the advent of AM technology, there has been an ever-increasing demand for AM-developed drug delivery kits with a host of specific product ranges. Drug delivery issues can be categorized under presurgical, postsurgical and nonsurgical planning procedures in the health care industry [81].

AM gathers data from a CT scan or an MRI about the condition of the patient and assists in designing a patient-specific drug dose and a preprogrammed drug release profile. Subsequently, a personalized drug administering protocol and the drug release requirement are prepared as a part of pre–drug delivery treatment plan. There are two advantages of AM-assisted drug delivery—(1) customized patient-specific drug delivery and (2) customized drug release profile. Drug delivery systems can be categorized as discussed in the following sections.

7.2.4.1 Oral Medications

This is the oldest, commonest and cheapest mode of drug delivery and is administered in the forms of tablets, capsules, syrups, lozenges, films and others. However, the disadvantages of oral medication are the concentration of the medicine, variation in the release profile and degradation of the medicine before acting due to low pH in the human digestive system. AM-designed oral medications are such that a single customized tablet or pill would combine all the medicines of patients suffering from chronic diseases (e.g., diabetes, heart disease, kidney disease, etc.). This would, in turn, considerably improve their compliance with the treatment protocol. Oral dose medication through AM consists of a customized complex structure, shape and size (tailored aesthetics—square, pyramidal, ring, cubical, etc.), a different pH-based drug release profile, and a combination of multiple drugs (fast-disintegrating forms, polypills) and tablets with material gradient [82–86]. Table 7.1 shows a few types of AM-fabricated oral drug delivery platforms that have been proposed by many researchers.

7.2.4.2 Vaginal and Rectal Medicine

Vaginally administered medicines in the form of tablets, suppositories, solutions, gels, pessaries and vaginal rings are available commercially to treat various conditions, such as contraception, infertility, osteoporosis and others. Rectally administered drugs come in the form of creams, rectal capsules, gels and suppositories. Both of these are widely used due to their benefits such as bypassing the gastrointestinal tract (reduced metabolic and enzymatic activity), ease of access, and for patients with high vomiting and difficulty swallowing. However, problems with rectally and vaginally administered drugs are their reduced absorption of the medicine and high variations depending on the individual [93–94]. AM techniques such as SLA and

TABLE 7.1
Few Examples of AM-Manufactured Oral Drug Delivery Platforms

Drug structure	Drug composition	Drug loaded with	Reference
Customized drug-loaded tablets	• Paracetamol • Progesterone • Ibuprofen	Mixing	[87]
Pellets	• Paracetamol • Ibuprofen	Mixing	[88]
Complex geometry	• Fenofibrate • N-acetyl-para-aminophenol (APAP)	Mixed with powdered polymer	[89]
Tablets with different pH-phase release profiles	• Chlorpheniramine maleate • Diclofenac	Mixed with powdered polymer	[90]
Tablet with material gradient	• APAP	Mixed with powdered polymer	[91]
Fast-disintegrating tablets	• Paracetamol	Mixed with powdered polymer	[92]

FDM have earlier produced non-dissolving rectal and vaginal suppositories of lidocaine, ibuprofen, diclofenac and ketoprofen with controlled drug release ability [95].

7.2.4.3 Intravenous Catheters

In order to inject intravenous medicines through the vein of a person, intravenous devices are used employing a needle or tube. They are generally used when the medicine injected needs to reach the bloodstream of the patient as quickly as possible (in the case of emergencies). Usually, a needle is inserted into the vein of the patient while a catheter is pushed over the needle. Subsequently, the needle is removed, and the catheter remains in the vein. AM techniques such as FDM have been used in order to manufacture patient-specific eluting catheters and bioresorbable catheters for personalized drug delivery [96].

7.2.4.4 Transdermal Medicine

Medicines administered through the skin of a patient are transdermal medicines. Generally, these types of medicine come in the form of creams, gels, ointments, patches and drug carriers. They have benefits such as being cheap, having the ability for self-administration, being easy to use, being noninvasive, and having a long-lasting drug release profile. However, their limitation is that they have a low ability to permeate the skin, making it difficult to efficient drug delivery. AM technology has facilitated the fabrication of uncoated and coated drug-loaded microneedle patches for transdermal drug delivery [97].

7.2.4.5 Implants and Scaffolds

Bioimplants coated with drugs with the ability to be released in a controlled manner are replaced with a missing part in the body. In addition to its functionality as implant materials, it also supplies drugs at a controlled release rate for the resident disease. The release action may be physical (absorption of the drug through a polymeric matrix or coating and slowly releasing the drug when inside the body) or chemical (chemical degradation). Bio-scaffolds are biocompatible materials used as a support for cell attachment, development and proliferation of tissue. These drug-loaded scaffolds are used in drug delivery with a controlled release rate. However, with technological advancements, the personalization and customization of these implants and scaffolds have become requirements that cannot be attained with traditional manufacturing techniques. AM has the ability to make these custom implants and scaffold materials based on patient-specific cases. Hence, titanium-based antibiotic-releasing implants and water-dissolvable 3D-printed molds for scaffolds have previously been prepared employing AM, such as the laser melting process [98–99].

7.3 ROLE OF AM IN POSTSURGICAL PLANNING

Postsurgical planning is also as important as presurgical planning. Postsurgical drug delivery and rehabilitation form an important regime for the patient to recover completely or adjust to their daily life. It has been mentioned before that precise drug delivery platforms mentioned earlier also form a huge part of postsurgical planning as it provides information to the patient above the exact drug use for full recovery or disease control. Drug delivery platforms manufactured through AM technology have been instrumental in postsurgical planning. Additionally, postsurgical planning also involves rehabilitation after a surgery, especially surgeries that would cause amputation or severe impairment to the patient's body parts. AM has also contributed greatly to the design and development of various orthoses and prostheses required for postsurgical rehabilitation of amputees or patients with physical disabilities. The contribution of AM on postsurgical planning and rehabilitation is discussed in the following sections.

7.3.1 Postsurgical Planning in Orthoses and Prostheses

Orthoses are artificial additional appliances added to the body in order to support the body parts for the objectives of support, stabilization and efficient movement. Prostheses are synthetic devices that are used to replace an anatomically missing limb or any other body part in the patient. Two types of orthoses and prostheses (O&P) are available commercially—prefabricated standard types and custom-made as per the patient's fit. Standard types are cheap and available off the shelf, but customized products provide a better fitting with the body, that is, ergonomic comfort. Researchers have also provided data that concludes that comfort and fit are the most important parameters for the satisfaction of O&P customers. In this regard, AM has huge potential to provide customized products at a low cost and rapid manufacturing time, thus providing a pathbreaking service to persons with physical disabilities. The following are types of O&P [100]:

Upper limb orthoses—Hand orthoses, wrist–hand orthoses, wrist orthoses, elbow–wrist–hand orthoses, elbow orthoses

Spinal orthoses—Cervical–thoracic lumbosacral orthoses, cervical orthoses, thoracic–lumbosacral orthoses, thoracic orthoses, lumbosacral orthoses, lumbar orthoses, sacroiliac orthoses

Lower limb orthoses—Foot orthoses (FOs), ankle–foot orthoses (AFOs), knee orthoses, knee–ankle–foot orthoses, hip orthoses, hip–knee–ankle–foot orthoses

Prostheses—Above elbow, below elbow, above knee, below knee

7.3.1.1 FOs

AM fabrication of personalized O&P employs three major steps: (1) Determine the geometry of the O&P based on the patient-specific limb/foot, (2) design and 3D modeling of the O&P through software and (3) fabrication through an AM technique.

Determining the geometry of O&P required based on the patient-specific limb through AM consists of methods such as optical scanning, CT and MRI, or a combination of two techniques can be used to achieve clarity in the geometry. Earlier research has shown that an AM-fabricated FO scan can efficiently distribute the pressure over the heel and arch. Pallari et al. also formulated a proposed a structure for the mass production of customized FOs [101]. Saleh and Dalgarno [102] conducted a comparative cost analysis between traditional and AM-fabricated FOs (using SLS and FDM) and concluded that the cost of AM-manufactured FOs is equivalent to that of the traditional plaster molding method. It was shown through the research of Sun et al. [103] that there was a 5% reduction in the front part of foot and heel pressure and a 5% increase in arch pressure on using shoe insoles produced through an AM technique (PolyJet®). Cook et al. [104] employed AM techniques to make a positive model to create a negative silicone mold to cast polyurethane (PU) foam as the inner layer of FO and create hard shells for personalized FOs in case of club foot. It was also observed through the study of Pallari et al. [105] that the gait constraints (cadence, velocity, cycle of time), along with the fit perception parameter were equivalent for standard commercially available custom FOs and AM-fabricated FOs (SLS technique). Moreover, the cost analysis also showed equivalent expenses for both types of products. Pallari et al. [106] in a subsequent study proposed the idea of adding sensors in FOs and developing a software platform specifically for mass production of AM-fabricated patient-specific FOs. In a comparative analysis between AM-fabricated insoles and regular insoles, it was observed that the former provided an even distribution of pressure across the entire foot [107–108]. In subsequent studies, it was also proved that AM-made custom insoles facilitated reduced heel discomfort, lower dorsiflexion at foot strike, overall better fit and reduced heel peak pressure, which finally lowered injury risks [109]. Earlier, a comparative cost analysis was performed by Saleh [110] for traditional, as well as AM techniques such as SLS, SLA, FDM, and inkjet 3D printing. The analysis revealed that the SLS technique showed the highest productivity rate and lowest cost, but the cost was still higher than conventional FOs. Chen et al. [111] showed that employing a sparse structure in FO design can lower the cost of manufacturing as well as reduce production time. Telfer et al. [112] showed that AM techniques had the capability of handling and designing complex FOs with higher functionality by fabricating FOs with adaptable components in order to alleviate pressure at the metatarsal heads. Several companies such as podfo®, 3DOrthotics and SOLS® have come up that today produce AM-fabricated FOs commercially.

7.3.1.2 AFOs

Steps required for AM fabrication of AFOs are (1) 3D scanning of ankle and foot, (2) using CAD software to add the two scans together at the interface, (3) designing the path and support structure of AFO and (4) fabricating the AFO using AM. Milusheva et al. [113–114] first proposed using AM for manufacturing AFOs in 2005 by making elastic elements that were exchangeable so that the customer could adjust the mechanical properties of the AFOs. Faustini et al. [115] made AFOs, with nylon 11, nylon 12 and glass fiber–reinforced nylon 12 composites with the SLS technique of AM, which provided comparable stiffness and higher damping properties than carbon fiber AFOs. Pallari et al. [105] proposed integration of sensors in AM-fabricated AFO. Additionally, they also employed finite element method (FEM) and topology optimization in designing AFOs manufactured via the SLS technique. Mavroidis et al. [116] deduced that the gait parameters (walking speed and length of each step) were equivalent while the support time for AFOs was doubled in the case of SLA-fabricated AFOs when compared with AFOs manufactured through traditional methods. Schrank and Stanhope [117] produced a highly accurate AFO via SLS technique using their proposed five-step customization structure encompassing foot alignment, leg segment and subject characterization. Telfer et al. [112] studied the effects of AFO stiffness on the ankle kinematics and, thereafter, produced an AFO with adjustable stiffness using AM. Creylman et al. [118] concluded that SLS-fabricated AFOs had equivalent performances with conventional AFOs after assessing gait parameters (unilateral drop foot gait and gait performance). Schrank et al. [119] quantitatively predicted, as well as experimentally validated, the bending stiffness of FDM-fabricated AFOs using CAD and FEM analysis. Chen et al. [120] deduced that the FDM method had the capability of producing AFOs with high stiffness and a lightweight design by conducting a comparative strain analysis among conventional polypropylene and polyethylene (PP-PE) copolymer AFO and two FDM-fabricated AFOs (one with polycarbonate/acrylonitrile butadiene styrene (PC-ABS) and other with ULTEMTM materials (ULTEM is an amorphous thermoplastic polyetherimide (PEI) material that combines exceptional mechanical, thermal, and electrical properties)). Harper et al. [121] found limited differences between standard carbon fiber AFOs and SLS-fabricated AFOs on conducting their evaluation of gait.

7.3.1.3   Prosthetic Sockets of the Lower Limb

In research from the University of Texas in the early 1990s, researchers used the SLS technique of AM in order to manufacture prosthetic sockets. Initially, they developed scaled-down sockets after 3D scanning a residual limb and designing through CAD software were conducted. AM-facilitated integration of the socket bottom to the fixture of the pylon. Finally, they built the scaled model in the next year [122–123]. Earlier, researchers have employed SLA and FDM techniques to manufacture prosthetic sockets after digitizing the 3D geometry of the residual limb. Freeman and Wontorick [124] found that SLA-fabricated sockets were sturdy enough to support the weight of the patient during fitting and were comparable to conventional sockets. However, they also found that the SLA sockets were not suitable for handling stresses and impact loads. Conventional processes involved manually building a positive mold with flexibility in shape and differences in wall thickness. However, with the advent of AM technology, the digitization of the scanning process and rapid manufacturing of sockets, with the ability to use various types of materials at a lower cost and shorter production time, has made the whole process very advantageous. Rogers et al. [125] and Stephens et al. [126] employed a double-walled prosthetic socket for the transtibial part and compared to a conventional socket. Their design showed higher ergonomic comfort and equivalent gait performance. In another study, Rogers et al. [127] demonstrated that SLS sockets provided satisfactory fits in all subjects with higher comfort, resulting in the subjects' ability to wear the prosthesis for a longer duration. However, the gait parameters were equivalent to traditionally manufactured ones.

In a study of prosthetic sockets conducted by researchers at the University of Texas, they incorporated transducers on prosthetic sockets in order to alleviate contact pressure and subsequently were successful in reducing 20% average pressure and 23–45% peak pressure. In another study, FEM was employed to predict the structural reliability of AM-fabricated sockets and this showed a satisfactory match with the experimental values. In 2010, SLS-fabricated sockets that had active actuators for inflatable/deflatable elements attached to the socket in order to compensate volumetric changes in the residual limb were first introduced [128]. A research group at the National University of Singapore manufactured a rapid socket manufacturing machine (RSMM) employing the FDM technology to manufacture PP prosthetic sockets that had good static loading strength and fatigue properties but had a 12–23% reduction in ultimate tensile strength values [129–130]. Clinical trials showed that these RSMM-fabricated PP prosthetic sockets had equivalent properties when compared with traditional sockets [131]. Herbert et al. [132] manufactured a plaster-based 3D-printed socket model providing good comfort to the subject, but no investigation on the mechanical properties of the socket was made. Researchers at National Cheng Kung University employed a novel vacuum forming tool for capturing the residual limb geometry under a vacuum and subsequently building a positive mold for 3D scanning and fabricating a socket [133]. They also increased the flexural properties of an FDM-fabricated socket by coating it with polyester resin [134–135]. A research group at the Massachusetts Institute of Technology built a 3D-printed socket having variations in the hardness at different locations. The hardness and tissue compliance had an inverse relationship at different contact points. The hardness required at different contact points was mapped based on MRI data. These sockets provided 10–20% relief in contact pressure and a 16% increase in the walking speed [136].

7.3.1.4 Miscellaneous Applications

AM has also been in fabricating personalized auricular prostheses [137–138], wrist splints [139], hand prosthetics and feet prosthetics. Paterson et al. [139] investigated different processes of AM, such as SLS, SLA, FDM and 3D printing, in order to build customized wrist splints. Earlier, Dalley et al. [140–141] built complex parts of hand prosthetics that were high in strength and lightweight. Zuniga et al. [142] built an AM-fabricated low-cost prosthetic hand for children of developing countries called the "Cyborg Beast" that had satisfactory hand fit. Leddy et al. [143] employed molds fabricated through AM to construct prosthetic hands with high stiffness and low weight. South et al. [144] used the SLS technique and topology optimization to manufacture prosthetic foot out of nylon 11 for higher energy storage and return. They compared both SLS-fabricated foot and carbon fiber foot and found that both had equivalent mechanical properties. Ventura et al. [145] also used SLS to build prosthetic ankles with stiffness variation. They observed that ankles with higher dorsiflexion and higher energy storage and return assists in lowering force the asymmetric loading of both legs and the residual limb's ground reaction force.

7.4 MAJOR FINDINGS THROUGH THE STUDY

The contribution of AM is paramount in the domains of medicine, specifically in pre- and postsurgical planning of treatment protocols and complex surgeries, including the following:

- Through this study, it is evident that additive manufacturing is being widely used in the pre- and postsurgical domains of medicine and surgery. The field of AM is continuously improving and advancing to create different innovations in the field of medicine, that is, cardiology, dental, orthopedics, implants, drug delivery, prosthetics and others.

- AM assists in presurgical planning by fabricating a physical model from a digitized 3D scan. This object can serve as a surgeon's practicing tool and teaching aid for health professionals, thus reducing the risks of operation and the need for secondary intervention.
- Through AM preplanned 3D models of the defect, surgical guides can also be built as a part of surgical preplanning, which results in reduced time and high accuracy in the case of complex surgeries.
- AM assists in formulating a customized surgical protocol presurgery by studying the 3D replica of the patient's defect.
- Surgeons and health professionals can now convert their requirements/ideas into a real 3D model that facilitates an extensive package to fabricate the customized implant, practice model, guides (presurgical planning) or drug delivery systems and prosthetics (postsurgery) as per the requirements of the patient. It saves time for the dental technician and provides improved opportunities to create a new dental product.
- AM facilitates digitized data acquisition and accurate fabrication of the object at a reduced time at a cheaper or comparable cost. It also facilitates the use of a variety of materials for fabrication, which provides the user to select the right material with the required mechanical properties.

7.5 CHALLENGES IN USING AM FOR PRE- AND POSTSURGICAL PLANNING

- *Deficiency in the advancement of design platforms:* Developments continue regarding updating existing software for better acquisition of scanning data, the creation of a virtual 3D geometry, the efficient conversion of an irregular or contoured surface into a solid model and the creation of trim lines. However, there is a continuous need for the software platforms available to be more user-friendly and efficient in converting the actual scanned data received through patient investigation into 3D models accurately. Although AM facilitates the design and fabrication of objects with high complexity and functionality, the design interface should not be limited by shape, sizes, contours and irregularities [146–148].
- *High initial cost:* Starting up an AM facility with all its equipment is expensive. The high initial investment cost is one of the barriers to extensively using AM for medical fields. However, with the increasing demand and mass production of AM facilities, it is expected that the cost of AM software and equipment will drop. [149]
- *Low deposition rate and material throughput:* Another barrier for faster production is reduced deposition rate layer by layer and low material throughput. However, with the increased use of designing innovations, such as topology optimization and sparse structure, better designs can be created that will guarantee material utilization in an optimized way with lower fabrication time. [110]

- *Limited access:* The variety of materials that can be printable commercially, the expensive cost of biocompatible materials, the limited conversion of *in vitro* products in actual clinical applications, the high price of research and development in the field of 3D printing, issues in image processing, problems in development and printing complex organs are some of the issues related to the accessibility of AM for the regular consumer.
- *Safety and durability:* The safety and durability of AM-fabricated objects are also necessary, especially if they are used repeatedly and loaded with stress, for example, implants and prosthetics. In this regard, a variety of materials have been used in AM techniques with varied parameters in order to achieve the required mechanical properties. However, for extensive commercial viability, longer and more extensive safety and durability studies, along with quality control of the products, must be conducted [150].
- *Cyber-physical system:* This is a system in which the health professional takes the 3D scan of the patient, prescribes the requirements of the 3D object (model, guides, prosthetics or implants) and sends it to a remote location where the design and optimization of the 3D model are conducted. If the design of the model is approved by the health professional, it is sent to an AM facility through the internet for manufacturing. Such types of facilities, where there is a distributed scanning, design and manufacturing facility, that is, cyber-physical system, are the need of the hour for the proper utilization of AM resources and their extensive use [100].

7.6 CONCLUSION

Technological advancements have taken place in the field of AM in leaps and bounds over the last few years, especially its application in the medical field. Its ability to manufacture accurate models, guides, equipment, implants, prosthetics, rehabilitation tools and drug delivery platforms and rehabilitation at a faster time and lesser cost along with properties comparable to the products made with traditional methods have created huge avenues for mass production and their extensive uses in the health industry. Three-dimensional scanning and modeling of complex structures and defects using advanced software have assisted surgeons in optimizing and efficiently planning their presurgical protocols as well as their postsurgical rehabilitation. As a part of presurgical planning, AM has facilitated the production of 3D models for practice and teaching; enhanced diagnostic visualization of the defect; the design and fabrication of surgical guides, stents and implants; doctor–patient detailed communication of the disease; and presurgical drug delivery platforms.

With AM's assistance, surgeons can detail all the surgical protocols presurgery with high accuracy and efficiency, which would lead to a successful and precise operative procedure with minimal patient stress and without the need for a secondary intervention. Any customized implant produced through AM is more reliable and replicable with the original anatomical form, which leads to patient comfort, increased implant functionality and, most important, better postsurgical rehabilitation. Similarly, the contribution of AM to the field of postsurgical planning is also significant: (1) It has facilitated the fabrication of customized postsurgical drug delivery platforms for precise drug delivery and their absorption, and (2) it has facilitated the design and fabrication of customized orthoses and prostheses for defective or missing limbs and body parts with precise body-prosthetic ergonomics, thus generating greater comfort with more durable and safe materials at a lower cost and in less time.

It is evident that AM technology has had a huge impact on the preoperative planning of cardiology, orthopedic and dental problems along with drug delivery platforms. Similarly, the contribution of AM in the customized postoperative planning and rehabilitation of patients through developing postsurgical drug delivery platforms and prosthetics is also paramount. Having stated that, it is also pertinent to be mentioned that the commercialization of AM technology in the medical field has its own challenges. Deficiencies in advanced design platforms to facilitate the efficient conversion of scanned data into models, high initial investments, lower deposition rates and material throughput, less variety of printable materials, expensive biocompatible materials, the high cost of research and development in the field of AM and issues related to the printing of complex organs and structures are challenges in the application of AM in the health industry that still need to be fixed. However, with the evolution of AM technology, it has been observed that AM has come leaps and bounds in tackling various setbacks in the medical field. Continuous investments in the research and development of AM technology, updating regulatory guidelines and structures for clinical applications, developing a cyber-physical system and continuous encouragement of the AM industry by extensively using their products would foster huge developments in the field of AM products that will serve the health industry.

REFERENCES

1. B.C. Gross, J.L. Erkal, S.Y. Lockwood, C. Chen, and D.M. Spence. Evaluation of 3D printing and its potential impact on biotechnology and the chemical sciences. *Anal Chem.* 86(7) (2014), pp. 3240–3253.
2. L.K. Cheung, M.C.M. Wong, and L.L.S. Wong. Refinement of facial reconstructive surgery by stereo model planning. *Ann R Aust College Dent Surg.* 16 (2002), pp. 129–132.
3. I. Gibson, L.K. Cheung, S.P. Chow, W.L. Cheung, S.L. Beh, M. Savalani, and S.H. Lee. The use of rapid prototyping to assist medical applications. *Rapid Prototyp J.* 12 (2006), pp. 53–58.
4. R. Bibb, D. Eggbeer, P. Evans, A. Bocca, and A Sugar. Rapid manufacture of custom fitting surgical guides. *Rapid Prototyp J.* 15 (2009), pp. 346–354.
5. T. Jukka, K.S. Paloheimo, J. Vehviläinen, R. Björkstrand, M. Salmi, E. Huotilainen, R. Kontio, S. Rouse, I. Gibson, and A.A. Mäkitie. A novel classification and online platform for planning and documentation of medical applications of additive manufacturing. *Surg Innovation.* 21 (2014), pp. 553–559.
6. M. Shuaib, L. Kumar, M. Javaid, A. Haleem, and M.I. Khan. A comparison of additive manufacturing technologies. *International Conference on Advance Production and Industrial Engineering, DTU Delhi* (2016). p. 353–60.
7. S.P. Krishnan, A. Dawood, R. Richards, J. Henckel, and A.J. Hart. A review of rapid prototyped surgical guides for patient-specific total knee replacement. *Bone Joint J.* 94 (2012), pp. 1457–1461.
8. V. Kumar, L. Kumar, and A. Haleem. Selection of rapid Prototyping technology using an ANP based approach. *IOSR J Mech Civ Eng.* 13 (2016), pp. 71–78.

9. M.Y. Lee, C.C. Chang, C.C. Lin, L.J. Lo, and Y.R. Chen. Custom implant design for patient with cranial defect. *IEEE Engineering in Medicine and Biology*. 21(2) (2002), pp. 38–44.

10. S. Singare, Q. Lian, W.P. Wang, F. Wang, Y. Liu, D. Li, and B. Lu. Rapid prototyping assisted surgery planning and custom implant design. *Rapid Prototyping J.* 15(1) (2009), pp. 19–23.

11. K. Ibrahim and L.M. Faller. Development of a customised rehabilitation device using additive manufacturing. *14th Pervasive Technologies Related to Assistive Environments Conference* (2021), pp. 354–358.

12. V. Ricotta, R.I. Campbell, T. Ingrassia, and V. Nigrelli. A new design approach for customised medical devices realized by additive manufacturing. *International Journal on Interactive Design and Manufacturing*. 14(4) (2020), pp. 1171–1178.

13. M. Feroze, K. Owais, C. Taylor, M. Montealegre-Gallegos, W. Manning, R. Matyal, and K.R. Khabbaz. Three-dimensional printing of mitral valve using echocardiographic data. *JACC Cardiovasc Imaging* 8 (2015), pp. 227–229.

14. M. Vukicevic, B. Mosadegh, J.K. Min, and S.H. Little. Cardiac 3D printing and its future directions. *JACC Cardiovasc Imaging* 10 (2017), pp. 171–184.

15. D.H. Ballard, A.P. Trace, S. Ali, T. Hodgdon, M.E. Zygmont, C.M. DeBenedectis, S.E. Smith, M.L. Richardson, M.J. Patel, S.J. Decker, and L. Lenchik. Clinical applications of 3D printing: Primer for radiologists. *Acad Radiol*. 25 (2018), pp. 52–65.

16. R. Faletti, M. Gatti, A. Cosentino, L. Bergamasco, E.C. Stura, D. Garabello, G. Pennisi, S. Salizzoni, S. Veglia, D. Ottavio, and M. Rinaldi. 3D printing of the aortic annulus based on cardiovascular computed tomography: Preliminary experience in preprocedural planning for aortic valve sizing. *J Cardiovasc Comp Tomogr*. 12(5) (2018), pp. 391–397.

17. J.P. Costello, L.J. Olivieri, L. Su, A. Krieger, F. Alfares, O. Thabit, M.B. Marshall, S.J. Yoo, P.C. Kim, R.A. Jonas, and D.S. Nath. Incorporating three-dimensional printing into a simulation-based congenital heart disease and critical care training curriculum for resident physicians. *Congenit Heart Disease*. 10 (2015), pp. 185–190.

18. D. Schmauss, S. Haeberle, C. Hagl, and R. Sodian. Three-dimensional printing in cardiac surgery and interventional cardiology: A single-centre experience. *Eur J Cardiothorac Surg*. 47 (2015), pp. 1044–1052.

19. C. Tanner. Is the end of donor transplants in sight? Scientists create a 3D printed silicone artificial heart that beats like the real organ. Mail online. 2017. Url: www.dailymail. co.uk/health/article-4704204/Scientists-create-3D-printed-silicone-artificial-heart.html. retrieved on 08.08.2021.

20. M.S. Sacks and A.P. Yoganathan. Heart valve function: A biomechanical perspective. *Phil Trans Roy Soc B: Biol Sci*. 362 (2007), 1369–2139.

21. W.R. Witschey, A.M. Pouch, and J.R. McGarvey. Three-dimensional ultrasound-derived physical mitral valve modelling. *Ann Thorac Surg*. 98 (2014), pp. 691–694.

22. T. Moore, E.J. Madriago, and E.S. Renteria. Co-registration of 3D echo and MR data to create physical models of congenital heart malformations. *J Cardiovasc Magn Reson*. 17(1) (2015), p. 198.

23. A. Haleem, M. Javaid, and A. Saxena. Additive manufacturing applications in cardiology: A review. *The Egyptian Heart Journal*. 70 (2018), pp. 433–441.

24. M.S. Kim, A.R. Hansgen, O. Wink, R.A. Quaife, and J.D. Carroll. Rapid prototyping: A new tool in understanding and treating structural heart disease. *Circulation*. 117 (2008), 2388–2394.

25. R. Sodian, S. Weber, M. Markert, M. Loeff, T. Lueth, F. C. Weis, S. Daebritz, E. Malec, C. Schmitz, and B. Reichart. Pediatric cardiac transplantation: Three dimensional printing of anatomic models for surgical planning of heart transplantation in patients with univentricular heart. *J Thorac Cardiovasc Surg*. 136 (2008), pp. 1098–1099.

26. R. Sodian, S. Weber, M. Markert, D. Rassoulian, I. Kaczmarek, T.C. Lueth, B. Reichart, and Sabine Daebritz. Stereolithographic models for surgical planning in congenital heart surgery. *Ann Thorac Surg.* 83 (2007), 1854–1857.

27. A.M. Noecker, J.F. Chen, Q. Zhou, R.D. White, M.W. Kopcak, M.J. Arruda, and B.W. Duncan. Development of patient-specific three dimensional pediatric cardiac models. *ASAIO J.* 52 (2006), pp. 349–353.

28. I. Shiraishi, Y. Kajiyama, M. Yamagishi, and K. Hamaoka. Images in cardiovascular medicine. Stereolithographic biomodelling of congenital heart disease by multislice computed tomography imaging. *Circulation.* 113 (2006), pp. 733–734.

29. K.J. Dickinson, J. Matsumoto, S.D. Cassivi, M. Reinersman, J.G. Fletcher, J. Morris, L. M. Song, and S.H. Blackmon. Individualizing management of complex oesophagal pathology using three dimensional printed models. *Ann Thorac Surg.* 100 (2015), pp. 692–697.

30. J. Gosnell, T. Pietila, B.P. Samuel, H.K.N. Kurup, M.P. Haw, and J.J. Vettukattil. Integration of computed tomography and three-dimensional echocardiography for hybrid three-dimensional printing in congenital heart disease. *J Digit Imaging.* 29 (2016), pp. 665–669.

31. M. Mathur, P. Patil, and A Bove. The role of 3D printing in structural heart disease: All that glitters is not gold. *JACC Cardiovasc Imaging* 8 (2015), pp. 987–988.

32. E. Perez-Arjona, M. Dujovny, H. Park, D. Kulyanov, A. Galaniuk, C. Agner, D. Michael, and F.G. Diaz. Stereolithography: Neurosurgical and medical implications. *Neurol Res.* 25 (2003), pp. 227–236.

33. B. Miller. *3-D Printer Creates Transformative Device for Heart Treatment.* Washington University in St Louis. (Online Article) http://news. wustl. edu/news/Pages/26554. aspx (2014).

34. K.M. Farooqi, O. Saeed, A. Zaidi, J. Sanz, J.C. Nielsen, D.T. Hsu, and U.P. Jorde. 3D printing to guide ventricular assist device placement in adults with congenital heart disease and heart failure. *JACC Heart Fail.* 4 (2016), pp. 301–311.

35. K. Torres, G. Staskiewicz, M. Sniezynski, A. Drop, and R. Maciejewski. Application of rapid prototyping techniques for modelling of anatomical structures in medical training and education. *Folia Morphol.* 70 (2011), pp. 1–4.

36. A. Haleem, M. Javaid, and A. Saxena. Additive manufacturing applications in cardiology: A review. *The Egyptian Heart Journal.* 70 (2018), pp. 433–441

37. I. Shiraishi, M. Yamagishi, K. Hamaoka, M. Fukuzawa, and T. Yagihara. Simulative operation on congenital heart disease using rubber-like urethane stereolithographic models based on 3D datasets of multislice computed tomography. *Eur J Cardiothorac Surg.* 37 (2010), pp. 302–306.

38. D. Schmauss, G. Juchem, S. Weber, N. Gerber, C. Hagl, and R. Sodian. Three-dimensional printing for perioperative planning of complex aortic arch surgery. *Ann Thorac Surg.* 97 (2014), pp. 2160–2163.

39. S. Jacobs, R. Grunert, F.W. Mohr, and V. Falk. 3D-Imaging of cardiac structures using 3D heart models for planning in heart surgery: A preliminary study. *Interact Cardiovasc Thorac Surg.* 7 (2008), pp. 6–9.

40. M.S. Sacks and A.P. Yoganathan. Heart valve function: A biomechanical perspective. *Phil Trans Roy Soc B: Biol Sci.* 362 (2007), pp. 1369–2139.

41. M. Vukicevic, B. Mosadegh, J.K. Min, and S.H. Little. Cardiac 3D printing and its future directions. *JACC Cardiovasc Imaging* 10 (2017), pp. 171–184.

42. M. Lazkani, F. Bashir, K. Brady, S. Pophal, M. Morris, and A. Pershad. Postinfarct VSD management using 3D computer printing assisted percutaneous closure. *Indian Heart J.* 67 (2015), pp. 581–585.

43. S.M. Green, A.J. Klein, S. Pancholy, S.V. Rao, D. Steinberg, R. Lipner, J. Marshall, and J.C. Messenger. The current state of medical simulation in interventional cardiology: A clinical document from the society for cardiovascular angiography and intervention's (SCAI) simulation committee. *Catheter Cardiovasc Interv.* 83 (2013), pp. 37–46.

44. L.J. Olivieri, A. Krieger, Y.H. Loke, D.S. Nath, P.C. Kima, and C.A. Sable. Three-dimensional printing of intracardiac defects from three-dimensional echocardiographic images: Feasibility and relative accuracy. *J Am Soc Echocardiogr.* 28 (2015), pp. 392–397.

45. D. Pacione, O. Tanweer, P. Berman, and D.H. Harter. The utility of a multi-material 3D printed model for surgical planning of complex deformity of the skull base and craniovertebral junction. *J Neurosurg.* 125(5) (2016), pp. 1194–1197.

46. A. Vaish and R. Vaish. 3D printing and its applications in Orthopedics. *Journal of Clinical Orthopaedics and Trauma.* 9 (2018), pp. S74–S79.

47. A. Pietrabissa, S. Marconi, A. Peri, L. Pugliese, E. Cavazzi, A. Vinci, M. Botti, F. Auricchio. From CT scanning to 3D printing technology for the preoperative planning in laparoscopic splenectomy. *Surg Endosc.* 30 (1) (2016), pp. 366–371.

48. R. Souzaki, Y. Kinoshita, S. Ieiri, M. Hayashida, Y. Koga, K. Shirabe, T. Hara, Y. Maehara, M. Hashizume, and T. Taguchi. Three-dimensional liver model based on preoperative CT images as a tool to assist in surgical planning for hepatoblastoma in a child. *Pediatr Surg Int.* 31(6) (2015), pp. 593–596.

49. Y.L. Yap, Y.S.E. Tan, H.K.J. Tan, Z.K. Peh, X.Y. Low, W.Y. Yeong, C.S.H. Tan, and A. Laude. 3D printed bio-models for medical applications. *Rapid Prototyping Journal.* 23(2) (2017), pp. 227–235.

50. K.C. Wong, S.M. Kumta, N.V. Geel, and J. Demol. One-step reconstruction with a 3D-printed, biomechanically evaluated custom implant after complex pelvic tumor resection. *Comput Aided Surg.* 20(1) (2015), pp. 14–23.

51. M. Javaid and A. Haleem. Additive manufacturing applications in medical cases: A literature based review. *Alexandria Journal of Medicine.* 54(4) (2018), pp. 411–422.

52. A. Pietrabissa, S. Marconi, A. Peri, L Pugliese, E. Cavazzi, A. Vinci, M. Botti, and F. Auricchio. From CT scanning to 3D printing technology for the preoperative planning in laparoscopic splenectomy. *Surg Endosc.* 30 (1) (2016), pp. 366–371.

53. Q. Han, Y. Qin, Y. Zou, C. Wang, H. Bai, T. Yu, L. Huang, and J. Wang. Novel exploration of 3D printed wrist arthroplasty to solve the severe and complicated bone defect of wrist. *Rapid Prototyping Journal.* 23(3) (2017), pp. 465–473.

54. A.L. Jardini, M.A. Larosa, R. Maciel Filho, C.A.D. Carvalho Zavaglia, L.F. Bernardes, C.S. Lambert, D.R. Calderoni, and P. Kharmandayan. Cranial reconstruction: 3D bio model and custom built implant created using additive manufacturing. *J Craniomaxillofac Surg.* 42(8) (2014), pp. 1877–1884.

55. T.M. Wong, J. Jin, T.W. Lau, C. Fang, C.H. Yan, K. Yeung, M. To, and F. Leung. The use of three dimensional printing technology in orthopaedic surgery: A review. *Journal of Orthopaedic Surgery.* 25 (1) (2017), pp. 1–7.

56. M. Salmi, J. Tuomi, K.S. Paloheimo, R. Björkstrand, M. Paloheimo, J. Salo, R. Kontio, K. Mesimäki, and A.A. Mäkitie. Patient-specific reconstruction with 3D modeling and DMLS additive manufacturing. *Rapid Prototyping Journal.* 18 (3) (2012), pp. 209–214.

57. B. Boonen, M.G. Schotanus, and N.P. Kort. Preliminary experience with the patient-specific templating total knee arthroplasty. *Acta Orthop.* 83(4) (2012), pp. 387–393.

58. A. Mahmoud and M. Bennett. Introducing 3-dimensional printing of a human anatomic pathology specimen: Potential benefits for undergraduate and postgraduate education and anatomic pathology practice. *Arch Pathol Lab Med.* 139(8) (2015), pp. 1048–1051.

59. C. Hurson, A. Tansey, B. O'Donnchadha, P. Nicholson, J. Rice, and J. McElwain. Rapid prototyping in the assessment, classification and pre-operative planning of acetabular fractures. *Injury.* 38(10) (2007), pp. 1158–1162.

60. A. Dawood, B.M. Marti, V. Sauret-Jackson, and A. Darwood. 3D printing in dentistry. *Br Dent J.* 219(11) (2015), pp. 521–529.

61. M. Esposito, Y. Ardebili, and H.V. Worthington. Interventions for replacing missing teeth: Different types of dental implants. *Cochrane Database Syst Rev* (2014). https://doi.org/ 10.1002/14651858.

62. K. Chawla. 3D bioprinting: Technology in dentistry. *Int J Dent Res Oral Sci*. 2(2) (2017), pp. 63–64.
63. S. Tunchel, A. Blay, R. Kolerman, E. Mijiritsky, and J.A. Shibli. 3D printing/additive manufacturing single titanium dental implants: A prospective multicenter study with 3years of follow-up. *Int J Dentistry*. 2016 (2016), pp. 1–9.
64. T.V. Flügge, K. Nelson, R. Schmelzeisen, and M.C. Metzger. Three-dimensional plotting and printing of an implant drilling guide: Simplifying guided implant surgery. *J Oral Maxillofac Surg*. 71 (2013), pp. 1340–1346.
65. U. Klammert, U. Gbureck, E. Vorndran, J. Rodiger, P. Meyer-Marcotty, and A.C. Kubler. 3D powder printed calcium phosphate implants for reconstruction of cranial and maxillofacial defects. *J Cranio-Maxillofacial Surg*. 38 (2010), pp. 565–570.
66. M. T. Chiang, T.I. Li, H. W. Yeh, C. C. Su, K.C. Chiu, M.P. Chung, R.Y. Huang, and Y.S. Shieh. Evaluation of missing-tooth effect on articular eminence inclination of temporomandibular joint. *J Dent Sci*. 10 (2015), pp. 383–387.
67. Q. Liu, M. Leu, and S. Schmitt. Rapid prototyping in dentistry: Technology and application. *Int J Adv Manuf Technol*. 29 (2006), pp. 317–335.
68. J.W. Evans and P.S. Desai. Applications for three-dimensional printing in dentistry. *J Multidiscip Care*. (Jul 2016).
69. D.C.N. Chan, K.B. Frazier, L. Tse, and D. Rosen. Application of rapid prototyping to operative dentistry curriculum. *J Dent Educ*. 68(1) (2004), pp. 64–70.
70. N. Van Assche, D. Van Steenberghe, M.E. Guerrero, E. Hirsch, F. Schutyser, M. Quirynen, and R. Jacobs. Accuracy of implant placement based on pre-surgical planning of three-dimensional cone-beam images: A pilot study. *Clin Periodontol*. 34 (2007), pp. 816–821.
71. J Xia, HH Ip, N Samman, D. Wang, C.S.B. Kot, R.W.K. Yeung, and H. Tideman. Computer-assisted three-dimensional surgical planning and simulation: 3D virtual osteotomy. *Int J Oral Maxillofac Surg*. 29(1) (2000), pp. 11–17.
72. H. Li, L. Song, J. Sun, J. Ma, and Z. Shen. Dental ceramic prostheses by stereolithography based additive manufacturing: Potentials and challenges. *Adv Appl Ceram*. 118 (2018), pp. 30–36.
73. A. Bhargav, V. Sanjairaj, V. Rosa, L.W. Feng, and Y.J. Fuh. Applications of additive manufacturing in dentistry: A review. *J Biomed Mater Res B Appl Biomater*. 106(5) (2018), pp. 2058–2064.
74. S.N. Kurenov, C. Ionita, D. Sammons, and T.L. Demmy. Three-dimensional printing to facilitate anatomic study, device development, simulation, and planning in thoracic surgery. *J Thorac Cardiovasc Surg*. 149 (2015), pp. 973–979.
75. A. Haleem and M. Javaid. Role of CT and MRI in the design and development of orthopaedic model using additive manufacturing. *J Clin Orthop Trauma*. 9(3) (2018), pp. 213–217.
76. R.P. Singh, R. Kataria, and S. Singhal. Performance evaluation of macor dental ceramic: An investigation with rotary ultrasonic machining. *Adv Dent Oral Health*. 8(2) (2018), pp. 1–6.
77. M. Takemoto, S. Fujibayashi, E. Ota, B. Otsuki, H. Kimura, T. Sakamoto, T. Kawai, T. Futami, K. Sasaki, T. Matsushita, and T. Nakamura. Additive-manufactured patient-specific titanium templates for thoracic pedicle screw placement: Novel design with reduced contact area. *Eur Spine J*. 25(6) (2015), pp. 1698–1705.
78. S. Negi, S. Dhiman, and R.K. Sharma. Basics and applications of rapid prototyping medical models. *Rapid Prototyp J*. 20 (2014), pp. 256–267.
79. V. Karageorgiou and D. Kaplan. Porosity of 3D biomaterial scaffolds and osteogenesis. *Biomaterials*. 26(27) (2005), pp. 5474–5491.
80. D. Mehrotra. Dentistry: Changing paradigm with growth of basic sciences. *J Oral Biol Craniofac Res*. 4(3) (2014), pp. 159.

81. A. Mohammeda, A. Elshaerb, P. Sareha, M. Elsayed, and H. Hassanina. Additive manufacturing technologies for drug delivery applications. *Int. J. Pharm.* 580 (2020), p. 119245.

82. A. Goyanes, M. Kobayashi, R. Martínez-Pacheco, S. Gaisford, and A.W. Basit. Fused-filament 3D printing of drug products: Microstructure analysis and drug release characteristics of PVA-based caplets. *Int. J. Pharm.* 514 (2016), pp. 290–295.

83. A. Goyanes, P. Robles Martinez, A. Buanz, A.W. Basit, and S. Gaisford. Effect of geometry on drug release from 3D printed tablets. *Int. J. Pharm.* 494 (2015), pp. 657–663.

84. S.A. Khaled, J.C. Burley, M.R. Alexander, and C.J. Roberts. Desktop 3D printing controlled release pharmaceutical bilayer tablets. *Int. J. Pharm.* 461 (2014.), pp. 105–111.

85. S.A. Khaled, J.C. Burley, M.R. Alexander, J. Yang, and C.J. Roberts. 3D printing of tablets containing multiple drugs with defined release profiles. *Int. J. Pharm.* 494 (2015), pp. 643–650.

86. T.C. Okwuosa, B.C. Pereira, B. Arafat, M. Cieszynska, A. Isreb, and M.A. Alhnan. Fabricating a shell-core delayed release tablet using dual FDM 3D printing for patient-centred therapy. *Pharmaceutical Research* 34 (2017), pp. 427–437.

87. F. Fina, A. Goyanes, C.M. Madla, A. Awad, S.J. Trenfield, J.M. Kuek, P. Patel, S Gaisford, and A.W. Basit. 3D printing of drug-loaded gyroid lattices using selective laser sintering. *Int. J. Pharm.* 547 (2018), pp. 44–52.

88. A. Awad, F. Fina, S.J. Trenfield, P. Patel, A. Goyanes, S. Gaisford, and A.W. Basit. 3D printed pellets (Miniprintlets): A novel, multi-drug. Controlled release platform technology. *Pharmaceutics* 11 (2019), p. 148.

89. M. Kyobula, A. Adedeji, M.R. Alexander, E. Saleh, R. Wildman, I. Ashcroft, P.R. Gellert, and C.J. Roberts. 3D inkjet printing of tablets exploiting bespoke complex geometries for controlled and tuneable drug release. *J. Control. Release* 261 (2017), pp. 207–215.

90. C.W. Rowe, W.E. Katstra, R.D. Palazzolo, B. Giritlioglu, P. Teung, and M.J. Cima. Multimechanism oral dosage forms fabricated by three dimensional printing™. *J. Control. Release* 66 (2000), pp. 11–17.

91. D.G. Yu, X.L. Yang, W.D. Huang, J. Liu, Y.G. Wang, and H. Xu. Tablets With Material Gradients Fabricated by Three-Dimensional Printing. *J. Pharm. Sci.* 96 (2007), pp. 2446–2456.

92. D.G. Yu, X.-X Shen, C. Branford-White, L.M. Zhu, K. White, and X.L. Yang. Novel oral fast-disintegrating drug delivery devices with predefined inner structure fabricated by Three-Dimensional Printing. *J. Pharm. Pharmacol.* 61 (2009), pp. 323–329.

93. K.K. Jain. Current status and future prospects of drug delivery systems. In: Jain, K.K. (Ed.), *Drug Delivery System*. Springer, New York, NY, (2014), pp. 1–56.

94. A. Hussain and F. Ahsan. The vagina as a route for systemic drug delivery. *J. Control. Release*. 103 (2005), pp. 301–313.

95. Y. Sun, X. Ruan, H. Li, H. Kathuria, G. Du, and L. Kang. Fabrication of non-dissolving analgesic suppositories using 3D printed moulds. *Int. J. Pharm.* 513 (2016), pp. 717–724.

96. J.A. Weisman, D.H. Ballard, U. Jammalamadaka, K. Tappa, J. Sumerel, H.B. D'Agostino, D.K. Mills, and P.K. Woodard. 3D printed antibiotic and chemotherapeutic eluting catheters for potential use in interventional radiology. In vitro proof of concept study. *Academic Radiology* 26 (2019), pp. 270–274.

97. C.L. Caudill, J.L. Perry, S. Tian, J.C. Luft, and J.M. DeSimone. Spatially controlled coating of continuous liquid interface production microneedles for transdermal protein delivery. *J. Control. Release*. 284 (2018), pp. 122–132.

98. S.C. Cox, P. Jamshidi, N.M. Eisenstein, M.A. Webber, H. Hassanin, M.M. Attallah, D.E.T. Shepherd, O. Addison, and L.M. Grover. Adding functionality with additive manufacturing: Fabrication of titanium-based antibiotic eluting implants. *Materials Science and Engineering: C* 64 (2016), pp. 407–415.

99. H. Hassanin, L. Finet, S.C. Cox, P. Jamshidi, L.M. Grover, D.E.T. Shepherd, O. Addison, and M.M. Attallah. Tailoring selective laser melting process for titanium drug delivering implants with releasing micro-channels. *Additive Manufacturing* 20 (2018), pp. 144–155.

100. R.K. Chen, Y. Jin, J. Wensman, and A. Shih. Additive manufacturing of custom orthoses and prostheses—a review. *Additive Manufacturing* 12 (2016), pp. 77–89.

101. J.H.P. Pallari, K.W. Dalgarno, and J. Woodburn. Mass customisation of foot orthosesfor rheumatoid arthritis. *Proceedings of the 19th Annual International SolidFreeform Fabrication Symposium* (2008), pp. 130–137.

102. J.M. Saleh and K.W. Dalgarno. Cost and benefit analysis of fused deposition modelling (FDM) technique and selective laser sintering (SLS) for fabrication of customised foot orthoses. In: *Innovative Developments in Design and Manufacturing*. CRC Press, Boca Raton, FL, (Sep 22, 2009), pp. 723–728.

103. S.P. Sun, Y. J. Chou, and C.C. Sue. Classification and mass production techniquefor three-quarter shoe insoles using non-weight-bearing plantar shapes. *Appl. Ergon.* 40(4) (2009), pp. 630–635.

104. D. Cook, V. Gervasi, R. Rizza, S. Kamara, and X.C. Liu. Additive fabrication ofcustom pedorthoses for clubfoot correction. *Rapid Prototyp. J.* 16(3) (2010), pp. 189–193.

105. J.H.P. Pallari, K.W. Dalgarno, and J. Woodburn. Mass customization of footorthoses for rheumatoid arthritis using selective laser sintering. *IEEE Trans. Biomed. Eng.* 57(7) (2010), pp. 1750–1756.

106. J.H.P. Pallari, K.W. Dalgarno, J. Munguia, L. Muraru, L. Peeraer, S. Telfer, and J. Woodburn. Design and additive fabrication of foot and ankle-foot orthoses. *Proceedings of the 21st Annual International Solid Freeform Fabrication Symposium* (2010), pp. 834–845.

107. A.S. Salles and D.E. Gyi. Delivering personalised insoles to the high street using additive manufacturing. *Int. J. Comput. Integr. Manuf.* 26(5) (2013), pp. 1–15.

108. A.S. Salles and D.E. Gyi. The specification of personalised insoles using additive manufacturing. *Work.* 41 (2012), pp. 1771–1774.

109. A.S. Salles and D.E. Gyi. An evaluation of personalised insoles developed using additive manufacturing. *J. Sports Sci.* 31(4) (2013), pp. 442–450.

110. J.M. Saleh. Cost modelling of rapid manufacturing based mass customisation system for fabrication of custom Foor orthoses. PhD Thesis, University of Newcastle (2013).

111. R.K. Chen, Y.A. Jin, J. Wensman, and A. Shih. Additive manufacturing of custom orthoses and prostheses—A review. *Addit. Manuf.* 12 (1 Oct, 2016), pp. 77–89.

112. S. Telfer, J. Pallari, J. Munguia, K. Dalgarno, M. McGeough, and J. Woodburn Embracing additive manufacture: Implications for foot and ankle orthosis design. *BMC Musculoskelet Disord.* 13 (2012), p. 84.

113. S. Milusheva, D. Tochev, L. Stefanova, and Y. Toshev. Virtual models and prototypeof individual ankle foot orthosis. *Proceedings of ISB XXth Congress – ASB29th Annual Meeting* (2005), p. 227.

114. S.M. Milusheva, E.Y. Tosheva, Y.E. Toshev, and R. Taiar. Ankle foot orthosis with exchangeable elastic elements. *Ser. Biomech.* 23(1) (2007), pp. 90–95.

115. M.C. Faustini, R.R. Neptune, R.H. Crawford, and S.J. Stanhope. Manufacture of passive dynamic ankle-foot orthoses using selective laser sintering. *IEEE Trans. Biomed. Eng.* 55(2) (2008), pp. 784–790.

116. C. Mavroidis, R.G. Ranky, M.L. Sivak, B.L. Patritti, J. DiPisa, A. Caddle, K. Gilhooly, L. Govoni, S. Sivak, M. Lancia, R. Drillio, and P. Bonato. Patient specific ankle-foot orthoses using rapid prototyping, *J. Neuroeng. Rehabil.* 8(1) (2011), pp. 1–11.

117. E.S. Schrank and S.J. Stanhope. Dimensional accuracy of ankle-foot orthoses constructed by rapid customization and manufacturing framework. *J. Rehabil.Res. Dev.* 48(1) (2011), pp. 31–42.

118. V. Creylman, L. Muraru, J. Pallari, H. Vertommen, and L. Peeraer. Gait assessment during the initial fitting of customized selective laser sintering ankle foot orthoses in subjects with drop foot. *Prosthet. Orthot. Int.* 37(2) (2013), pp. 132–138.

119. E.S. Schrank, L. Hitch, K. Wallace, R. Moore, and S.J. Stanhope. Assessment of a virtual functional prototyping process for the rapid manufacture of passive-dynamic ankle-foot orthoses, *J. Biomech. Eng.* 135(10) (2013), pp. 101011–101017.

120. R.K. Chen, L. Chen, B.L. Tai, Y. Wang, A.J. Shih, and J. Wensman. Additive manufacturing of personalized ankle-foot orthosis. *Proceedings of Transactions of the North American Manufacturing Research Institution of SME (NAMRC42)*. (2014).

121. N.G. Harper, E.M. Russell, J.M. Wilken, and R.R. Neptune. Selective laser sintered versus carbon fiber passive-dynamic ankle-foot orthoses: A comparison of patient walking performance. *J. Biomech. Eng.* 136 (9) (2014), p. 091001.

122. W.E. Rogers, R.H. Crawford, J.J. Beaman, and N.E. Walsh. Fabrication of prosthetic sockets by selective laser sintering. *Solid Freeform Fabrication Symposium Proceedings* 6 (1991), pp. 158–163.

123. W.E. Rogers, R.H. Crawford, V. Faulkner, and J.J. Beaman. Fabrication of an integrated prosthetic socket using solid freeform fabrication. *7th World Congress of the International Society for Prosthetics and Orthotics* (1992), p. b12.

124. D. Freeman and L. Wontorcik. Stereolithography and prosthetic test socket manufacture: A cost/benefit analysis. *J. Prosthet. Orthot.* 10(1) (1998), pp. 17–20.

125. B. Rogers, S. Stephens, A. Gitter, G. Bosker, and R. Crawford. Double-wall, transtibial prosthetic socket fabricated using selective laser sintering: A case study. *J Prosthet. Orthot.* 12(3) (2000), pp. 97–103.

126. S. Stephens, R. Crawford, W. Rogers, A. Gitter, and G. Bosker. Manufacture of compliant prosthesis sockets using selective laser sintering. *11th Freeform Fabrication Symposium* (2000), pp. 565–577.

127. B. Rogers, A. Gitter, G. Bosker, M. Faustini, M. Lokhande, and R. Crawford. Clinical evaluation of prosthetic sockets manufactured by selective laser sintering. *2001 Solid Freeform Fabrication Symposium Proceedings* (2001), pp. 505–512.

128. J.T. Montgomery, M.R. Vaughan, and R.H. Crawford. Design of an actively actuated prosthetic socket. *Rapid Prototyp. J.* 16(3) (2010), pp. 194–201.

129. J.C.H. Goh, P.V.S. Lee, and P. Ng. Structural integrity of polypropylene prosthetic sockets manufactured using the polymer deposition technique. *Proc. Inst. Mech. Eng. H.* 216(6) (2002), pp. 359–368.

130. P. Ng, P.S.V. Lee, and J.C.H. Goh. Prosthetic sockets fabrication using rapid prototyping technology. *Rapid Prototyp. J.* 8(1) (2002), pp. 53–59.

131. F.E.H. Tay, M. Manna, and L.X. Liu. A CASD/CASM method for prosthetic socket fabrication using the FDM technology. *Rapid Prototyp. J.* 8(4) (2002), pp. 258–262.

132. N. Herbert, D. Simpson, W.D. Spence, and W. Ion. A preliminary investigation into the development of 3D printing of prosthetic sockets. *J. Rehabil. Res. Dev.* 42(2) (2005), pp. 141–146.

133. W.C. Chuang, H.H. Hsieh, L.H. Hsu, H.J. Ho, J.T. Chen, and M.J. Tzeng. A system for supporting the design of total surface bearing transtibial sockets. *Comput. Aided Des. Appl.* 8(5) (2011), pp. 723–734.

134. L.H. Hsu, G.F. Huang, C.T. Lu, C.W. Lai, Y.M. Chen, I.C. Yu, and H.S. Shih. The application of rapid prototyping for the design and manufacturing of transtibial prosthetic socket. *Mater. Sci. Forum* 594 (2008), pp. 273–280.

135. L.H. Hsu, G.F. Huang, C.T. Lu, D.Y. Hong, and S.H. Liu. The development of a rapid prototyping prosthetic socket coated with a resin layer for transtibial amputees. *Prosthet. Orthot. Int.* 34(1) (2010), pp. 37–45.

136. D.M. Sengeh and H. Herr. A variable-impedance prosthetic socket for a transtibial amputee designed from magnetic resonance imaging data. *J. Prosthet. Orthot.* 25(3) (2013), pp. 129–137.

137. K. Subburaj, C. Nair, S. Rajesh, S.M. Meshram, and B. Ravi. Rapid development of auricular prosthesis using CAD and rapid prototyping technologies. *Int. J. Oral Maxillofac. Surg.* 36(10) (2007), pp. 938–943.

138. P. Liacouras, J. Garnes, N. Roman, A. Petrich, and G.T. Grant. Designing and manufacturing an auricular prosthesis using computed tomography,3-dimensional photographic imaging, and additive manufacturing: A clinical report. *J. Prosthet. Dent.* 105(2) (2011), pp. 78–82.

139. A.M. Paterson, R. Bibb, R.I. Campbell, and G. Bingham. Comparing additive manufacturing technologies for customised wrist splints. *Rapid Prototyp. J.* 21(3) (2015), pp. 230–243.

140. S.A. Dalley, T.E. Wiste, T.J. Withrow, and M. Goldfarb. Design of a multifunctional anthropomorphic prosthetic hand with extrinsic actuation. *IEEE/ASME Trans. Mechatron.* 14 (6) (2009), pp. 699–706.

141. S.A. Dalley, T.E. Wiste, H.A. Varol, and M. Goldfarb. A multi-grasp hand prosthesis for transradial amputees. *2010 Annual International Conference of the IEEE Engineering in Medicine and Biology Society* (2010), pp. 5062–5065.

142. J. Zuniga, D. Katsavelis, J. Peck, J. Stollberg, M. Petrykowski, A. Carson, and C. Fernandez. Cyborg beast: A low-cost 3d-printed prosthetic hand for children with upper-limb differences. *BMC Res. Notes* 8 (2015) pp. 10.

143. M.T. Leddy, J.T. Belter, K.D. Gemmell, and A.M. Dollar. Lightweight custom composite prosthetic components using an additive manufacturing-based molding technique. In: *2015 37th Annual International Conference of the IEEE Engineering in Medicine and Biology Society (EMBC)*, IEEE, (2015), pp. 4797–4802.

144. B.J. South, N.P. Fey, G. Bosker, and R.R. Neptune. Manufacture of energy storage and return prosthetic feet using selective laser sintering. *J. Biomech. Eng.* 132(1) (2010), pp. 015001–1–6.

145. J.D. Ventura, G.K. Klute, and R.R. Neptune. The effects of prosthetic ankle dorsiflexion and energy return on below-knee amputee leg loading. *Clin. Biomech.* 26(3) (2011), pp. 298–303.

146. Q. Yan, H. Dong, J. Su, J. Han, B. Song, Q. Wei, and Y. Shi. A review of 3D printing technology for medical applications. *Engineering.* 4(5) (2018), pp. 729–742.

147. J.H.P. Pallari, K.W. Dalgarno, J. Munguia, L. Muraru, L. Peeraer, S. Telfer, and J. Woodburn. Design and additive fabrication of foot and ankle-foot orthoses. *Proceedings of the 21st Annual International Solid Freeform Fabrication Symposium* (2010), pp. 834–845.

148. B. Rogers, G.W. Bosker, R.H. Crawford, M.C. Faustini, R.R. Neptune, G. Walden, and A.J. Gitter. Advanced trans-tibial socket fabrication using selective laser sintering. *Prosthet. Orthot. Int.* 31(1) (2007), pp. 88–100.

149. A.S. Salles and D.E. Gyi. Delivering personalised insoles to the high street using additive manufacturing. *Int. J. Comput. Integr. Manuf.* 26(5) (2013), 386–400.

150. N. Herbert, D. Simpson, W.D. Spence, and W. Ion. A preliminary investigation into the development of 3D printing of prosthetic sockets. *J. Rehabil. Res. Dev.* 42(2) (2005), pp. 141–146.

8 Additive Manufacturing in Biomedical Engineering
Present and Future Applications

Vidyapati Kumar[1], Chander Prakash[2], Atul Babbar[3], Shubham Choudhary[4], Ankit Sharma[5] and Amrinder Singh Uppal[6]

[1] Department of Mechanical Engineering, Indian Institute of Technology, Kharagpur 721302, India

[2] School of Mechanical Engineering, Lovely Professional University, Phagwara 144001, India

[3] Department of Mechanical Engineering, Shree Guru Gobind Singh Tricentenary University, Gurugram 122505, India

[4] Department of Mechanical Engineering, Ajay Kumar Garg Engineering College, Ghaziabad-201009, India

[5] Chitkara College of Applied Engineering, Chitkara University, Rajpura 140401, India

[6] Merla Wellhead Solution, 51 Esplanade Blvd Suite 600, Houston, TX 77060, USA

CONTENTS

8.1 Introduction 144
8.2 AM 145
    8.2.1 Steps Involved in Production through the AM Process 146
8.3 Biomedical Application of AM 148
    8.3.1 Medical Models 148
    8.3.2 Implants 150
    8.3.3 Medical Device Parts, Tools and Instruments 151
    8.3.4 Medical Aids, Splints, and Prostheses 151
    8.3.5 Biomanufacturing 152

DOI: 10.1201/9781003217961-8

8.4   Discussion and Conclusion.. 153
      8.4.1   Limitations of Previous Reviews 153
      8.4.2   Rarely Used Processes—DED, SL 154
      8.4.3   Prevalent Techniques—PBF, ME, VP... 154
      8.4.4   Techniques Prevalent in Some Application Areas—MJ, BJ............. 155
8.5   Conclusion and Future Possibilities.. 155
References... 156

8.1   INTRODUCTION

In the current environment, advanced three-dimensional (3D) printing technology has acquired widespread appeal due to its several advantages over traditional and nontraditional manufacturing (AM) processes, including cost reduction, speed, design flexibility, one-step manufacturing, and sustainable development. AM is the layer-by-layer creation of a 3D item from a computer-aided-design (CAD) model or a digital 3D model, which simplifies the process of machining and eliminates superfluous material from a bigger stock. This technique is unusual in that it immediately converts the material to its final shape with minimal material waste while achieving the requisite geometric proportions. Due to the availability of a larger range of 3D-printing processes [1–4], this AM process is used for a specific material and application, making it a challenging effort to determine the appropriate AM technique. Depending on the material used for printing, different methods offer different surface finishes, high-dimensional precision, and postprocessing needs. AM has applications in a variety of fields, including aerospace, structural, biomedical, and complicated component production, among others. Furthermore, AM has drawn a lot of interest because of its versatility in quickly making cost-effective, surgical tools and patient-specific bio-implants [5–8]. AM has been successfully used to repair or fabricate human body tissues such as dental implants, artificial livers, and artificial cardiovascular systems, but it is not restricted to orthopedic implants; it may also be used to fabricate medical electronic and microfluidic devices. Stress shielding occurs in this circumstance owing to a mechanical mismatch between metal implants and native body parts or organs, resulting in organ or part resorption failure and implant failure. This form of implant failure is more common in implants that are made using traditional manufacturing techniques. As a result, it is critical to create an AM technique that demonstrates to be a feasible option for fabricating prostheses with regulated strength and porosity that match the characteristics of natural bone and organs, reducing the risk of stress shielding. The ability to create highly personalized medical implants utilizing 3D-printing technology has provided a once-in-a-lifetime chance to address particular body component issues [9–11]. As a demand-based manufacturing approach, AM's ability to manufacture complex-shaped implants has made the technique considerably more affordable and cost-effective. AM does not require any tools for product fabrication, resulting in the same cost per component in this process, but in traditional machining, the cost of tooling plays a larger role in determining the cost of AM components [12–26]. The economic study established a case for using 3D printing to fabricate body implants

[27]. Different kinds of processes and techniques have been implemented to fabricate the necessary parts for AM equipment [28–59].

8.2 AM

It is feasible to create objects with complex architecture in a short amount of time using AM techniques. 3D product model data generated by CAD is necessary for this purpose. AM techniques do not need the modeling of machining technology processes, tool and mold design, particular machining equipment, distribution and warehousing operations, and so forth [16, 60–63]. Only the fundamentals of manufacturing processes and how the machine applies a material are required.

Rapid prototyping and rapid production are two major applications of AM technology. Figure 8.1 depicts the various types of AM processes and their types.

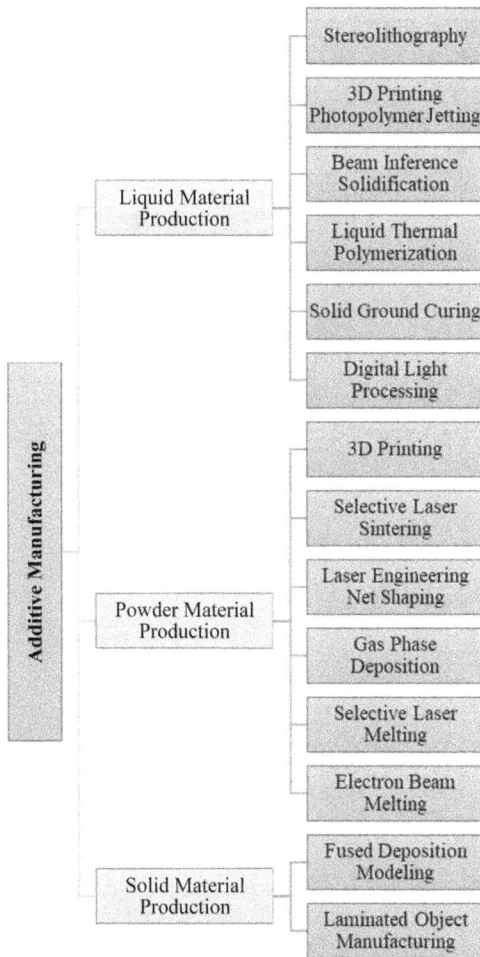

FIGURE 8.1 Classification of AM process.

8.2.1 Steps Involved in Production through the AM Process

The process of AM entails a number of processes that go from a virtual CAD model to a real item as shown in Figure 8.2. These are the procedures to follow:

1. **CAD:** All prototyped components must start with a software model that correctly represents the external geometry. It's possible to utilize almost any professional CAD solid modeling program, but the output must be a 3D solid or surface rendering. Reverse-engineering equipment may be used to create this image.
2. **Conversion to STL format:** STL stands for stereolithography, and almost every AM machine understands the STL file format, which has become the de facto industry standard, and nearly any CAD system can generate one. This file is used to calculate the slices and specifies the externally enclosed surfaces of the original CAD model.
3. **Machine transfer and STL file manipulation:** The part's STL file must be transferred to the AM machine. It's conceivable that the file will be altered in some manner in order to bring it to the appropriate dimensions, placement, and alignment for building.

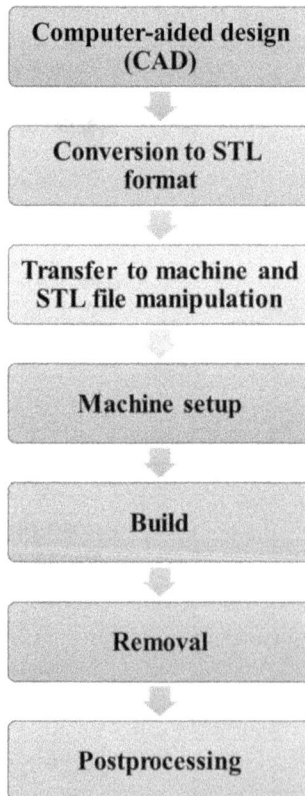

FIGURE 8.2   Steps of the AM process.

4. **Installation of machinery:** Prior to beginning the construction process, the machine must be correctly set up. These options would be related to construction characteristics such as material limitations, energy supply, layer thickness, and timings, among others.

5. **Build:** The method of manufacturing the component is highly automated, and the equipment can work without observation for the most part.

6. **Removal:** The pieces must be removed when the machine has finished the construction. This may need contact with the machinery, which may have protective interlocks in place to guarantee that, for instance, the operating temperature is kept below a certain level or that no actively moving parts are present.

7. **Postprocessing:** After components have been removed from equipment, they may need further cleaning before they are ready for use. Parts may be weak or have supporting features that need to be deleted at this time. This often requires patience and dexterity of the hands. They may, however, need further processing before being used or assembled with other mechanical or electrical components to create a completed model.

The issue of what the benefits of AM are in comparison to conventional methods and technology is frequently raised. Most of the time, the issue is if it is cheaper to produce, but the entire component and methodology life cycle ought to be examined. Genuine production costs can't be used as the primary criterion for success. Table 8.1 outlines some of the medical and dentistry advantages of AM. Identical advantages may frequently be seen in domains other than medicine and dentistry, such as the industrial sector, where a database system of manufacturing spare parts has a significant correlation with the digital storage of dental data.

There are seven distinct types of AM methods, according to the American Society for Testing and Materials (ASTM) and International Organization for Standardization (ISO) [1]:

- Powder bed fusion (PBF)
- Material extrusion (ME)
- Vat photopolymerization (VP)
- Material jetting (MJ)
- Binder jetting (BJ)
- Sheet lamination (SL)
- Directed energy deposition (DED)

Each area contains a large number of suppliers, services, and material possibilities, which might be troublesome because standard language is still not used in most research, and procedures are frequently referred to by trade names. Table 8.2 displays the details of the processing categories, along with a brief description, as well as the most frequent material, brand titles, and how successfully the procedure is utilized to make plastics, metals or ceramics. Some methods, such as DED, VP, and MJ for metals, are still in the developing stage, while others, such as SL of ceramics or DED of plastics and ceramics, appear to be nonexistent. There may be scientific research and trials of these, but there are no industrial suppliers. New processes and component

TABLE 8.1

Medical and Dentistry Advantages of AM

Authors	Outcomes	Application Domain
Ballard et al. [64]	Savings in both money and time	Maxillofacial and orthopedic incision
Choonara et al. [65]	Personalization	Transplantation
Mahmoud et al. [66]	Monetary reductions	Patho-biological samples for academics
Tack et al. [67]	Time reductions, quality diagnostic outcomes, lowered radioactivity	Surgery
Ballard et al. [68]	Utilization of antibiotic therapy	Implantation
Lin et al. [69]	Customization, monetary savings	Dentistry
Javaid et al. [70]	Customization, digital storage, and cost and time reductions	Dentistry
Aho et al. [71]	Personalization	Pharmaceutical
Salmi et al. [72]	Reduction in labor-intensive activity	Dentistry accessories
Aquino et al. [73]	Just-in-time production, customization	Pharmaceutical
Javaid et al. [74]	Customization, reliability, savings in both money and time, completely autonomous and digital production	Orthopedical area
Emelogu et al. [75]	Opportunities in the supply chain	Implantation
Haleem et al. [76]	Capacity to work with a variety of components	Medical
Murr et al. [77]	Capacity to create intricate symmetries	Implantation
Peltola et al. [78]	Implant-formation template	Implantation
Ramakrishnaiah et al. [79]	Better osseointegration and stability with a rough and porous surface roughness	Dentistry Implantation
Nazir et al. [80]	Variations in design, supply chain options, and complicated geometries	Medical instruments
Yang et al. [81]	Increased anatomical knowledge and surgical precision	Surgery
Gibson et al. [82]	Using a surgeon as a designer has the potential to be really innovative	Surgery

composition are frequently created in response to demand, which typically emphasizes big firms and a significant need. In most cases, this results in the identification of a widely utilized component that may be used in a number of applications.

8.3 BIOMEDICAL APPLICATION OF AM

8.3.1 Medical Models

Health care designs, which are centered on human physiology, can be utilized for surgical preparation and mentoring before and after the surgery, medical student

TABLE 8.2
Details of the Processing Categories of AM

Additive Manufacturing Process	Outline	Structure of Component	Plastics	Metals	Ceramics	Trademarks
PBF	Regions of a powder bed are fused using heat energy.	Powdered	✓✓✓	✓✓✓	✓	SLS, DMLS, SLM
ME	a substance that is sprayed via a jet	Glue, granules, and wire	✓✓✓	✓✓	✓✓	FDM, FFF
VP	Light is utilized for curing the liquid photopolymer in a vat	liquefied	✓✓✓	✓	✓✓	SLA, DLP
MJ	Globules of particles are sprayed in a controlled manner	liquefied	✓✓✓	✓	✓	PolyJet, NJP
BJ	In a regulated way, a liquefied adhesive material is applied	Powdered	✓✓✓	✓	✓	3DP, CJP
SL	Material sheets are glued together.	sheets	✓✓	✓✓	✗	LOM, UAM
DED	Concentrated thermal radiation is used to melt components together while depositing	Powdered, wire form	✗	✓✓✓	✓	LENS, EBAM

Note: PBF, powder bed fusion; ME, material extrusion; VP, vat photopolymerization; MJ, material jetting; BJ, binder jetting; SL, sheet lamination; DED, directed energy deposition; SLS, selective laser sintering; DMLS, direct metal laser sintering; SLM, selective laser melting; FDM, fused deposition modeling; FFF, fused filament fabrication; DLP, digital light projection; 3DP, 3D printing; CJP, ColorJet printing; LOM, laminated object manufacturing; UAM, ultrasonic additive manufacturing; LENS, laser-engineered net shaping.

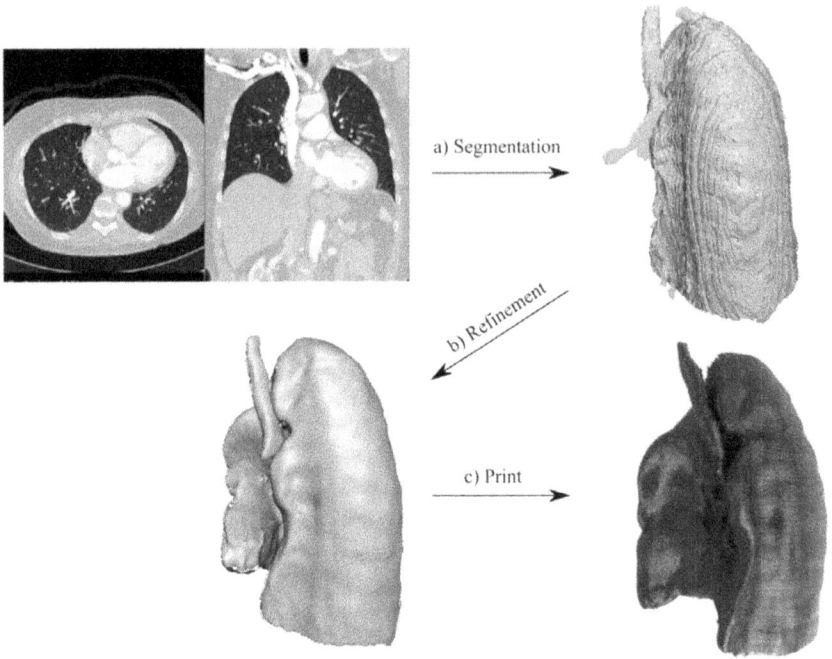

FIGURE 8.3   Process workflow for manufacturing medical models [85].

training and patient and family education [67, 83]. The shape may be changed by removing only the most intriguing portions or stretching it upward or downward. A kinesthetic reaction near the bone may be useful if prototypes are utilized for teaching, such as bone drilling. Health care designs are frequently utilized in the craniomaxillofacial region; however, there are several cases from other bones frameworks, such as the backbone and pelvis [67, 84]. It may be necessary to sterilize the models if they are used in the operating room, but the material option is generally fairly flexible, highlighting the fact that this is among the most well-known uses. Figure 8.3 shows a general medical model production method workflow, which starts with patient physiology captured using imaging techniques such as computed tomography (CT), magnetic resonance imaging (MRI) or ultrasound and ends with segmentation algorithms constructing a 3D model geometry for AM [85]. Postprocessing, such as eliminating support structures, is frequently required following AM.

8.3.2   IMPLANTS

Implants are made in an additive or indirect way to restore damaged or missing tissue [86–87]. Dental applications such as crowns and bridges are also included in this category [88]. Tissue compatibility is required, and the criteria are stringent, with lengthy approval processes. Cell adhesion may be affected by surface characteristics. Some of the most recent research [89–90] have looked at material embedding

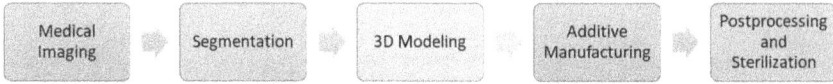

FIGURE 8.4   Process workflow for implants.

techniques into implants as a sort of a medication distribution network. AM is a good option for customized implants, and a typical method involves capturing a patient's anatomy in the same way as medical models do. Then, to allow patient-specific fitting, this digital 3D prototype of the human morphology is employed as a designing inspiration [91]. The PBF technique is utilized to produce the majority of typical implants, which requires numerous postprocessing procedures such as honing the structures, grinding, and thermal treatment options. Implants must be disinfected before being used in a therapeutic setting. Figure 8.4 depicts a typical AM process flow for implants, commencing with medical imaging and segmentation and progressing to 3D modeling, postprocessing and sterilizing.

8.3.3   MEDICAL DEVICE PARTS, TOOLS AND INSTRUMENTS

Medical devices, equipment, as well as components enable or improve clinical operations. They may utilize patient-specific sizes and variations in drilling guides, for instance [92], and they may be invasive and need sterilization since they can come into contact with the water, lipids, cells, and organ systems for a short time period. This category includes specialized equipment and periodontal equipment [93–95]. The VP method is used to create molds for vacuum-forming transparent orthodontic aligners, which is one of the most well-known and effective businesses in this area. When patient-specific dimensions are utilized, the process is similar to that of implantation and before surgical models from healthcare image acquisition or 3D scans. If a human-focused geometrical or alignment is not needed, 3D modeling may be done from idea to implementation or utilizing a 3D design of the sufferer's physiology. Postprocessing includes support removal, heat treatments, milling, and sterilizing. Figure 8.5 depicts a typical production flow used to create tools, instruments, and components for medical devices. Obtaining an imprint of the patient's teeth, 3D scanning it, 3D modeling, VP AM, postprocessing and using the component as a mold for soft orthodontic aligners are just a few examples of stages in the process.

8.3.4   MEDICAL AIDS, SPLINTS, AND PROSTHESES

AM parts are not part of the human body, and they may be coupled with conventional equipment to aid with modification. Protracted and postsurgery stabilizers, mobility aides, fixators, prosthetic implants, customized orthotics and orthopedic activities all fall into this group [96–98]. Medical imaging may be the first step, followed by segmentation, 3D scanning or 3D measuring, all of which may give data for the 3D-rendering transition stage. Complementary production methods for AMs, such as computer numerical control (CNC) technology, are extensively used [99].

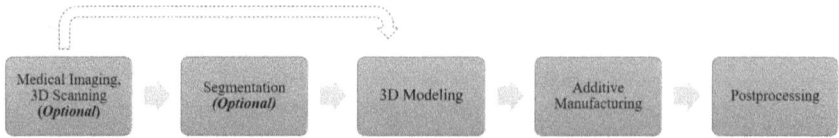

FIGURE 8.5   Process workflow for medical device parts, tools and instruments.

Depending on the purpose, postprocessing may involve supporter removals, thermal treatment options, and decoration or glazing. Figure 8.6 depicts a typical AM workflow for medical aids, supporting guides, splints, and prostheses. An excellent example is a movable external support for a pilon fracture that was built using 3D modeling and additive manufacturing components to place the hinge such that it regulates the movement under force near the ankle's free mobility.

8.3.5   BIOMANUFACTURING

AM and tissue engineering are combined in biomanufacturing [100]. A wide range of polymeric materials, ceramic materials, and composites are used since they must be physiologically friendly and regularly active with the body. Cell specialization may be influenced by porous structures with culture and a 3D matrix. It may be osteoinductive, osteoconductive, or resorbable depending on the material [101–103]. Contours may be modified to fit certain faults [104]. The patient's geometry must be recorded via medical imaging or 3D scanning for customized shapes. Micro- and macrostructures are modeled in the 3D-modeling phase, and porous structures are frequently employed for cell attraction and proliferation. It's common to need a sterile technique or things that can be sanitized after printing. It's possible that cell development in vitro and in vivo studies will be required before final application. Figure 8.6 shows a patient's anatomy using CT and segmentation and then 3D modeling and AM of an orbital floor resorbable implant. After manufacturing, the implant is sterilized.

The applications mentioned in the preceding section make use of a variety of AM techniques. For the hard-to-find application areas for particular processes, a search was conducted first using ISO/ASTM terminology with a mix of AM medical application keywords in a specific class and then using trade names or other widely used names for the processes, such as the manufacturer name. The goal was to locate at least a few instances for each category, as well as to figure out which regions lacked certain applications and procedures, and why. Scopus, Web of Science and Google Scholar were the databases utilized for the search. There has been earlier research on PBF of metallic implants [105–106], AM of medical equipment [93], biomaterials in medical AM [107], and medical phantoms and regenerated tissue and organ applications using AM [108], to name a few. Previous research has either failed to classify AM processes or has only looked at a single one. Various optimization [109–113] and selection strategies [114] may also be utilized to ensure optimum biomaterial selection and manufacture for application as implants, scaffolds and prosthetics devices.

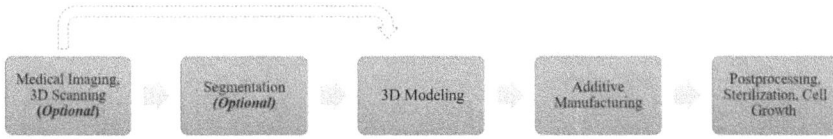

FIGURE 8.6 Process workflow for medical aids, supportive guides, splints and prostheses.

TABLE 8.3

Search Terminologies in the Application Area of Medical or Dental or Implants or Surgery or Clinical

AM Process	Process Term
PBF	PBF is an abbreviation for powder bed fusion, often known as SLS (selective laser sintering) or DMLS (direct metal laser sintering).
ME	ME is sometimes referred to as material extrusion, FFF (fused filament fabrication), or FDM (fused deposition modeling).
VP	Vat photopolymerization or stereolithography (SLA)
MJ	Material jetting or Polyjet or nanoparticle jetting
BJ	It is also known as binder jetting or Colorjet printing.
SL	SL is an abbreviation for sheet lamination, which is also known as laminated object manufacturing (LOM).
DED	It is known as directed energy deposition or LENS (laser-engineered net shaping).

Some studies simply looked at the materials that were used, while others only looked at the applications themselves, with no mention of the AM procedures or materials. The search emphasis was then moved to additional processes and applications when at least three specific application classes and processes were discovered. Table 8.3 shows some specific search terms.

8.4 DISCUSSION AND CONCLUSION

8.4.1 LIMITATIONS OF PREVIOUS REVIEWS

Many evaluations of AM's medicinal uses have been published [70, 74, 93, 115–122]. The majority of them concentrate on specific application areas, such as surgical tools [93], orthopedics [74], and cardiology [115], or on specific materials, such as metals for prosthodontic applications [122]. Some researchers have looked at different AM techniques, such as ME and BJ for making medicines [123] or ME, BJ, VP or PBF methods for creating ceramics for dental purposes [118]. Furthermore, other researchers focused just on the general applications of AM [119] or the entire process chain advances, such as the design phase. There are studies that focus on applications and even categorize them in specific AM methods, such as VP, ME and PBF [116–117], but there is none for the others. There are reviews in dentistry that categorize different AM processes, such as ME, BJ, VP, PBF, MJ and [70, 120], or that focus specifically on metallic implants in dentistry that use the PBF process [121].

The limitations are generally that the utilized AM processes are not specified at all, that trade names and the like are used to represent the technology or that the reviews do not relate the applications to the specific AM processes. This is the most significant barrier to systematic reviews and statistics. The names FFF, FDM, and filament freeform fabrication, for example, are used in the literature to describe the ME process. These words are linked because Stratasys registered and trademarked FDM, forcing other manufacturers to coin a new phrase. Other disciplines in AM face similar difficulties. Materials, on the other hand, are typically thoroughly defined, with metals such as titanium alloys, thermoplastics and photopolymers being the most prevalent.

8.4.2 Rarely Used Processes—DED, SL

DED is mostly utilized in implants, but even still, it's rare. This might be due to the lack of precision and poor surface quality. Typically, the procedure is limited to metals. One prospective use would be to investigate mending parts for medical equipment, as it has already been done in other sectors [124]. However, rigorous medical device laws may limit usage because each repair may require its own clearance procedure if the repair method is too identical in all situations. Metals, such as titanium alloys, are commonly employed in directed energy deposition for implants, which restricts its usage in medical models, for example. SL is only used for clinical prototypes or phantoms [125–126], which tends to indicate its ability to create full-color, realistic-looking models [127]. Other industries that utilize a fresh product as a sheet have a tough time working with it since fresh material samples are seldom in the shape of strips. On the metallic front, the idea is to integrate dissimilar metallic materials in distinct layers that might broaden options, such as giving functional capacity to particular implants and medical equipment via bimetal components [128–130]. On the marketplace, there are only two producers of SL machines: metal-based Fabrisonic and paper-based, which appears to be under administration.

8.4.3 Prevalent Techniques—PBF, ME, VP

PBF, MEX, and VP are all well-known techniques utilized in medical and dental applications [105, 131–132]. This may be because these are perhaps the most used procedures in the organization; there is inexpensive research equipment accessible, and they are easily available as starting ingredients to investigate in powder, resin, pellet or paste form. In addition, new materials may be mixed with older ones. Metals, particularly titanium alloys, are perhaps the most often used components for implantation, while polymers such as polyamide, acrylonitrile butadiene styrene (ABS), nylon, and other photocurable resins are used for a variety of purposes. The ME of reinforced composites would be an attractive material when minimal weight is needed, such as for prostheses, and there are new advances in metal extrusion that may work in a variety of applications [133–136].

8.4.4   Techniques Prevalent in Some Application Areas—MJ, BJ

Implants and biomanufacturing do not require MJ. This might be due to the technology's difficulty, as the material must be forced through many tiny nozzles, comparable to inkjet 2D printing. MJ, on the other hand, is a very precise technique, making it ideal for medical models that require great precision. Material jetting may also create components with various materials and colors, as shown in medical models [137].

BJ is not used in the medical device category for equipment, instruments, or components. The explanation for this might be that components created using BJ are typically weaker than those made with other techniques [138]. It's a great technique for medical models since it allows you to utilize colors and doesn't require any support structures; plus, it's quick and inexpensive [139, 140]. The gypsum-based powders ZP150 and ZP151 are the most prevalent. Metals and biomaterials are also employed in the process. HP and Desktop Metal are now working on BJ-based manufacturing systems for metal components, which would allow the BJ method to be used for tools, instruments and medical device parts [141–143].

8.5   CONCLUSION AND FUTURE POSSIBILITIES

AM is a fast-developing invention utilized in a variety of fields to create personalized and customized biomedical implants and prosthetic devices. Various kinds of AM technologies have been addressed, along with their appropriate processes and procedures for manufacturing in the field of biomedical engineering. It is proposed that future research on dentistry and clinical uses of AMs, as well as research on the industrial side, use a common nomenclature [144]. This would make it possible to compare the use of various AM techniques in a more systematic manner. Current and future advancements in additive manufacturing techniques, devices and materials will enable more medical and dental applications. Some processes, such as sheet lamination, may become obsolete in the future, or new competitors may enter the market. Multimetals, on the other hand, can benefit from metal SL. With the ability to produce metal components, several techniques, for example, BJ and MJ, offer a lot of prospects in medical and dental applications. DED has the ability to repair metal components and extrude composite materials. In multimaterial components, material extrusion and material jetting will be possible. The development and capabilities of AM technologies (Table 8.2) were used to identify research gaps and, as a result, future research opportunities, which were compared to results from the literature.

Future medical AM research opportunities using various methods can be envisioned in the following areas:

1. DED can be employed to repair medical components, particularly tools, instruments and parts for clinical equipment.
2. SL can be used to manufacture multimetal elements in medicine, especially for equipment and instruments.

3. Material extrusion can also include composite and multimaterial components, which are used in medical aids and medical rehabilitation devices such as prostheses.
4. BJ and MJ can also be employed in the case of implants and tools, instruments, medical models and biomanufacturing.

REFERENCES

1. Labonnote N, Rønnquist A, Manum B, Rüther P. Additive construction: State-of-the-art, challenges and opportunities. *Automation in Construction*. 2016:347–66.
2. Bose S, Ke D, Sahasrabudhe H, Bandyopadhyay A. Additive manufacturing of biomaterials. *Progress in Materials Science*. 2018;93:45–111.
3. Wang X, Jiang M, Zhou Z, Gou J, Hui D. 3D printing of polymer matrix composites: A review and prospective. *Composites Part B: Engineering*. 2017:442–58.
4. Herzog D, Seyda V, Wycisk E, Emmelmann C. Additive manufacturing of metals. *Acta Materialia*. 2016;117:371–92.
5. Zuback JS, DebRoy T. The hardness of additively manufactured alloys. *Materials*. Nov 11, 2018;11:2070.
6. Kumar V, Chakraborty S. Analysis of the surface roughness characteristics of EDMed components using GRA method. *Proceedings of the International Conference on Industrial and Manufacturing Systems (CIMS-2020)* 2022 (pp. 461–78). Springer, Cham.
7. Chakraborty S, Das PP, Kumar V. Application of grey-fuzzy logic technique for parametric optimization of non-traditional machining processes. *Grey Systems: Theory and Application*. 2018;8:46–68.
8. Sharma A, Kumar V, Babbar A, Dhawan V, Kotecha K, Prakash C. Experimental investigation and optimization of electric discharge machining process parameters using grey-fuzzy-based hybrid techniques. *Materials*. 2021;14:5820.
9. Ni J, Ling H, Zhang S, Wang Z, Peng Z, Benyshek C, Zan R, Miri AK, Li Z, Zhang X, Lee J. Three-dimensional printing of metals for biomedical applications. *Materials Today Bio*. Jun 1, 2019;3:100024.
10. Chakraborty S, Kumar V. Development of an intelligent decision model for non-traditional machining processes. *Decision Making: Applications in Management and Engineering*. 2021;4:194–214.
11. Kumar V, Diyaley S, Chakraborty S. Teaching-learning-based parametric optimization of an electrical discharge machining process. *Facta Universitatis, Series: Mechanical Engineering*. 2020;18:281–300.
12. Prakash C, Kansal HK, Pabla BS, Puri S. Processing and characterization of novel biomimetic nanoporous bioceramic surface on β-Ti implant by powder mixed electric discharge machining. *Journal of Materials Engineering and Performance* [Internet]. Springer US; 2015;24:3622–33. Available from: http://link.springer.com/10.1007/s11665-015-1619-6
13. Prakash C, Kansal HK, Pabla BS, Puri S. Powder mixed electric discharge machining: An innovative surface modification technique to enhance fatigue performance and bioactivity of β-Ti implant for orthopedics application. *Journal of Computing and Information Science in Engineering*. 2016;16:1–9.
14. Singh S, Singh N, Gupta M, Prakash C, Singh R. Mechanical feasibility of ABS/HIPS-based multi-material structures primed by low-cost polymer printer. *Rapid Prototyping Journal* [Internet]. 2019;25:152–61. Available from: www.emeraldinsight.com/doi/10.1108/RPJ-01-2018-0028

15. Prakash C, Singh S, Pabla BS, Uddin MS. Synthesis, characterization, corrosion and bioactivity investigation of nano-HA coating deposited on biodegradable Mg-Zn-Mn alloy. *Surface and Coatings Technology* [Internet]. Elsevier B.V; 2018;346:9–18. Available from: https://doi.org/10.1016/j.surfcoat.2018.04.035

16. Prakash C, Singh S, Kopperi H, Ramakrihna S, Mohan SV. Comparative job production based life cycle assessment of conventional and additive manufacturing assisted investment casting of aluminium: A case study. *Journal of Cleaner Production* [Internet]. Elsevier Ltd; 2021;289:125164. Available from: https://doi.org/10.1016/j.jclepro.2020.125164

17. Prakash C, Singh S, Ramakrishna S, Królczyk G, Le CH. Microwave sintering of porous Ti—Nb-HA composite with high strength and enhanced bioactivity for implant applications. *Journal of Alloys and Compounds*. 2020;824.

18. Prakash C, Singh S, Verma K, Sidhu SS, Singh S. Synthesis and characterization of Mg-Zn-Mn-HA composite by spark plasma sintering process for orthopedic applications. *Vacuum* [Internet]. Elsevier; 2018;155:578–84. Available from: https://doi.org/10.1016/j.vacuum.2018.06.063

19. Prakash C, Singh S, Singh M, Verma K, Chaudhary B, Singh S. Multi-objective particle swarm optimization of EDM parameters to deposit HA-coating on biodegradable Mg-alloy. *Vacuum* [Internet]. Elsevier Ltd; 2018;158:180–90. Available from: https://doi.org/10.1016/j.vacuum.2018.09.050

20. Singh S, Singh M, Prakash C, Gupta MK, Mia M, Singh R. Optimization and reliability analysis to improve surface quality and mechanical characteristics of heat-treated fused filament fabricated parts. *International Journal of Advanced Manufacturing Technology*. 2019;102:1521–36.

21. Sharma A, Jain V. Experimental investigation of cutting temperature during drilling of float glass specimen. *IOP Conference Series: Materials Science and Engineering*. 2020;715(1):012050. IOP Publishing.

22. Sharma A, Jain V, Gupta D. A novel investigation study on float glass hole surface integrity & tool wear using chemical assisted rotary ultrasonic machining. *Materials Today: Proceedings* [Internet]. 2020;26:632–7. Available from: https://linkinghub.elsevier.com/retrieve/pii/S2214785319342324

23. Sharma A, Jain V, Gupta D. Effect of pre and post tempering on hole quality of float glass specimen: For rotary ultrasonic and conventional drilling. *Silicon*. 2021;13:2029–39.

24. Sharma A, Jain V, Gupta D. Comparative analysis of chipping mechanics of float glass during rotary ultrasonic drilling and conventional drilling: For multi-shaped tools. *Machining Science and Technology*. Jul 4, 2019;23(4):547–68.

25. Sharma A, Jain V, Gupta D. Characterization of chipping and tool wear during drilling of float glass using rotary ultrasonic machining. *Measurement*. Nov 1, 2018;128: 254–63.

26. Sharma A, Jain V, Gupta D. Comparative analysis of chipping mechanics of float glass during rotary ultrasonic drilling and conventional drilling: For multi-shaped tools. *Machining Science and Technology*. 2019;23:547–68.

27. Bandyopadhyay A, Bose S, Das S. 3D printing of biomaterials. *MRS Bulletin*. 2015;40:108–14.

28. Babbar A, Rai A, Sharma A. Latest trend in building construction: Three-dimensional printing. *Journal of Physics: Conference Series*. 2021;1950:012007.

29. Khanduja P, Bhargave H, Babbar A, Pundir P, Sharma A. Development of two-dimensional plotter using programmable logic controller and human machine interface. *Journal of Physics: Conference Series*. 2021;1950:012012.

30. Singh G, Babbar A, Jain V, Gupta D. Comparative statement for diametric delamination in drilling of cortical bone with conventional and ultrasonic assisted drilling techniques. *Journal of Orthopaedics* [Internet]. Elsevier B.V.; 2021;25:53–8. Available from: https://doi.org/10.1016/j.jor.2021.03.017

31. Babbar A, Jain V, Gupta D, Agrawal D, Prakash C, Singh S, et al. Experimental analysis of wear and multi-shape burr loading during neurosurgical bone grinding. *Journal of Materials Research and Technology* [Internet]. 2021; Available from: https://linkinghub.elsevier.com/retrieve/pii/S2238785421001861

32. Babbar A, Jain V, Gupta D, Agrawal D. Histological evaluation of thermal damage to Osteocytes: A comparative study of conventional and ultrasonic-assisted bone grinding. *Medical Engineering & Physics* [Internet]. Elsevier Ltd; 2021;90:1–8. Available from: https://doi.org/10.1016/j.medengphy.2021.01.009

33. Singh S, Prakash C, Pramanik A, Basak A, Shabadi R, Królczyk G, et al. Magneto-rheological fluid assisted abrasive nanofinishing of β-Phase Ti-Nb-Ta-Zr alloy: Parametric appraisal and corrosion analysis. *Materials* [Internet]. 2020;13:5156. Available from: www.mdpi.com/1996-1944/13/22/5156

34. Sharma A, Jain V, Gupta D, Babbar A. A review study on miniaturization. In *Advanced Manufacturing and Processing Technology* [Internet]. First edition. Boca Raton, FL: CRC Press, 2021, pp. 111–31. Available from: www.taylorfrancis.com/books/9781000193169/chapters/10.1201/9780429298042-5

35. Babbar A, Jain V, Gupta D, Prakash C, Sharma A. Fabrication and machining methods of composites for aerospace applications. In *Characterization, Testing, Measurement, and Metrology* [Internet]. First edition. Boca Raton, FL: CRC Press, 2020, pp. 109–24. Available from: www.taylorfrancis.com/books/9781000193336/chapters/10.1201/9780429298073-7

36. Babbar A, Jain V, Gupta D, Sharma A. Fabrication of microchannels using conventional and hybrid machining processes. In *Non-Conventional Hybrid Machining Processes* [Internet]. First edition. Boca Raton, FL: CRC Press, 2020, pp. 37–51. Available from: www.taylorfrancis.com/books/9780429642746/chapters/10.1201/9780429029165-3

37. Sharma A, Grover V, Babbar A, Rani R. A trending nonconventional hybrid finishing/machining process. In *Non-Conventional Hybrid Machining Processes* [Internet]. First edition. Boca Raton, FL: CRC Press, 2020, pp. 79–93. Available from: www.taylorfrancis.com/books/9780429642746/chapters/10.1201/9780429029165-5

38. Sharma A, Babbar A, Jain V, Gupta D. Influence of cutting force and drilling temperature on glass hole surface integrity during rotary ultrasonic drilling. *Advances in Production and Industrial Engineering* [Internet]. 2021:369–78. Available from: http://link.springer.com/10.1007/978-981-15-5519-0_28

39. Babbar A, Sharma A, Chugh M. Application of flexible sintered magnetic abrasive brush for finishing of brass plate. *Optimization in Engineering Research*. 2020;1:36–47.

40. Babbar A, Jain V, Gupta D. Preliminary investigations of rotary ultrasonic neurosurgical bone grinding using Grey-Taguchi optimization methodology. *Grey Systems: Theory and Application* [Internet]. Emerald Publishing Limited; 2020 [cited 2020 Jun 30];10:479–93. Available from: https://doi.org/10.1108/GS-11-2019-0054

41. Babbar A, Sharma A, Bansal S, Mago J, Toor V. Potential applications of three-dimensional printing for anatomical simulations and surgical planning. *Materials Today: Proceedings* [Internet]. Elsevier Ltd; 2020;33:1558–61. Available from: https://doi.org/10.1016/j.matpr.2020.04.123

42. Babbar A, Jain V, Gupta D. In vivo evaluation of machining forces, torque, and bone quality during skull bone grinding. *Proceedings of the Institution of Mechanical Engineers, Part H: Journal of Engineering in Medicine* [Internet]. 2020;234:626–38. Available from: http://journals.sagepub.com/doi/10.1177/0954411920911499

43. Baraiya R, Babbar A, Jain V, Gupta D. In-situ simultaneous surface finishing using abrasive flow machining via novel fixture. *Journal of Manufacturing Processes* [Internet]. Elsevier; 2020;50:266–78. Available from: https://doi.org/10.1016/j.jmapro.2019.12.051

44. Babbar A, Jain V, Gupta D. Thermogenesis mitigation using ultrasonic actuation during bone grinding: A hybrid approach using CEM43°C and Arrhenius model. *Journal of the Brazilian Society of Mechanical Sciences and Engineering* [Internet]. Springer Berlin Heidelberg; 2019;41:401. Available from: https://doi.org/10.1007/s40430-019-1913-6

45. Babbar A, Kumar A, Jain V, Gupta D. Enhancement of activated tungsten inert gas (A-TIG) welding using multi-component TiO2-SiO2-Al2O3 hybrid flux. *Measurement* [Internet]. Elsevier Ltd; 2019;148:106912. Available from: https://doi.org/10.1016/j.measurement.2019.106912

46. Kumar M, Babbar A, Sharma A, Shahi AS. Effect of post weld thermal aging (PWTA) sensitization on micro-hardness and corrosion behavior of AISI 304 weld joints. *Journal of Physics: Conference Series* [Internet]. 2019;1240:012078. Available from: https://iopscience.iop.org/article/10.1088/1742-6596/1240/1/012078

47. Babbar A, Sharma A, Jain V, Jain AK. Rotary ultrasonic milling of C/SiC composites fabricated using chemical vapor infiltration and needling technique. *Materials Research Express* [Internet]. IOP Publishing; 2019;6:085607. Available from: https://doi.org/10.1088/2053-1591/ab1bf7

48. Sharma A, Babbar A, Jain V, Gupta D. Enhancement of surface roughness for brittle material during rotary ultrasonic machining. *Chang G, editor. MATEC Web of Conferences* [Internet]. 2018;249:01006. Available from: www.matec-conferences.org/10.1051/matecconf/201824901006

49. Singh S, Prakash C. Effect of cryogenic treatment on the microstructure, mechanical properties and finishability of β-TNTZ alloy for orthopedic applications. *Materials Letters* [Internet]. 2020;278:128461. Available from: https://linkinghub.elsevier.com/retrieve/pii/S0167577X20311666

50. Prakash C, Uddin MS. Surface modification of β-phase Ti implant by hydroaxyapatite mixed electric discharge machining to enhance the corrosion resistance and in-vitro bioactivity. *Surface and Coatings Technology* [Internet]. Elsevier B.V; 2017;326:134–45. Available from: http://dx.doi.org/10.1016/j.surfcoat.2017.07.040

51. Singh S, Singh G, Prakash C, Ramakrishna S. Current status and future directions of fused fi lament fabrication. *Journal of Manufacturing Processes* [Internet]. Elsevier; 2020;55:288–306. Available from: https://doi.org/10.1016/j.jmapro.2020.04.049

52. Prakash C, Kansal HK, Pabla BS, Puri S, Prakash C, Kansal HK, et al. Experimental investigations in powder mixed electric discharge machining of Ti—35Nb—7Ta—5Zr β—titanium alloy. *Materials and Manufacturing Processes* [Internet]. Taylor & Francis; 2017;32:274–85. Available from: http://dx.doi.org/10.1080/10426914.2016.1198018

53. Prakash C, Kansal HK, Pabla BS, Puri S. On the influence of nanoporous layer fabricated by PMEDM on β-Ti implant: Biological and computational evaluation of bone-implant interface. *Materials Today: Proceedings.* Jan 1, 2017;4(2):2298–2307.

54. Prakash C, Kansal HK, Pabla BS, Puri S. To optimize the surface roughness and microhardness of β-Ti alloy in PMEDM process using non-dominated sorting genetic algorithm-II. 2015 2nd International Conference on Recent Advances in Engineering and Computational Sciences, RAECS, 2015.2016.

55. Prakash C, Kansal HK, Pabla BS, Puri S. Multi-objective optimization of powder mixed electric discharge machining parameters for fabrication of biocompatible layer on β-Ti alloy using NSGA-II coupled with Taguchi based response surface methodology. *Journal of Mechanical Science and Technology.* Sep 2016;30(9):4195–204.

56. Prakash C, Singh S, Farina I, Fraternali F, Feo L. Physical-mechanical characterization of biodegradable Mg-3Si-HA composites. *PSU Research Review.* 2018;2:152–74.

57. Prakash C, Kansal HK, Pabla BS, Puri S. Potential of silicon powder-mixed electro spark alloying for surface modification of β-phase titanium alloy for orthopedic applications. *Materials Today: Proceedings*. 2017:10080–3.

58. Prakash C, Kansal HK, Pabla BS, Puri S. On the influence of nanoporous layer fabricated by PMEDM on β-Ti implant: Biological and computational evaluation of bone-implant interface. *Materials Today: Proceedings*. 2017:2298–307.

59. Prakash C, Kansal HK, Pabla BS, Puri S. Experimental investigations in powder mixed electric discharge machining of Ti—35Nb—7Ta—5Zrβ-titanium alloy. *Materials and Manufacturing Processes*. 2017;32:274–85.

60. Singh S, Prakash C, Ramakrishna S. 3D printing of polyether-ether-ketone for biomedical applications. *European Polymer Journal* [Internet]. Elsevier; 2019;114:234–48. Available from: https://doi.org/10.1016/j.eurpolymj.2019.02.035

61. Babbar A, Jain V, Gupta D, Prakash C, Singh S, Sharma A. 3D Bioprinting in pharmaceuticals, medicine, and tissue engineering applications. In *Advanced Manufacturing and Processing Technology* [Internet]. First edition. Boca Raton, FL: CRC Press, 2021, pp. 147–61. Available from: www.taylorfrancis.com/books/9781000193169/chapters/10.1201/9780429298042-7

62. Aliyu AA, Abdul-Rani AM, Ginta TL, Prakash C, Axinte E, Razak MA, et al. A review of additive mixed-electric discharge machining: Current status and future perspectives for surface modification of biomedical implants. *Advances in Materials Science and Engineering* [Internet]. 2017;1–23. Available from: www.hindawi.com/journals/amse/2017/8723239/

63. Singh S, Prakash C, Singh M, Mann GS, Gupta MK, Singh R, et al. Poly-lactic-Acid: Potential material for bio-printing applications. *Biomanufacturing*. 2019:69–87.

64. Ballard DH, Mills P, Duszak R, Weisman JA, Rybicki FJ, Woodard PK. Medical 3D printing cost-savings in orthopedic and maxillofacial surgery: Cost analysis of operating room time saved with 3D printed anatomic models and surgical guides. *Academic Radiology*. 2020;27:1103–13.

65. Choonara YE, Du Toit LC, Kumar P, Kondiah PPD, Pillay V. 3D-printing and the effect on medical costs: A new era? *Expert Review of Pharmacoeconomics and Outcomes Research*. 2016;16:23–32.

66. Mahmoud A, Bennett M. Introducing 3-dimensional printing of a human anatomic pathology specimen: Potential benefits for undergraduate and postgraduate education and anatomic pathology practice. *Archives of Pathology and Laboratory Medicine*. 2015;139:1048–51.

67. Tack P, Victor J, Gemmel P, Annemans L. 3D-printing techniques in a medical setting: A systematic literature review. *BioMedical Engineering Online*. Dec 2016;15(1):1–21.

68. Ballard DH, Tappa K, Boyer CJ, Jammalamadaka U, Hemmanur K, Weisman JA, et al. Antibiotics in 3D-printed implants, instruments and materials: Benefits, challenges and future directions. *Journal of 3D Printing in Medicine*. 2019;3:83–93.

69. Lin L, Fang Y, Liao Y, Chen G, Gao C, Zhu P. 3D printing and digital processing techniques in dentistry: A review of literature. *Advanced Engineering Materials*. Jun 2019;21(6):1801013.

70. Javaid M, Haleem A. Current status and applications of additive manufacturing in dentistry: A literature-based review. *Journal of Oral Biology and Craniofacial Research*. 2019:179–85.

71. Aho J, Bøtker JP, Genina N, Edinger M, Arnfast L, Rantanen J. Roadmap to 3D-printed oral pharmaceutical dosage forms: Feedstock filament properties and characterization for fused deposition modeling. *Journal of Pharmaceutical Sciences*. 2019:26–35.

72. Salm M, Paloheimo KS, Tuomi J, Ingman T, Mäkitie A. A digital process for additive manufacturing of occlusal splints: A clinical pilot study. *Journal of the Royal Society Interface*. 2013;10.

73. Aquino RP, Barile S, Grasso A, Saviano M. Envisioning smart and sustainable healthcare: 3D Printing technologies for personalized medication. *Futures*. 2018;103:35–50.
74. Javaid M, Haleem A. Current status and challenges of Additive manufacturing in orthopaedics: An overview. *Journal of Clinical Orthopaedics and Trauma*. 2019;10:380–6.
75. Emelogu A, Marufuzzaman M, Thompson SM, Shamsaei N, Bian L. Additive manufacturing of biomedical implants: A feasibility assessment via supply-chain cost analysis. *Additive Manufacturing*. 2016;11:97–113.
76. Haleem A, Javaid M. 3D printed medical parts with different materials using additive manufacturing. *Clinical Epidemiology and Global Health*. 2020;8:215–23.
77. Murr LE, Gaytan SM, Medina F, Lopez H, Martinez E, MacHado BI, et al. Next-generation biomedical implants using additive manufacturing of complex cellular and functional mesh arrays. *Philosophical Transactions of the Royal Society A: Mathematical, Physical and Engineering Sciences*. 2010;368:1999–2032.
78. Peltola MJ, Vallittu PK, Vuorinen V, Aho AAJ, Puntala A, Aitasalo KMJ. Novel composite implant in craniofacial bone reconstruction. *European Archives of Oto-Rhino-Laryngology*. 2012;269:623–8.
79. Ramakrishnaiah R, Al kheraif AA, Mohammad A, Divakar DD, Kotha SB, Celur SL, et al. Preliminary fabrication and characterization of electron beam melted Ti—6Al—4V customized dental implant. *Saudi Journal of Biological Sciences*. 2017;24: 787–96.
80. Nazir A, Azhar A, Nazir U, Liu YF, Qureshi WS, Chen JE, Alanazi E. The rise of 3D printing entangled with smart computer aided design during COVID-19 era. *Journal of Manufacturing Systems*. Jul 1, 2020;60:774–86.
81. Yang T, Lin S, Xie Q, Ouyang W, Tan T, Li J, et al. Impact of 3D printing technology on the comprehension of surgical liver anatomy. *Surgical Endoscopy*. 2019;33:411–7.
82. Gibson I, Srinath A. Simplifying medical additive manufacturing: Making the surgeon the designer. *Procedia Technology*. 2015;20:237–42.
83. Lee Ventola C. Medical applications for 3D printing: Current and projected uses. *P and T*. 2014;39:704–11.
84. Salmi M. Possibilities of preoperative medical models made by 3D printing or additive manufacturing. *Journal of Medical Engineering*. 2016;2016:1–6.
85. Bücking TM, Hill ER, Robertson JL, Maneas E, Plumb AA, Nikitichev DI. From medical imaging data to 3D printed anatomical models. *PLoS One*. 2017;12.
86. Salmi M, Tuomi J, Paloheimo K, Paloheimo M, Björkstrand R, Mäkitie AA, et al. Digital design and rapid manufacturing in orbital wall reconstruction. *Innovative Developments in Design and Manufacturing—Advanced Research in Virtual and Rapid Prototyping*. 2010:339–42.
87. Wang X, Xu S, Zhou S, Xu W, Leary M, Choong P, et al. Topological design and additive manufacturing of porous metals for bone scaffolds and orthopaedic implants: A review. *Biomaterials*. 2016:127–41.
88. Tahayeri A, Morgan MC, Fugolin AP, Bompolaki D, Athirasala A, Pfeifer CS, et al. 3D printed versus conventionally cured provisional crown and bridge dental materials. *Dental Materials*. 2018;34:192–200.
89. Akmal JS, Salmi M, Mäkitie A, Björkstrand R, Partanen J. Implementation of industrial additive manufacturing: Intelligent implants and drug delivery systems. *Journal of Functional Biomaterials*. 2018;9.
90. Prasad LK, Smyth H. 3D printing technologies for drug delivery: A review. *Drug Development and Industrial Pharmacy*. 2016:1019–31.
91. Hieu LC, Bohez E, Vander Sloten J, Phien HN, Vatcharaporn E, Binh PH, et al. Design for medical rapid prototyping of cranioplasty implants. *Rapid Prototyping Journal*. 2003;9:175–86.

92. Liu K, Zhang Q, Li X, Zhao C, Quan X, Zhao R, et al. Preliminary application of a multi-level 3D printing drill guide template for pedicle screw placement in severe and rigid scoliosis. *European Spine Journal*. 2017;26:1684–9.

93. Culmone C, Smit G, Breedveld P. Additive manufacturing of medical instruments: A state-of-the-art review. *Additive Manufacturing*. 2019:461–73.

94. Kontio R, Bjorkstrand R. Designing and additive manufacturing a prototype for a novel instrument for mandible fracture reduction. *Surgery: Current Research*. 2012;01.

95. Chin SJ, Wilde F, Neuhaus M, Schramm A, Gellrich NC, Rana M. Accuracy of virtual surgical planning of orthognathic surgery with aid of CAD/CAM fabricated surgical splint—A novel 3D analyzing algorithm. *Journal of Cranio-Maxillofacial Surgery*. 2017;45:1962–70.

96. Herbert N, Simpson D, Spence WD, Ion W. A preliminary investigation into the development of 3-D printing of prosthetic sockets. *Journal of Rehabilitation Research and Development*. 2005;42:141–6.

97. ten Kate J, Smit G, Breedveld P. 3D-printed upper limb prostheses: A review. *Disability and Rehabilitation: Assistive Technology*. 2017:300–14.

98. Paterson AM, Donnison E, Bibb RJ, Ian Campbell R. Computer-aided design to support fabrication of wrist splints using 3D printing: A feasibility study. Hand Therapy. 2014;19:102–13.

99. Rosicky J, Grygar A, Chapcak P, Bouma T, Rosicky J. Application of 3D scanning in prosthetic and orthotic clinical practice. *Proceedings of the 7th International Conference on 3D Body Scanning Technologies*. Nov 30, 2016, pp. 88–97.

100. Bártolo PJ, Chua CK, Almeida HA, Chou SM, Lim ASC. Biomanufacturing for tissue engineering: Present and future trends. *Virtual and Physical Prototyping*. 2009;4:203–16.

101. Danna NR, Leucht P. Designing resorbable scaffolds for bone defects. *Bulletin of the Hospital for Joint Diseases*. 2019;77:39–44.

102. Babbar A, Jain V, Gupta D, Agrawal D. Finite element simulation and integration of CEM43 °C and Arrhenius Models for ultrasonic-assisted skull bone grinding: A thermal dose model. *Medical Engineering and Physics*. 2021;90:9–22.

103. Babbar A, Jain V, Gupta D, Singh S, Prakash C, Pruncu C. Biomaterials and fabrication methods of scaffolds for tissue engineering applications. *3D Printing in Biomedical Engineering*, Dr. Sunpreet Singh, Dr. Chander Prakash, Prof. Rupinder Singh, Eds. 2020, pp. 167–86, Springer, Singapore.

104. Zadpoor A. Design for additive bio-manufacturing: From patient-specific medical devices to rationally designed meta-biomaterials. *International Journal of Molecular Sciences*. 2017;18:1607.

105. Lowther M, Louth S, Davey A, Hussain A, Ginestra P, Carter L, et al. Clinical, industrial, and research perspectives on powder bed fusion additively manufactured metal implants. *Additive Manufacturing*. 2019:565–84.

106. Babbar A, Sharma A, Kumar R, Pundir P, Dhiman V. Functionalized biomaterials for 3D printing: An overview of the literature. *Additive Manufacturing with Functionalized Nanomaterials*. 2021:87–107.

107. Tappa K, Jammalamadaka U. Novel biomaterials used in medical 3D printing techniques. *Journal of Functional Biomaterials*. Mar 2018;9(1):17.

108. Wang K, Ho CC, Zhang C, Wang B. A Review on the 3D printing of functional structures for medical phantoms and regenerated tissue and organ applications. *Engineering*. 2017;3:653–62.

109. Kumar V, Das PP, Chakraborty S. Grey-fuzzy method-based parametric analysis of abrasive water jet machining on GFRP composites. *Sādhanā*. 2020;45:106.

110. Chakraborty S, Das PP, Kumar V. A grey fuzzy logic approach for cotton fibre selection. *Journal of The Institution of Engineers (India): Series E*. 2017;98.

111. Babbar A, Prakash C, Singh S, Gupta MK, Mia M, Pruncu CI. Application of hybrid nature-inspired algorithm: Single and bi-objective constrained optimization of magnetic abrasive finishing process parameters. *Journal of Materials Research and Technology.* 2020;9:7961–74.

112. Singh D, Babbar A, Jain V, Gupta D, Saxena S, Dwibedi V. Synthesis, characterization, and bioactivity investigation of biomimetic biodegradable PLA scaffold fabricated by fused filament fabrication process. *Journal of the Brazilian Society of Mechanical Sciences and Engineering.* 2019;41.

113. Babbar A, Sharma A, Singh P. Multi-objective optimization of magnetic abrasive finishing using grey relational analysis. *Materials Today: Proceedings.* Jan 1, 2022;50:570–5.

114. Chakraborty S, Kumar V, Ramakrishnan KR. Selection of the all-time best world XI test cricket team using the TOPSIS method. *Decision Science Letters.* 2019;8:95–108.

115. Haleem A, Javaid M, Saxena A. Additive manufacturing applications in cardiology: A review. *Egyptian Heart Journal.* 2018:433–41.

116. Thompson A, McNally D, Maskery I, Leach RK. X-ray computed tomography and additive manufacturing in medicine: A review. *International Journal of Metrology and Quality Engineering.* 2017;8:17.

117. Calignano F, Galati M, Iuliano L, Minetola P. Design of additively manufactured structures for biomedical applications: A review of the additive manufacturing processes applied to the biomedical sector. *Journal of Healthcare Engineering.* 2019;2019:1–6.

118. Galante R, Figueiredo-Pina CG, Serro AP. Additive manufacturing of ceramics for dental applications: A review. *Dental Materials.* 2019:825–46.

119. Ramola M, Yadav V, Jain R. On the adoption of additive manufacturing in healthcare: A literature review. *Journal of Manufacturing Technology Management.* 2019;30:48–69.

120. Bhargav A, Sanjairaj V, Rosa V, Feng LW, Fuh YH J. Applications of additive manufacturing in dentistry: A review. *Journal of Biomedical Materials Research Part B: Applied Biomaterials.* 2018;106:2058–64.

121. Revilla-León M, Sadeghpour M, Özcan M. A review of the applications of additive manufacturing technologies used to fabricate metals in implant dentistry. *Journal of Prosthodontics.* 2020:579–93.

122. Revilla-León M, Meyer MJ, Özcan M. Metal additive manufacturing technologies: Literature review of current status and prosthodontic applications [Verfahren zur additiven Metallfertigung: Literaturreview zum aktuellen Status und zu den prothetischen Einsatzmöglichkeiten]. *International Journal of Computerized Dentistry.* 2019;22:55–67.

123. Trivedi M, Jee J, Silva S, Blomgren C, Pontinha VM, Dixon DL, et al. Additive manufacturing of pharmaceuticals for precision medicine applications: A review of the promises and perils in implementation. *Additive Manufacturing.* 2018:319–28.

124. Oh WJ, Lee WJ, Kim MS, Jeon JB, Shim DS. Repairing additive-manufactured 316L stainless steel using direct energy deposition. *Optics and Laser Technology.* 2019;117:6–17.

125. Szymor P, Kozakiewicz M, Olszewski R. Accuracy of open-source software segmentation and paper-based printed three-dimensional models. *Journal of Cranio-Maxillofacial Surgery.* 2016;44:202–9.

126. Jahnke P, Schwarz S, Ziegert M, Schwarz FB, Hamm B, Scheel M. Paper-based 3D printing of anthropomorphic CT phantoms: Feasibility of two construction techniques. *European Radiology.* 2019;29:1384–90.

127. Olszewski R, Tilleux C, Hastir JP, Delvaux L, Danse E. Holding eternity in one's hand: First three-dimensional reconstruction and printing of the heart from 2700 years-old Egyptian mummy. *Anatomical Record.* 2019;302:912–6.

128. Ward AA, Cordero ZC. Junction growth and interdiffusion during ultrasonic additive manufacturing of multi-material laminates. *Scripta Materialia.* 2020;177:101–5.

129. Babbar A, Jain V, Gupta D, Prakash C. Experimental investigation and parametric optimization of neurosurgical bone grinding under bio-mimic environment. *Surface Review and Letters.* Jul 28, 2021:2141005.

130. Sharma A, Kalsia M, Uppal AS, Babbar A, Dhawan V. Machining of hard and brittle materials: A comprehensive review. *Materials Today: Proceedings.* Aug 4, 2021.

131. Kaza A, Rembalsky J, Roma N, Yellapu V, Delong W, Stawicki S. Medical applications of stereolithography: An overview. *International Journal of Academic Medicine.* 2018;4:252.

132. Feuerbach T, Kock S, Thommes M. Characterisation of fused deposition modeling 3D printers for pharmaceutical and medical applications. *Pharmaceutical Development and Technology.* 2018;23:1136–45.

133. Ait-Mansour I, Kretzschmar N, Chekurov S, Salmi M, Rech J. Design-dependent shrinkage compensation modeling and mechanical property targeting of metal FFF. *Progress in Additive Manufacturing.* 2020;5:51–7.

134. Adumitroaie A, Antonov F, Khaziev A, Azarov A, Golubev M, Vasiliev VV. Novel continuous fiber bi-matrix composite 3-D printing technology. *Materials.* 2019;12:3011.

135. Gibson MA, Mykulowycz NM, Shim J, Fontana R, Schmitt P, Roberts A, et al. 3D printing metals like thermoplastics: Fused filament fabrication of metallic glasses. *Materials Today.* 2018;21:697–702.

136. Wolff M, Mesterknecht T, Bals A, Ebel T, Willumeit-Römer R. FFF of Mg-alloys for biomedical application. *Minerals, Metals and Materials Series.* 2019:43–9.

137. Spencer SR, Kay Watts L. Three-dimensional printing in medical and allied health practice: A literature review. *Journal of Medical Imaging and Radiation Sciences.* 2020:489–500.

138. Miyanaji H, Rahman KM, Da M, Williams CB. Effect of fine powder particles on quality of binder jetting parts. *Additive Manufacturing.* 2020;36.

139. Huang SJ, Ye CS, Zhao HP, Fan ZT. Parameters optimization of binder jetting process using modified silicate as a binder. *Materials and Manufacturing Processes.* 2020;35:214–20.

140. Babbar A, Jain V, Gupta D, Prakash C, Singh S, Sharma A. 3D bioprinting in pharmaceuticals, medicine, and tissue engineering applications. *Advanced Manufacturing and Processing Technology.* 2020:147–61.

141. Ziaee M, Crane NB. Binder jetting: A review of process, materials, and methods. *Additive Manufacturing.* 2019:781–801.

142. Babbar A, Jain V, Gupta D. Thermo-mechanical aspects and temperature measurement techniques of bone grinding. *Materials Today: Proceedings.* 2019:1458–62.

143. Babbar A, Jain V, Gupta D, Prakash C, Singh S, Sharma A. Effect of process parameters on cutting forces and osteonecrosis for orthopedic bone drilling applications. *Characterization, Testing, Measurement, and Metrology.* 2020:93–108.

144. Chhaya MP, Poh PSP, Balmayor ER, Van Griensven M, Schantz JT, Hutmacher DW. Additive manufacturing in biomedical sciences and the need for definitions and norms. *Expert Review of Medical Devices.* 2015;12:537–43.

9 Additive Manufacturing of Biomaterials

Classification, Techniques, and Application

Sudip Dasgupta1 and Sambit Ray[1]
[1] Department of Ceramic Engineering, National
Institute of Technology, Rourkela, India

CONTENTS

9.1 Introduction... 166
9.2 Types of AM Processes Based on Material Used 167
9.3 Powder-Based Techniques for AM 170
9.4 AM through Deposition of Material 170
9.5 Nanofabrication 171
9.6 Powder-Based Techniques for AM 171
    9.6.1 Selective Laser Sintering 172
    9.6.2 Laser Powder Bed Fusion 173
    9.6.3 EBM.. 173
9.7 Application of AM Techniques in the Biomedical Field 174
    9.7.1 Metals 174
    9.7.2 Ceramics 178
    9.7.3 Composite 180
    9.7.4 Polymers 181
    9.7.5 Extrusion-Based Technique 182
9.8 AM of 3D Ceramic Scaffolds Post Sintering.. 183
9.9 Printing of 3D Ceramic Scaffolds at Ambient/Low Temperatures 183
9.10 Post-Functionalized 3D-Printed Ceramic Scaffolds.................................... 184
9.11 3D Printing of Hydrogel Scaffolds 184
9.12 Cell-Embedded Hydrogel Scaffolds—3D Printing 185
9.13 Extrusion-Based 3D Printing—Non-Hydrogel-Based Polymer.................. 185
    9.13.1 High-Temperature-Processed Polyester Scaffolds for
         3D Printing.. 185
    9.13.2 Posttreatment of Polyester Scaffolds 3D-Printed at
         High Temperatures.. 186
    9.13.3 Natural and Synthetic Polymer for Bone Tissue Engineering:
         Scaffolds 3D-Printed at Room/Low Temperatures............ 187

DOI: 10.1201/9781003217961-9

9.13.4 Bone Regeneration by 3D-Printed Scaffolds of Synthetic/Natural
Polymer: Electrostatic Field-Assisted Micro-Extrusion 188
9.13.5 Synthetic Natural Polymer- and Inorganic-Based Composites
for Bone Tissue Regeneration 188
9.14 Vat Photopolymerization Techniques 189
9.15 Clinical Applications 190
9.15.1 Patient Variability 190
9.15.2 Shoulder and Other Joint Replacements 190
9.15.3 Fracture Fixation 191
9.15.4 Large Bone Defects 191
9.15.5 Surgical Guides 192
9.16 Research Direction and Future Scope 192
9.17 Summary 193
References 194

9.1 INTRODUCTION

In contrast to traditional subtractive manufacturing methods, additive manufacturing (AM), also known as three-dimensional (3D) printing, is a method of fabricating 3D objects by selectively joining materials in a layer-by-layer assembly as directed by computer-fed digital information from a 3D computer-aided-design (CAD) model. As a result, the AM process differs significantly from traditional manufacturing procedures such as machining, forging, casting, and other bulk processing methods. A number of materials, including polymers, ceramics, metals, and composites, can be produced into bespoke shapes and architecture using AM processes, ranging from highly dense to macro/micro-porous characteristics. AM-derived 3D-printed products can be used in a variety of industries, including turbine blade manufacture, jewellery creation, mold construction, tissue engineering, and more [1–4]. No molds, fixtures, or tooling is required to produce parts or objects using AM techniques, which is why AM techniques can successfully meet the criteria for the design and manufacturing of next-generation orthopedic implants. Although medical product customization in terms of shape, size, and architecture existed long before AM was introduced, the lack of surface tooling for producing unique designs in AM makes it more cost-effective for the fabrication of patient-specific orthopedic implants. Finally, the ability to introduce porous architecture into AM-derived objects allows for better bone ingrowth and osteointegration while maintaining superior mechanical performance. Understanding the state of the art of orthopedic applications of AM-derived implants for the economical production of efficiently customized objects with complex design and architecture is the key aspect of the current review. In particular, in the biomedical field, 3D printing has brought about a revolution primarily because of two factors; one is technological aspects, including its versatility, automation, accurate control over the fabrication steps, and easy handling, and the second factor is the characteristics of AM-derived products, such as their maneuverable structure, size, shape, architecture, and properties that are highly demanded in biomedical applications. Moreover, unlike traditional processes, economic production of low volume batches is feasible through AM process, which is a unique advantage for pilot plant–type projects.

TABLE 9.1

Advantages and Challenges in AM (reference table taken from [5])

Advantages	Challenges
• No limitation for geometry of the construct • No requirement of any other tools for creating parts of the construct • Less waste of materials since processing requires is done near net shapes • Ease to adjust the design and the intricacy of the construct • Ease to optimize the construct design and parts with better mechanical strength	• Requires postprocessing step for better surface finishing • Slower build rate for high volume manufacturing • Relatively expensive printer equipment • Limited adaptability which limits the build volume

As research in the field of 3D-printing technology and its associated products in the biomedical arena has grown rapidly worldwide, well-written review articles on AM and allied processes particularly relevant to biomedical engineering have been documented elsewhere [6–9]. Bone tissue engineering based on scaffold design holds exciting promises and has enormously been investigated [10]. Providing a conducive microenvironment for specific cells to attach, proliferate and differentiate is the ultimate objective of a tissue-engineered scaffold. AM processes enable the users to produce as desired scaffolds with customized shapes, architecture, and functionality for the effective and rapid regeneration of neo-tissues [11]. Bone scaffolds prepared by AM techniques can mimic the hierarchical organization of bone structure both in the macro- and microscopic scale, which is difficult to achieve by traditional fabrication processes [12]. Moreover, few AM methods can produce customized scaffolds, ready to serve as an excellent carrier for local, sustained delivery of drugs, and/or relevant biomolecules [13]. Furthermore, the thus-produced scaffold surface can be modified with bioactive molecules and cell-specific ligands to enhance its bioactivity and osteogenic properties. Three-dimensionally printed functional tissue engineering scaffolds (Figure 9.1) can be fabricated from a blended paste of functionally active nanoparticles and/or biomolecules with a solution of synthetic/natural polymers. Recent advances in the research and development of AM-derived bone tissue engineering scaffolds are highlighted in this review. Different AM processes to selectively design and fabricate patient-specific porous structures capable of osteointegrating with the surrounding bone tissue are discussed. In the end, the existing lacuna between current research and commercial demands, critical challenges in achieving so, and future research directions in AM-derived orthopedic implants are presented.

9.2 TYPES OF AM PROCESSES BASED ON MATERIAL USED

Depending on the materials used, a variety of AM processes have been developed since 1980. According to the ISO/ASTM 52900 standard, there are seven different processes for AM, and the categories are shown in Table 9.2 with a brief description of each method. Figure 9.2 categorizes AM process according to the materials used in biomedical applications. Figure 9.3 shows different precursors used in additive manufacturing techniques.

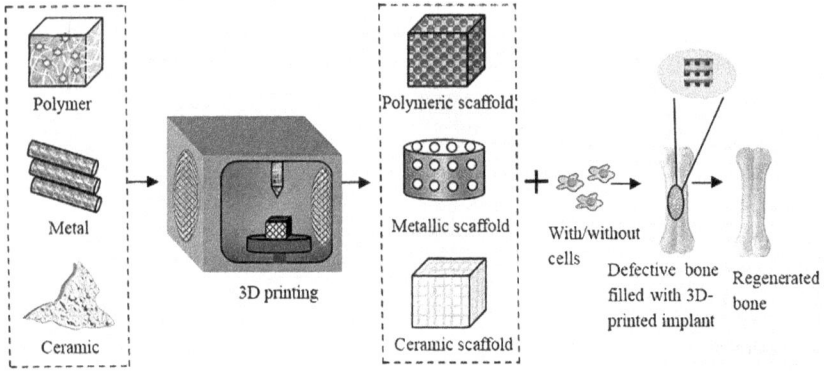

FIGURE 9.1   Symmetrical diagram for the 3D-printing/AM process.

TABLE 9.2
Commercially Available Machines for AM Processes [5]

Sl. No.	Materials in AM	Category	Commercial 3D Printing Technologies and Vendors
1	Solid	Material Extrusion	Fused Deposition Modeling from Stratasys
		Sheet Lamination	Mcor Technologies
2	Powder	Directed Energy Deposition	➤ Laser Engineered Net Shaping by Optomec Inc.
			➤ Direct Metal Deposition by DM3D
			➤ Electron Beam Welding by Sciaky Inc.
		Binder Jetting	➤ Zcorp
			➤ ExOne
			➤ Voxeljet
		Powder Bed Fusion	➤ SLS by 3D Systems
			➤ EBM by Arcam AB
			➤ DMLS by EOS
			➤ SLM by SLM solutions
3	Liquid	VAT polymerization	➤ Stereolithography from 3D systems
			➤ Bioplotters by Envisiontec
			➤ DDM Systems for Large Area Maskless Photopolymerization
		Material Jetting	➤ Object from Stratasys
			➤ Solidscape 3D Printers from Solidscape
			➤ Multijet Fusion Technology from HP

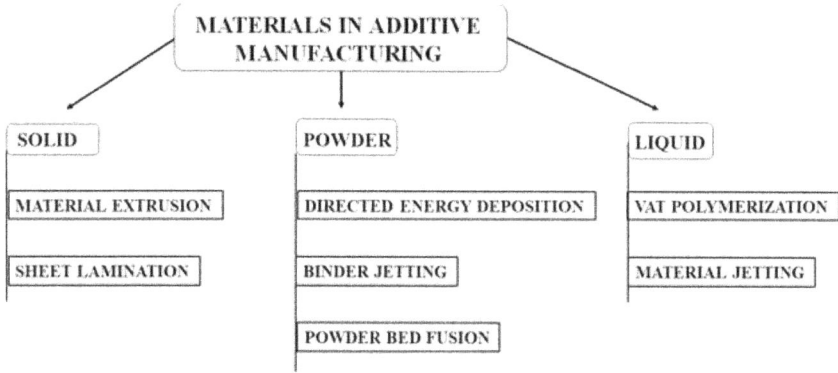

FIGURE 9.2 Categorizing AM processes according to the materials used in biomedical applications.

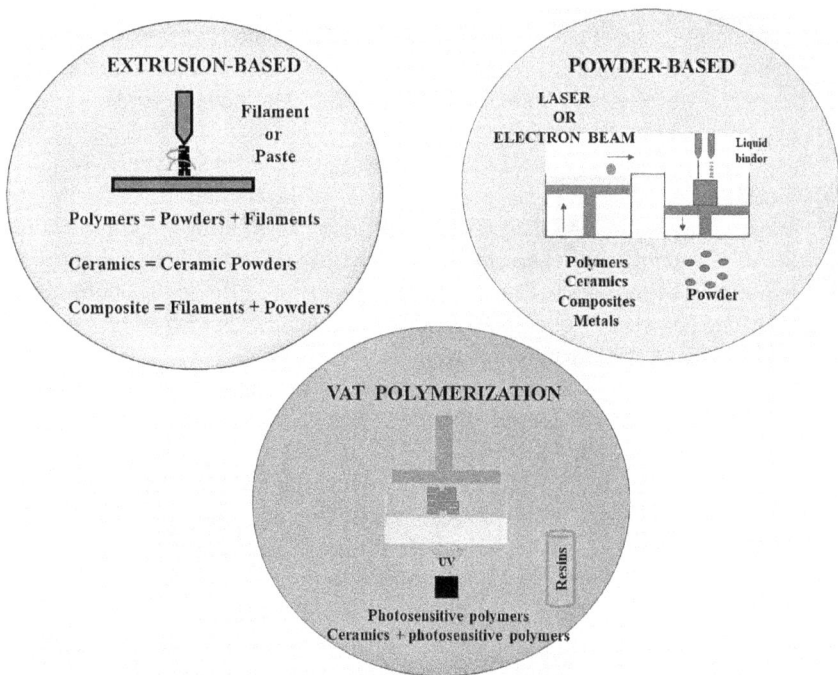

FIGURE 9.3 Different precursors used in AM techniques.

9.3 POWDER-BASED TECHNIQUES FOR AM

A powder bed in each layer can form the basis for the preparation of 3D constructs by the following two processes. The difference between the two processes lies in the anchoring of powders to fabricate 3D objects.

Jetting of Binder—In this technique, a layer of binder is spread in the form of a droplet jet to anchor each layer of the powder bed in three directions. Thus, the layer of binder remains sandwiched between two successive layers of powder bed, and only after one successful layering of binder over a powder bed is a fresh powder bed applied on top of the binder surface [14–15].

Fusion of the Powder Bed—In this technique, each layer of powder is melted or fused together on exposure to a laser or electron beam, and only after joining of powder particles by melt solidification or fusion technique in one layer is the successive layer of powder bed on top applied [14, 16].

9.4 AM THROUGH DEPOSITION OF MATERIAL

In these techniques, the deposition of material layers takes place by the use of nozzles.

Direct Energy Deposition—This technique works on the principle of the deposition of a continuous stream of metal onto the substrate surface with the help of a nozzle, where a laser source melts each layer continuously for solidification to occur layer by layer [14,].

Material Extrusion—Thermoplastics are generally used in this case, which are melted into a semiliquid state, and the layer-by-layer deposition of semiliquid material takes place on the printing head after the solidification of the bottom layer. The semiliquid characteristics of the plastic layers help it solidify and bond by the process of fusion followed by curing in the ambient atmosphere [17]. The co-printing of composite pastes and hydrogels with embedded living cells is also possible with this technique.

Material Jetting (MJ)— Liquid resin in the form of a jet is sprayed layer-wise in this process. A layer is cured with ultraviolet (UV) light before the next layer is printed on top of it [14, 18].

Bioprinting—To print living cells on a 3D scale with the help of different AM-based processes is called bioprinting. This does not fall under the category of any specific AM technique. In this process, the suspension of specific cells in a bio-ink is used for its deposition by a nozzle-based technique, namely, material extrusion or jetting, or by a nozzle-free technique driven by a laser. In the later process, the cell membrane facing the printing surface is coated with a bio-ink, and a laser source is focused on it to transfer forward the droplet of cells on the side of the membrane [19]. High resolution in microscale and the existence of very little shear stress on the cell due to the absence of an orifice are the advantages of this technique [20]. Drop-on-demand (DOD) inkjet bioprinting is another technique for cell-based printing. In contrast to printing of normal ink, inkjet technology involves the printing of living cells associated with biological factors. A cell-containing bio-ink in the form of nanodroplets is ejected and then deposited with very high precision to aggregate into fibers. The fibers are then crosslinked before the next layer is deposited to generate the 3D architecture [21–22]. In this process, the resolution in the vicinity of 100 μm or so can be obtained due to the ejection of a submicron volume of the droplets [23].

Stereolithography (SLA)—In this technique, the print bed is scrolled down into a vat containing a photocurable liquid resin, and then the bed is lifted up to be exposed onto either UV or visible light focused on the bed–resin interface to crosslink the resin [24]. After each step of photopolymerization of resin on exposure to UV or visible light, the bed is again dipped into the vat to deposit a fresh layer of resin, and the process is thus repeated [14, 24].

Sheet Lamination—This process deals with cutting sheets of material, such as paper, plastic, or metal, either with the help of a laser or a blade. In this case, each sheet is sliced into pieces as per the model derived from computer-aided design (CAD). After cutting all the sheets, these are stacked on top of each other and anchored in 3D with the application of a binder. Finally, the 3D inner design is obtained after the sections are cut and removed [14, 25].

9.5   NANOFABRICATION

Nanofabrication is a process mostly suitable for electronics and medicine where a construct less than 100 nm in dimension is fabricated with the help of either a top-down or a bottom-up approach [26]. Although it is not recognized as a conventional AM technique, nanofabrication employs principles similar to AM processes. A "top-down" approach revolves around deconstructing a larger material to form the desired nanostructure, akin to carving a statue out of a block of stone and other traditional machining methods [26]. The "top-down" approach suffers from poor reproducibility of resulting nanostructures due to a lack of accurate control of the parameters in the fabrication process [26]. The second category of nonmanufacturing processes is the "bottom-up" approach, where primary material, is either self-organized or "printed" to generate nanostructures [26] and may have a resolution even at the atomic scale. This additive nature of the "bottom-up" approach is quite similar to most of the other AM processes. A number of applications are possible with nanofabrication technique that covers biomedicine and tissue engineering, such as preserving vaccine's immunogenicity; the minimization of immuno-rejection; the production of biomaterials superior in mechanical and biological performances; controlled and sustained local delivery of drug; the removal of toxins and waste from circulation; and others [27].

9.6   POWDER-BASED TECHNIQUES FOR AM

In powder-based fusion techniques, an object is created in powder-based AM methods by depositing thin layers of powder materials by carving the object's cross section in each layer. Due to their benefits in combining flexibility, easy upscaling, and (often) good material qualities of their outputs, powder-based AM methods have found significant application for a variety of metallic, polymeric, and ceramic materials. The ability to repeat these procedures is dependent on the deposition of uniform layers, which has a direct impact on the quality of the finished products. As a result, powder qualities such as particle size distribution, shape, and roughness, as well as process-related properties like powder flowability and packing density must be carefully examined. Due to these constraints, these techniques have so far been unable to find commercial applications for specific applications [5, 28–29].

Binder jetting and powder bed fusion (PBF) are different types of powder-based AM methods. DED is a group of AM processes that adds material alongside the heat input simultaneously. The heat input can either be a laser or electron beam or a plasma arc to melt the materials as they are deposited and simultaneously fused to form a 3D scaffold. The material feedstock is either metal powder or wire. Powders result in lower deposition efficiency compared with metal wires as only a part of the total powder would be melted and bonded to the substrate. Like the electron PBF (E-PBF), electron beam systems in DED require a vacuum, would not have high oxidation issues and laser system and, on the other hand, would require other methods to introduce inert gases. Powder DED machines often have inert gas blown together with the powder from the nozzles, thereby sheathing the melted region, reducing the oxidization rate. Powder DED systems can use single or multiple nozzles to eject the metal powder. Using multiple nozzles allows the possibility of mixing different materials to get functionally graded materials (FGMs). Laser-engineered net shaping (LENS) is an example of such a procedure. PBF techniques, such as selective laser melting (SLM) and electron beam melting (EBM), use thermal energy to selectively fuse portions of a powder bed.

Binder jetting is a method of joining powder materials by depositing a selective liquid bonding agent. In this process, selective powder material or materials are overlaid into a layer and selectively joined by a binder, which is typically a polymeric liquid. As the desired 3D construct is established, each layer is bonded with the binder that can be heated to cure or set the binder, and the printed part or parts can be removed by a process called "depowdering". Thus, the resulting green body created is then subjected to postprocessing techniques, such as sintering or infiltration, to obtain specific properties. Parameters such as binder selection, binder deposition mechanism, powder–binder interaction, printing capability, printing process parameters (speed, layer thickness, roller speed), densification kinetics of complex structure, postprocessing procedure (sintering, post–heat treatment, surface finishing), and binder burnout characteristics are all factors to consider. Binder jetting has recently been used for electrochemical energy storage, food technology, solid oxide fuel cells, sand-casting molds, waveguide circuits and antennas, concrete construction, renewable bio-based materials, ceramic scaffolds, biopolymers, sandstone production, and biomedical applications and drug delivery.

9.6.1 SELECTIVE LASER SINTERING

Selective laser sintering, or SLS, is a form of powder bed technology that uses a laser beam to selectively sinter thin layers (from about 60–100 μm or more) of thermoplastic powders [30]. Following the completion of a layer, the construction table is lowered by the layer height, fresh powder is distributed over the building bed, and a new layer is defined and sintered [31]. During the process, the build chamber, as well as the powder bed, can be heated or preheated prior to local melting with the laser. The SLS method now can be applied to a wide variety of available thermoplastic powders [32]. Today in the medical sector, SLS is mostly utilized to create visualization models, surgical equipment, and customized implants [33]. Herlin et al. [34] devised a polyamide guide to position the osteotomized bone pieces during a zygomatic osteotomy. In another study, nylon powders were used to create pilot models for preoperative planning and testing [35]. Shishkovsky and Scherbakov conducted studies on the effect of mixing of oxide ceramics and a poly(ether ether ketone) (PEEK) and poly-ε-caprolactone (PLC) compound to fabricate porous scaffolds for tissue engineering applications [36]. Also, several researchers have established tissue-specific scaffold fabrication via the SLS technique [37–41]. In most of the studies, by examining various microstructure and postprinting functionalization, the majority of them exhibited the efficacy of maintaining cell development.

9.6.2 LASER POWDER BED FUSION

Laser powder bed fusion, or L-PBF, commonly known as selective laser melting (SLM), is a process that utilizes a high-energy-density laser, mostly a ytterbium fiber laser. According to the input data, the laser fuses specified areas in a single layer and creates a 3D model part by part and layer-wise. In an inert environment, fine metallic powders are layered on a substrate plate to begin the fabrication process. The platform then lowers itself and a new layer is added after selective melting. This process continues until a desired shape or scaffold of particular dimensions is obtained. Parameters such as laser power, scanning speed, hatching distance, and layer thickness are all common parameters that affect volumetric energy density, mechanical properties, and surface roughness of the parts in L-PBF process [42]. Stainless steel, cobalt chromium (Co-Cr alloys), nickel (Ni)-based alloys, aluminum (Al-Si-Mg alloys), and titanium (Ti6Al4V alloy) are some of the most commonly available alloys for the process [43].

9.6.3 EBM

Electron beam melting (EBM), or electron powder bed fusion (E-PBF), is an AM process for metal powders. In this process, the powder layer is preheated. To the preheated powder, the energy from an electron is then focused in a form of a beam to melt the powder [44]. Hence, the EBM system comprises a combined mechanics of welding machine hardware with electron microscopes operational bases [45]. ARCAM AB owns the rights for EBM® technology [45]. The EBM system works under a vacuum to avoid the beam being deflected by the air molecules. When the process is completed, a soft agglomeration of powder occurs in the scaffold that can be removed in a postprocessing method, such as sandblasting [46]. Because no oxygen is present inside the isolated chamber throughout the melting process, the wasted powder can be recycled numerous times as the chemical composition or physical attributes remains the same. CoCr and Ti6Al4VELI are the most commonly used alloy materials for medical implants fabrication via EBM. Various patient-specific and customized scaffolds and implants with high biocompatibility and osteointegration properties have been developed and studied by many researchers [47–52]. One of the successful examples is the large-scale production of titanium acetabular cups, which are manufactured by two well-known and established companies: Lima Ltd and Ala Ortho Srl.

9.7 APPLICATION OF AM TECHNIQUES IN THE BIOMEDICAL FIELD

9.7.1 METALS

Implants for dental and orthopedic implants, hip and knee replacements, cardiovascular valves, and numerous other surgical equipment are among the biomedical applications of metallic materials. Most commonly used metallic materials for the fabrication of medical devices and implants are 316 L stainless steel (SS), cobalt–chromium (CoCr) alloys, tantalum (Ta), and titanium (Ti) alloys [53–55]. Parameters such as mechanical, biological, and corrosion performance in the physiological milieu of the body determine the reliability of the application of different biomedical implants and medical devices [5]. The demands placed on these metallic materials vary depending on the biomedical applications. For example, metallic materials with elastic moduli closer to those of human bone are required for bone implant applications. Hence, according to the specific applications, these metallic, materials should have high specific strengths, low Young's moduli, good wear characteristics, strong corrosion strength, and biocompatibility [56–57]. Mismatch in elastic moduli of metallic implants and the host or the surrounding bone can result in the resorption around metallic implants, stress-shielding, and eventually complete implant loosening. In this case, revision surgeries to remove or replace the metallic implants are usually required, which are unpleasant and costly for the patients. Casting, powder metallurgy, space holder technology, and foaming can all be used to make biomedical devices out of these metallic materials; however, these traditional methods are not only expensive and time-consuming because they require many energy-intensive processing steps, but they also require secondary processing and complex assemblies to achieve the desired shape. As a result, new technologies are required to create complex metallic structures with decreased rigidity without compromising the critical requirements of the scaffolds. The anchoring of orthopedic implants in natural bone and their interaction with the surrounding tissues are critical to their clinical effectiveness. To stimulate new bone ingrowth, orthopedic tissue engineering implants should have a structure comparable to that of natural bone. Metallic implants can be reliably fixed in the host tissues by matching the native bone's architecture, that is, to that of cortical bone and cancellous bone. Extremely porous metallic structure scaffolds can escape the stress-shielding effect as they demonstrate high strength with low stiffness with certain modifications in their microstructures. The Young's modulus of cancellous bone is substantially lower (22.4–132.32 MPa) than that of cortical bone (7.7–21.8 GPa) [58–59]. For these reasons, it has been demonstrated that lightweight porous structures increase bone ingrowth, which is useful in the long-term fixation of orthopedic implants, when compared to fully dense materials. Critical needs for metallic bone implants, such as form, shapes, sizes, and mechanical qualities, are determined by the implants' intended functions, as well as the patient's age and physical features. SLM and EBM are new AM technologies that are capable of producing intricate and patient-specific porous metallic scaffolds without the need for additional postprocessing [58, 60]. Ti alloys have better biocompatibility, corrosion resistance, and superb mechanical properties, which make them widely used in orthopedic implants [61]. The best-studied biomedical Ti alloy, Ti-6Al-4V, has an identical elastic modulus to human bone and is reasonably inexpensive [62–64]. But cytotoxicity tests using Ti-6Al-4V scaffolds show that Al and V ions are released in the human body, affecting cell growth and causing cytotoxicity [65]. However, using pure Ti, as a good bio-metal, results in preventing hazardous ions from being released into the environment [66]. The researchers discovered that pure Ti scaffolds having a dodecahedral unit structure have superior fatigue cycle strength and ductility than that of Ti-6Al-4V [53, 67]. Certain alloying elements, such as Nb and Zr, enhance the biocompatibility, as well as improve the biological and mechanical properties of the Ti alloy [68–69].

In a study in 2020, Liang *et al.* on Ti-25Nb porous scaffolds having hydrophilic surface structure found that the scaffolds upregulate the expression of phagocytes M2 type and enhance the activity of anti-inflammatory phagocytes. Luo *et al.* in 2020 established a functional relationship among the porosity, yield strength, and the elastic modulus of the Ti-30Nb-5Ta-8Zr scaffold and cortical bone in terms of fatigue strength, compression, and tensile characteristics. Wauthle *et al.* in 2015 and Wang *et al.* in 2019 were able to fabricate three different types of porous metal scaffolds of Ta, pure Ti, and Ti-6Al-4V and reported that Ta porous scaffolds exhibit the same cell proliferation, survival, and osteogenic qualities as Ti scaffolds. Also Ta scaffolds exhibited better toughness and fatigue limit than Ti-6Al-4V scaffolds. Scaffolds made of 316L SS have good mechanical properties, which are similar to the trabecular bone mechanical properties. However, SS, on the other hand, has a larger elastic modulus than that of Ti alloy and Ta, which can easily lead to stress shielding [70–71]. Thus, it is crucial for 316L SS porous scaffold to establish a balanced relationship between strength and elastic modulus by adjusting the pore size and porosity of the scaffolds. The effect of pore size and porosity on the elastic modulus, yield strength, and permeability of 316L SS porous scaffolds was investigated by Ma *et al.* in 2019. The authors reported a functional link between the previously mentioned parameters and the forecasted scaffold's permeability. The superelasticity and shape memory properties of NiTi alloy make it a good candidate for biological applications [72–73]. Nonetheless, the Ni ions in the alloys are cytotoxic, which can cause concern among individuals. Habijan *et al.*, in 2013, cultured human mesenchymal stem cells (hMSC) on NiTi scaffolds with varying porosity and surface morphology. They discovered that the porous scaffold released more Ni than the dense sample, but both were below the cytotoxic concentration. They also discovered that adjusting the spot diameter can improve the surface morphology of the scaffold and that reducing the spot diameter can limit the discharge of Ni ions. They believe NiTi scaffolds are suitable carriers for hMSCs, but process parameters and postprocessing must be fine-tuned before *in vivo* investigations can be conducted. The Co-Cr alloys are frequently used in orthopedic surgery, particularly in hip and knee replacements, because of their superior biocompatibility, corrosion resistance, and wear resistance [74]. Co-Cr alloy, on the other hand, has poor osseointegration and biomechanical qualities when compared to Ti-6Al-4V alloys. Shah *et al.*, in 2016, used EBM to make Co-Cr and Ti-6Al-4V porous scaffolds and investigated *in vivo* application. The authors reported that the Co-Cr scaffold has a lower bone-implant bonding rate than the Ti-6Al-4V scaffold, but they have equivalent bone cell density and dispersion in freshly produced bone. Caravaggi *et al.*, in 2019, used SLM to fabricate Co-Cr scaffolds with various porous architectures and discovered that the elastic modulus of the porous structure is about 32 GPa, which is comparable to the elastic modulus of human bone. Also, the number of cells on the porous structure continued to increase over the course of a week in cell culture trials, demonstrating that the Co-Cr alloy was biocompatible.

Biodegradable metallic biomaterials have been in development for a long time, fabricating biodegradable metallic biomaterials with a fully interconnected porosity and topologically ordered design has been difficult until recently, when direct metal printing made it possible [75–77]. However, the number of materials from which biodegradable porous metallic biomaterials may be fabricated using AM is still restricted, and much more research is needed to advance the subject. Furthermore, the long-term in vivo effects of biodegradable metals are still unknown [78]. However, the local and systemic effects of metallic biodegradable biomaterials require more room for research on the size distribution of the biodegraded products to the immune system reaction and in vivo cytocompatibility toward these products. Also, the mechanical and biodegradation profile, as well as the features of biodegradation products, could theoretically be changed via topological design at the microscale [79].

Furthermore, the enormous surface area of topologically organized volume-porous biomaterials could be exploited to speed up the biodegradation process, allowing for the utilization of metals such as zinc (Zn) or iron (Fe) that disintegrate too slowly. The link between microscale topological design and biodegradation profile, on the other hand, is mainly unknown. Fe is a necessary component of the human body that is also biocompatible. The biggest difficulty with Fe is that it degrades at a slower rate in the human body, which can slow down the rate at which bone tissue grows [80]. Li *et al.*, in 2019, fabricated Fe scaffolds with pore sizes of 600 m (S0.4), 600–800 m (Dense-out), 800–600 m (Dense-in), and 800–600 m (S0.2). The authors reported that the S0.2 and Dense-out scaffolds had the same structure in the center, but the Dense-out scaffold lost more weight in the middle than the S0.2 scaffold as shown in Figure 9.4. The researchers hypothesized that the flow velocities in the center of the Dense-out scaffolds were higher than those on the periphery and that the rate of deterioration of Fe can be influenced by adding alloy components to the scaffolds. Carluccio *et al.*, in 2019, developed porous Fe and Fe-Mn (manganese) scaffolds. The authors reported that the corrosion rate of Fe-Mn scaffold is substantially higher than that of pure Fe. They theorized that a galvanic cell forms between the various metal scaffolds speed up the breakdown of Fe-Mn alloys. Mammalian cells respond well to the Fe-Mn alloy scaffold, which has good biocompatibility and vitality. Magnesium (Mg)-alloy porous scaffolds degrade more quickly, causing them to be completely degraded before bone tissue has fully grown into them. Surface

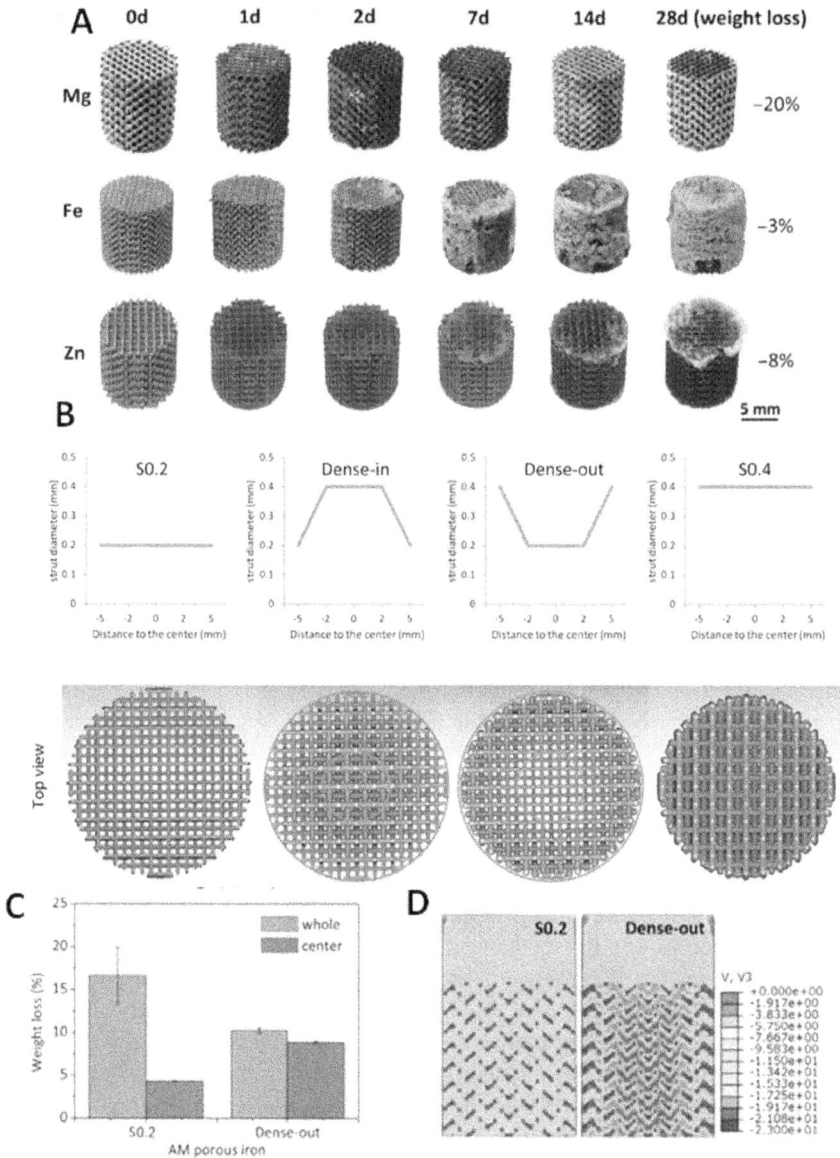

FIGURE 9.4 (a) The morphologies of different Mg, Fe, and Zn porous biodegradable samples after in vitro immersion; (b) the graded structure of porous scaffolds; (c) the S0.2 and Dense-out for 28 days; and (d) the flow distribution in S0.2 and Dense-out sample according to the computational fluid dynamics (CFD) modeling. (Image taken from [81–82].)

modifications (plasma electrolytic oxidation) and heat treatment processes were used by Kopp *et al.* in 2019 to reduce the rate of degradation of the Mg scaffold.

It was observed that Mg hydroxide and oxide develop on the scaffold surface, slowing the rate of deterioration in the simulated bodily fluid. Because Mg is more active, it might cause issues like difficulty in preparation, powder splashing, cracks, and so on. The rate at which Mg scaffolds degrade can result in the formation of hydrogen, which can have a deteriorating effect on cell proliferation. Zn alloys have attracted the interest of many researchers as their breakdown rate is similar to that of bone tissue, which is favorable to bone tissue mending [83–84]. Li *et al.*, in 2020, fabricated diamond-structured Zn scaffolds and discovered that the mechanical properties are similar to cancellous bone. After 28 days of dynamic and static immersion in vitro, the volume loss is 7.8% and 3.6%, respectively. Also, after soaking, the mechanical characteristics of Zn scaffolds improved when degradation of the scaffold was initiated.

High-entropy alloys are rapidly becoming a focus of research due to their greater comprehensive properties when compared to standard metals and alloys. These alloys are no longer based on a single component but rather a combination of metals to improve qualities including strength, corrosion resistance, and biocompatibility [85]. Motallebzadeh *et al.*, in 2019, developed high-entropy TiZrTaHfNb and $Ti_{1.5}ZrTa_{0.5}Hf_{0.5}Nb0.5$ alloys and compared their characteristics to those of 316L, Co-Cr-Mo, and Ti6Al4V alloys. The authors reported that high entropy alloys have better wear and corrosion resistance and that the higher mechanical properties were attributed to the high entropy alloy's "cocktail effect". Nagase *et al.*, in 2020, used a mix of Ti-Nb-Ta-Zr-Mo and Co-Cr-Mo alloy systems to produce innovative $TiZrHfCr_{0.2}Mo$ and $TiZrHfCo_{0.07}Cr_{0.07}Mo$ high-entropy alloys for metallic biomaterials. The results of the experiments revealed that the newly produced high entropy has a biocompatibility that is comparable to pure Ti.

9.7.2 CERAMICS

Tooling and molding are the most typical methods for shaping ceramics, but additive technologies have reduced the complications related to macroscale fabrications. AM processes have the advantage of quickly customizing parts with extremely complicated geometries and interconnected porosity with a balance in maintaining the mechanical behavior of ceramic materials [86]. Recently, 3D printing of ceramic materials such as tricalcium phosphate (TCP), hydroxyapatite, calcium sulfate, alumina, porcelain, and ceramic composites have gathered the attention of the researchers for the fabrication of bone and teeth [87–88]

Castilho *et al.*, in 2013, studied the effect of 3D-printing orientation on microstructure and mechanical properties of β-TCP by using Spectrum Z510 Z Corp. The β-TCP powder was sieved, synthesized, and ball-milled to obtain a size of <160 μm, which was mixed with 20% (v/v) phosphoric acid. The findings show that low-temperature 3D printing is a dependable method for creating personalized synthetic scaffolds and that when combined with topology optimization design, it can be a potent tool for fabricating patient-specific bone implants. From the study, it was concluded that the printing direction had a significant effect on the mechanical properties of the 3D-printed scaffold (with printing in the *y*-direction indicating the highest mechanical strength, toughness, and stiffness); however, structural properties, such as geometric accuracy and porosity, were not affected. Vlasea, Toyserkani, and Pilliar, in 2015, fabricated 3D interconnected macroporous β-TCP scaffolds with regulated internal architecture by 3D printing that showed good mechanical strength after microwave sintering. Authors reported maximum compressive strengths of 10.95 ± 1.28 MPa and 6.62 ± 0.67 MPa for scaffolds sintered in microwave and conventional furnaces with 500-mm planned pores (approximately 400 mm after sintering). In another study, Vorndran *et al.* in 2008 outlined the fabrication of porous 3D-printed β-TCP with 5 wt% hydroxypropyl methylcellulose that had a low printing resolution, low specific surface area, and a compressive strength of about 1.2 ± 0.2 MPa. Different postprocessing conditions affecting the densification behavior of the final product were studied by Bertol, Schabbach, and Loureiro dos Santos in 2017, including immersing the printed samples in various solutions, such as a binder, Ringer's solution, or phosphoric acid, or sintering at temperatures ranging from 800–1500 °C for 3D printed α-TCP scaffolds. The densified scaffolds formed contained a variety of phases, including calcium-deficient hydroxyapatite, brushite, monetite, and unreacted α-TCP, according to phase analysis data. The mechanical properties achieved are still low, but the high porosity presented in α-TCP scaffolds with different phases can potentially result in greater bone ingrowth. Porosity, density, phase stability, mechanical behavior, and biocompatibility of binder-jetted scaffolds composed of β-TCP were described by Santos *et al.* in 2012. The authors studied the scaffolds sintered at 1250 °C and at 1400 °C, which had an apparent density of $55 \pm 2\%$ and $46 \pm 9\%$, water adsorption of $84 \pm 8\%$ and $57 \pm 2\%$, and compressive strength of 2.36 ± 0.05 MPa and 8.66 ± 0.11 MPa, respectively.

Hydroxyapatite (HA) is a derivative of tricalcium phosphate with the same Ca:P ratio of 1.67 as bone structure, so it has better biocompatibility compared with other CaPs compounds. Seitz *et al.*, in 2005, produced binder-jetted HA scaffolds and showed that the 3D-printed parts sintered at 1250 °C could have various levels of porosity based on the designed microchannels where the comprehensive strength of approximately 22 MPa was reported for the dense structure. Another derivative of calcium phosphate is tetracalcium phosphate (TTCP), with a Ca:P ratio of 2. As stated earlier, the higher the Ca:P ratio, the lower degradation can be expected for the CaPs compounds; therefore, TTCP has the highest biocompatibility among the CaPs widely used for bone matrix. Also, dicalcium phosphate (DCP) is another common calcium phosphate bioceramic with a Ca:P ratio of 1. Vorndran *et al.*, in 2008, proposed binder jetting from two different mixtures made of powders with a Ca:P ratio of 1.7 (method A) and TTCP/DCP composite (method B) to study the printability, densification, and mechanical behavior of the 3D-printed scaffolds. Porous scaffolds produced by method A showed a higher print resolution with a porosity of 56% and compressive strength of 7.4 ± 0.7 MPa while method B showed a porosity of 60% with compressive strength of 1.2 ± 0.2 MPa. Klammert *et al.*, in 2010, reported applying an acid solution as a binder on calcium phosphate to print TTCP or DCP powders using binder jet 3D printing (BJ3DP) for cranial and maxillofacial defect fixations. Afterward, hydrothermal treatment of the implants (refers to Figure 9.5) caused the brushite compound to convert to monetite with a high print resolution and part accuracy. In another study, Habibovic *et al.*, in 2008, a low-temperature direct 3D printing was employed to fabricate brushite and monetite implants with various shapes.

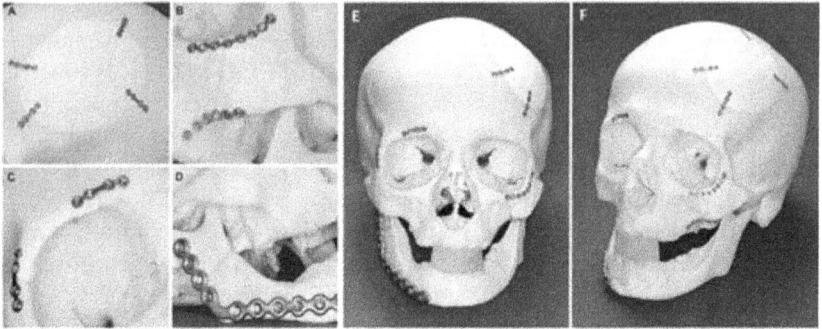

FIGURE 9.5   The hydrothermal treatment of the brushite compound to convert to monetite in cranial and maxillofacial fixation areas. (Image reference taken from [89].)

Calcium sulfate ($CaSO_4$) is an inorganic compound used as a biomaterial in bone tissue engineering. One main drawback of the scaffold structures made from calcium sulfate is the low mechanical performance due to the brittle character. Also, the presence of organic compounds in the initial powder, as well as the binder solution, can cause high toxicity levels in products. Asadi-Eydivand *et al.*, in 2016, studied the optimization of binder jetting of calcium sulfate and the resulting mechanical strength of the porous parts. Results demonstrated that printing in the x-direction with a minimum layer thickness of 89 µm and a delay time of 300 ms could lead to the highest quality scaffold prototypes in terms of dimensional accuracy, a compressive strength of 0.75 MPa, Young's modulus of 47.15 MPa, and a total porosity of 67.7%. In other words, target porosity and optimal mechanical strength correlated with the lowest layer thickness. Vaezi and Chua, in 2011, reported the influence of binder jet processing parameters such as layer thicknesses and printing orientations on the physical and mechanical properties of 3D-printed scaffolds. A layer thickness of 0.1125 mm and printing in the *x*-direction were the best printing conditions, leading to the highest compressive strength, toughness, and Young's modulus. Furthermore, microscopy and µCT analyses demonstrated that scaffolds printed with a layer thickness of 0.1125 mm in the *x*-direction had more dimensional accuracy with designed microchannels interconnectivity and porosity.

9.7.3   COMPOSITE

Ceramic composites have been used for various biomedical applications. The composition of ceramic matrix composites can be made based on a wide variety of ceramic and metal materials. Typically, different calcium phosphates (CaPs) have been blended for scaffold fabrication. Although HA shows outstanding biocompatibility, the biodegradation rate is too low; thus, it is generally combined with TCP for tailoring its biodegradability. Al2O3/Al composite is another composite material that is intensively studied. Since the ratio of the coarse to the fine powders needs to be optimized to attain a proper flowability of the mixture with maximum packing density, Zhou *et al.*, 2014, reported the effect of using coarse and fine powders in 3D printing of calcium sulfate/CaP scaffolds to gain advantages from bimodal powder mixtures. The influence of CaP particle size, calcium phosphate–to–calcium sulfate ratio (CaP:CaSO$_4$), and type of CaP used (which was TCP and HA) on the binder jetting process was investigated. As expected from the fine powder particles of ≤20 µm, a heterogeneous powder bed was reported with low powder bed density. Besides, some other characteristics such as slow drop penetration speed, large drop penetration depth, low wetting ratio, poor green mass, and low green strength are the main consequences of low powder bed density. Based on powder physical reactivity, the addition of β-TCP may compromise the CaSO$_4$–water reactivity as β-TCP:CaSO$_4$ powder combinations had significantly lower wetting ratios and green strengths when compared with the HA:CaSO$_4$ powder combinations. Castilho *et al.*, in 2014, reported 3D printing from an HA-TCP mixture to produce porous scaffolds for bone defects fixation. To cure the binder-jetted scaffolds, phosphoric acid was applied during 3D printing. The designed scaffolds had interconnected microchannels of 300 µm and a dimensional accuracy of >96.5%. Based on the microstructural observation and mechanical properties, a mixture of HA and TCP with a ratio of 1.83 resulted in a desired porosity level of 67 ± 0.8% for the sintered sample and a compressive strength of about 0.4 MPa. It was also found that the postprocessing treatment as infiltrating with poly(lactide-co-glycolide) (PLGA) could enhance the mechanical strength up to about 3.4 MPa with toughness about four times higher than only sintered scaffolds. Interestingly, the infiltrated scaffolds provided higher cell viability using osteoblastic cells MG63 compared with pure TCP control. In another study, binder-jetted bone tissue using a powder blended of HA-40 wt% TCP. The open porosity level of the final scaffolds was 53.1 ± 1.5% with desirable surface features for osteoclastic activation. Khalyfa *et al.*, 2007, blended TTCP (as a reacting agent with an aqueous citric acid binder) and β-TCP (as a biodegradable filler) to produce bone scaffolds. Scaffolds with a porosity level of about 38% and compressive strength of 0.7 MPa were binder-jetted where the strength increased up to the order of magnitude after a posttreatment using dianhydro-D-glucitol (bis(dilactoyl)-methacrylate)). Moreover, in vitro testing using MC3T3-E1 cells confirmed the biocompatibility of the binder jetted scaffolds. Recently, various additives including magnesia (MgO), strontia (SrO), zinc oxide (ZnO), and silica (SiO$_2$) have been used to enhance the physical and biological behavior of CaP scaffolds [428,604,608]. Fielding *et al.* used binder jetting technology to fabricate scaffolds with various interconnected microchannels sizes [90]. A remarkable enhancement of density, compressive strength and better bioactivity in vitro using osteoblast cells was attained in the β-TCP scaffolds doped with SiO$_2$ and ZnO.

9.7.4 POLYMERS

In general, polymers can be divided into two groups, natural and synthetic polymers. Natural polymers, such as chitosan, collagen, and gelatin, exhibit better biocompatibility and biodegradation properties than synthetic polymers. Depending on the degree of crosslinking, natural polymers can be degraded within 2 to 24 weeks by natural enzymes, without releasing any acidic by-products [91]. Even though the compressive modulus of these natural polymers ranges from 0.005 MPa–90 MPa compares to the cancellous bone compressive modulus, which is higher than 100 MPa [92–93], these polymers are used as additives or to make composites for their osteoinductive properties. Moreover, these polymers, when included, exhibit better cell and protein adhesion and hence better biomimetism. Preclinical in vivo studies done on mice and rats have shown that a combination of silk fibroin and chitosan can be used alone to heal craniofacial defects. For sterilization, generally, ethylene oxide sterilization is used for natural polymers as the process is suitable for heat-sensitive materials. Both electron-beam irradiation and autoclaving are not used as these processes can accelerate the degradation process and can hamper the crosslinking of the material [94–95]. On the other hand, synthetic polymers are man-made polymers that can be biodegradable and nonbiodegradable. Biodegradable polymers, such as poly-ε-caprolactone (PCL), PLGA, poly(lactic acid) (PLA), and poly(propylene fumarate) (PPF), or nonbiodegradable, such as PEEK and polyether ketone ketone (PEKK). Biodegradable polymers have better dimensional resolutions and better printability because of their low melting point (~60°C for PCL and ~175°C for PLA) [96], which makes these materials suitable for 3D printing without the installation of a complex heating system [97]. The degradation rate of these polymers can be tuned according to the application, and the degradation by-products are nontoxic, for example, PLA and PLGA, and release comparatively less acid, for example, PCL [98–99]. Moreover, these polymers exhibit better biocompatibility, osteoconductive, radiolucent, and histocompatible properties with better mechanical properties with compressive strength of the order of 2–39 MPa compared to the native bone compressive strength of 2–12 MPa and compressive modulus of 52–318 MPa subjected to the scaffold porosity [100–101] However, they are not highly biomimetic when used alone since they are unable to induce bone formation by themselves. Most clinical applications include craniomaxillofacial bone reconstruction and preclinical applications such as in load-bearing sites: femoral and tibiae defects. For sterilization, UV exposure, γ-irradiation, and β-irradiation are used. However, autoclaving, ethylene oxide, and plasma sterilization can result in shrinkage of the material and can induce toxicity.

9.7.5 EXTRUSION-BASED TECHNIQUE

Extrusion-based AM is one of the most widely used techniques for mass production of scaffolds with microscale structure and multiple material porous bioactive structures. In this process, there is a constant flow of material or materials in the form of a slurry or paste or thick ink, which is dispensed layer by layer by the extrusion nozzle controlled by a movable extrusion head. The entire 3D motion system is controlled by a computer that has a range of construction method inputs by different software(s). Also, the technique ensures the 3D bioconstruction of unique biological feature scaffolds with minimum biomaterial waste. Extrusion-based AM process can be divided into two different categories: processes that include material melting and process that don't involve material melting. The primary extrusion-based AM techniques are based on melting processes that include FDM, precision extrusion deposition, 3D fiber deposition, precise extrusion manufacturing, and multiphase jet solidification.

And the most often utilized extrusion-based AM technique without material melting includes pressure-assisted microsyringe (PAM), low-temperature deposition manufacturing, 3D bio-plotting, robocasting, direct-write assembly, and solvent-based extrusion freeforming.

One of the first methods based on polymer melts extrusion for 3D printing with a high-strength functional part was the FDM process. Polymeric material/filament is used as a feedstock, which is then pushed into the liquefier section and eventually extruded from a computer-controlled nozzle. For the manufacturing of biomaterials, a variety of modified FDM systems have been developed depending on the 3D microstructure and different pore sizes.

9.8 AM OF 3D CERAMIC SCAFFOLDS POST SINTERING

Particularly, CaP-based bioceramic scaffolds exhibit mechanical, structural, and compositional similarity to bone apatite in the extracellular matrix of native bone tissue. To take advantage of their beneficial properties, AM-derived 3D bioceramic scaffolds have been applied in bone tissue engineering on a wide scale. A vastly explored technique is to print "green body" with customized shape, geometry, pore size, and architecture followed by postprocess sintering at a suitable temperature [102]. This allows burnt removal of all organic phases, leaving behind pure ceramic scaffolds and enhancement of mechanical strength and Young's modulus of the sintered body by anchorages between ceramic phases. A microextrusion-based 3D-printing technique was employed by Seidenstuecker *et al.* fabricated bioglass/β-TCP green body scaffolds using dextrin as a binder that were later subjected to sintering at high temperatures [103]. Thus, the prepared scaffolds, although found to be not compatible for load-bearing applications because of the exhibition of a lower mechanical strength of 0.17–0.64 MPa, elicited enhanced osteogenic properties for their possible applications as bone filler [104]. In a similar work, Chen *et al.* prepared a lithium–calcium–silicate crystal-based bio-glass ceramic scaffold through extrusion-based AM process and postprocessing sintering for osteochondral interface regeneration that exhibited the dual properties of cartilage and bone regeneration [105]. The scaffolds were provided a strong interface to support both osteogenic and chondrogenic differentiation of mesenchymal stem cells (MSCs) in *in vitro* and *in vivo* as well [106].

9.9 PRINTING OF 3D CERAMIC SCAFFOLDS AT AMBIENT/LOW TEMPERATURES

A nonsintered ceramic scaffold can also be processed by extrusion-based AM technique to stimulate regeneration of bone tissue. In this case, binders in the form of an organic or natural polymer are employed to anchor green ceramic bodies, ceramic powders that remain in the 3D-printed implants under application conditions. Biphasic calcium phosphate nanoparticles (nBCPs) and PVA-based composite 3D scaffold containing platelet-rich fibrin were printed by Song et al. using an extrusion-based method at low temperatures [107]. Enhanced osteogenic activity, such as bone marrow–derived MSCs (BMSCs) adhesion, proliferation, and osteogenic differentiation, was observed *in vitro* and a greater degree of new bone information *in vivo* when the prepared scaffold was implanted in a rabbit model was exhibited. In a separate study, by employing a Fab@home 3D printer, graphene oxide/alginic acid/TCP (GO/AA/TCP)–containing scaffolds were manufactured to resemble the natural architecture of cancellous bone to facilitate nutrient exchange and neovascularization [108]. Because of the presence of GO, the scaffolds exhibited greater porosity without any deleterious effect on mechanical strength. Thus, prepared scaffolds exhibited higher bioactivity as evident from their greater capacity for biomineralization and the differentiation of osteoprecursor cell lines.

9.10 POST-FUNCTIONALIZED 3D-PRINTED CERAMIC SCAFFOLDS

After the fabrication of ceramic scaffolds, surface functionalization, including coating and adsorption of functional agents and/or biomolecules, has been vastly used to endow the scaffolds with enhanced surface properties. Robocasting technique was persuaded to print 3D scaffolds from a paste containing 60 vol% HA and 40 vol% β-TCP and then subjected to sintering [109]. A dip-coating method was adopted to further coat the sintered scaffolds with PCL/calcium peroxide (CPO) composite for the in situ generation of oxygen locally at the site of implantation.

The coated scaffolds could provide great potential for promoting bone ingrowth with improved osteoblast cell viability and proliferation under hypoxic conditions. Kim et al. incorporated bone morphogenetic protein-2 (BMP-2)-loaded PLGA nanoparticles on the surface of a 3D-printed HAp scaffold using a PCL emulsion coating method [110]. BMP-2/PLGA nanoparticles were uniformly distributed on the scaffold surface and BMP-2 was released gradually. Moreover, PCL coating improved the compressive strength of the scaffold. *In vitro* cell proliferation, adhesion, osteogenic differentiation, and *in vivo* new bone formation were all improved with PCL-BMP-2/PLGA nanoparticle-coated scaffold.

9.11 3D PRINTING OF HYDROGEL SCAFFOLDS

Extrusion-based 3D printing is one of the versatile techniques for preparing bone tissue–engineered 3D scaffolds because of its intrinsic capacity to encapsulate cells and biomolecules in situ [111]. A gelatin/PVA solution was utilized in the form of bio-ink to print scaffolds for hard tissue engineering on a plate kept at low temperature [112]. By a similar approach, sodium alginate was blended with a poly (ethyleneimine) solution in the form of a polyelectrolyte complex and reinforced with silica gel to produce osteoinductive scaffolds through 3D bioprinting. A paste from a combination of collagen, decellularized extracellular matrix (ECM), and silk fibroin was extruded to produce micro/nanoporous biocomposite scaffolds through 3D printing at low temperatures [113]. Such fabricated scaffolds, however, registered a compressive strength and a modulus considerably lower compared to that of human cancellous bone, favorable micro- and nanoporous architecture, and compositional similarity to ECM-promoted adhesion, proliferation, and differentiation of osteoprogenitor cells when cultured *in vitro* onto the scaffolds. Compositionally and functionally graded hydrogel scaffolds from a combination of N-acryloyl glycinamide, and *N*-[tris(hydroxymethyl) methyl] acrylamide was prepared by Gao et al for osteochondral tissue engineering by employing an extrusion-based 3D-printing technique [114]. MSCs cultured onto these functionally graded scaffolds were differentiated into chondrogenic and osteogenic lineage *in vitro* in a spatiotemporal scale. Furthermore, these scaffolds promoted new bone tissue formation and cartilage regeneration simultaneously *in vivo* to exhibit its potential for application in osteochondral tissue engineering. In another work, a direct 3D-printing method was employed for a gelatin/alginate solution as a printing ink to produce scaffolds that were further surface-modified through a uniform biomimetic coating of nanoapatite [115]. Thus, the produced scaffolds exhibited good mechanical properties, higher than that of human cancellous bone, promising a potential for the desirable protein adsorption and superior osteogenic properties when rat BMSCs were cultured onto it. The same research group printed 3D scaffolds from an alginate/PVA paste in which bovine serum albumin (BSA) and recombinant human BMP-2 (rhBMP-2) were encapsulated into alginate microparticles followed by crosslinking in $CaCl_2$ solution to support enough mechanical strength in the fabricated scaffolds against sudden collapse [116]. The formulation of bio-inks by crosslinking between appropriate peptide and alginate with the help of EDC/NHS coupling and 3D printing of such a bio-ink by extrusion-based techniques to prepare hybrid bone tissue–engineering scaffolds was studied by Heo *et al.* [117]. Human adipose tissue-derived stem cells supported in vitro osteogenesis onto these scaffolds. *In vivo* studies also demonstrated its high bone regeneration capacity, although the mechanical performance of such scaffolds was not investigated.

9.12 CELL-EMBEDDED HYDROGEL SCAFFOLDS—3D PRINTING

Osteoblast cells were seeded onto nanocomposite constructs from poly(ethylene glycol) diacrylate (PEGDA)/hyaluronic acid/nanoclay-based bio-inks and printed using a two-channel 3D bioprinting method [118]. With more than 95% viable osteoblast cells incorporated into PEG/clay constructs within a short time, it elicited a high long-term osteogenic capacity because of the release of bioactive ions, including Mg and Si ions, that promoted differentiation of interacting cells *in vitro* and *in vivo*. MC3T3-E1 pre-osteoblastic cells were embedded in chitosan- and chitosan-hyaluronic acid–based bio-ink and 3D-printed via extrusion-based technique as reported by Demirtas et al [119]. Cells embedded in chitosan/hyaluronic acid-based constructs exhibited promising osteogenic capacity as well. Better rheological behavior was shown by chitosan-based hydrogels in comparison to alginate-based hydrogels, which was attributed superior printable properties in the former and presented the bio-ink formulation as a better candidate for producing cell-embedded hydrogel scaffolds suitable for the purpose of regeneration of bone tissues.

9.13 EXTRUSION-BASED 3D PRINTING— NON-HYDROGEL-BASED POLYMER

9.13.1 HIGH-TEMPERATURE-PROCESSED POLYESTER SCAFFOLDS FOR 3D PRINTING

Other than ceramic components and hydrogels, polyesters can also be used as one of the major sources of printing inks to produce scaffolds for bone tissue regeneration by virtue of an extrusion-based 3D-printing technique, such as FDM. PLA, PLGA, and

PCL, being biocompatible as well as biodegradable polyesters, are often exploited in the form of wires or pellets to produce scaffolds for bone tissue engineering [120, 121]. Polyester wires and pellets are continuously fed into the heated chamber fitted with a metal nozzle and then are melted, extruded, and deposited in a customizable pattern as programmed through a CAD model. Because of heat dissipation at room temperature, the extruded patterns quickly solidify, and then the next extruded layer is deposited on top to form a layer-by-layer assembly of polyester scaffolds, intended for application in bone tissue engineering. FDM-derived poly(l-lactic acid) (PLLA) scaffolds were fabricated by Gremare et al., and the physicochemical and biological properties of such scaffolds were assessed [122]. After culturing osteoblastic cells into them, the scaffolds exhibited supportive osteogenic properties. Similarly, FDM was employed to produce PLGA scaffolds with controlled macroporous architecture [101]. The geometry and porous architecture of PLGA scaffolds could be tailored by controlling the inner diameter of the metallic nozzle, the extrusion pressure, the temperature, the printing angles, and the layer thickness. In addition to exhibiting favorable osteogenic potential, the fabricated PLGA scaffolds registered compressive strength values ranging between 15–23 MPa, with varying degrees of macroporosity, that diminished with increasing total porosity as usual.

Although FDM is a versatile technique for producing scaffolds with customized sizes, geometries, and porous architectures, the inability to exhibit superior bioactive properties by FDM-derived scaffolds plays spoilsport to its favorable osteogenic response and accelerated rate of bone regeneration [123].

9.13.2 Posttreatment of Polyester Scaffolds 3D-Printed at High Temperatures

Despite possessing favorable biodegradable properties essential for bone tissue engineering applications, the smooth strut surface in FDM-derived polyester scaffolds is a challenge to overcome for enhanced cellular attachment and cellular ingrowth into such scaffolds. In this regard, graphene incorporation into PCL scaffolds at high temperatures and extruded and 3D-printed by the FDM method showed promise by enhancing surface hydrophilicity and cellular attachment and ingrowth into it [124]. A pristine graphene elicited a favorable effect on osteoblast proliferation and viability. In order to impart higher roughness and hydrophilicity onto the scaffold's strut, PCL scaffolds were ultrasonicated in acetone and/or NaOH solution [125], and a higher rate of adsorption of osteogenic biomolecules, such as BMP-2 onto the scaffold's surface, was observed, although a little negative effect on mechanical properties was detected. In respect of *in vitro* biological properties, such surface-treated scaffolds exhibited higher proliferation and improved osteogenic differentiation of human MSCs. Porogen in the form of PEG was also used to impart surface porosity and hence hydrophilicity in FDM-derived polyester scaffolds. PCL/PEG scaffolds were fabricated by using FDM, followed in order to remove water-soluble PEG posttreatment to generate microporous topography on the strut surface [126]. In this way, the wettability, as well as cellular proliferation, was considerably enhanced on PCL/PEG scaffolds. Other strategies for surface modification include coating layers of hydrophilic molecules and different other biomolecules onto the strut surface to stimulate favorable cellular responses. After fabricating PLA scaffolds via the FDM technique, Teixeira *et al.* [127] directly immersed the scaffolds into mussel-inspired polydopamine (PDA) solution for 24 h [127], and then type I collagen was conjugated to the PDA-coated PLA scaffolds via EDC/NHS-mediated crosslinking mechanism for 48 h. Pre-osteoblast cells cultured onto the PDA/collagen-modified PLA scaffolds not only exhibited higher cellular attachments as shown by significant upregulation of expression of adhesive plaques of vinculin and F-actin cytoskeleton but also enhanced cellular ingrowth and osteogenic differentiation. In a separate study conducted by Ritz *et al.* [128], both collagen I and stromal-derived factor-1 (SDF-1) incorporated PLA scaffolds were fabricated by FDM technique in a cage- and disc-like geometry. A steady SDF-1 release was observed in PLA cage-like scaffolds to stimulate angiogenesis by the growth of endothelial cells and neovascularization *in vivo*, showcasing such PLA scaffolds' capability in enhancing bone tissue regeneration and repair.

9.13.3 NATURAL AND SYNTHETIC POLYMER FOR BONE TISSUE ENGINEERING: SCAFFOLDS 3D-PRINTED AT ROOM/LOW TEMPERATURES

For in situ delivery of biomolecules, room temperature or cryogenic temperature extrusion and 3D printing of natural and synthetic polymer is considered a viable option for producing scaffolds for application in bone tissue engineering [129]. Different organic solvents, such as 1,4-dioxane and dimethyl sulfoxide (DMSO), are employed to dissolve the synthetic polymer in the formation of bio-inks in which different bioagents such as biomolecules, drugs, and even bioceramic particles are loaded. By tailoring the processing parameters, multifunctional scaffolds loaded with different growth factors could be printed and processed. Alendronate (ALN)-infiltrated PCL/ALN scaffolds were fabricated by extrusion-based 3D printing using DMSO as a solvent [130]. The ALN release lasted for a continuous 4-week stretch from PCL scaffolds, and no apparent toxicity against MG-63 cells was observed; instead, osteoblast activity and matrix mineralization were enhanced. Furthermore, compared to a pure PCL scaffold, ALN-incorporated PCL scaffolds exhibited enhanced capability of forming new bone when placed inside a rat tibial defect model. In a separate study, P(DLLA-TMC), a thermo-responsive shape memory polymer, was dissolved in dichloromethane (DCM) and mixed with an aqueous solution of rhBMP-2 to formulate water-in-oil emulsion inks, and the scaffolds were printed by a 3D extrusion method [131]. The fabricated scaffold appeared soft at 37 °C though exhibiting excellent room temperature compressive strength and showed great potential for stimulating bone regeneration in a minimally invasive way. Yang *et al.* prepared macroporous scaffolds with a hierarchical structure using extrusion-based 3D printing at room temperature from PLLA/PCL/DCM-based water-in-oil emulsion as inks in which silicon dioxide nanoparticles were employed as emulsifiers [132]. The water phase in such an emulsion was very low—only 30:70 in volume ratio—that made it feasible to produce homogeneously distributed microporous (20-μm) struts in the scaffolds with high open porosity of 98.3%. Improved osteoblast adhesion and proliferation were observed on the scaffolds' surface, highlighting its capability to repair and regenerate bone tissue in an efficient manner.

9.13.4 Bone Regeneration by 3D-Printed Scaffolds of Synthetic/Natural Polymer: Electrostatic Field-Assisted Micro-Extrusion

Another important 3D-printing technique to produce tissue engineering scaffolds is electrospinning, which operates on the principle of electrostatic field-assisted micro-extrusion [133]. Ristovski et al. directly deposited an ordered scaffold with 200 layers by virtue of the near-field melt electrospinning technique [134]. A fiber spacing of 1 mm with a diameter in the range of 40 μm was obtained in the electrospun scaffold that induced efficient cell attachment and homogeneous cell distribution. The results showed that a regular microstructure in the electrospun mat could be possible during the fabrication of scaffolds by controlling the parameters by using electrostatic actuation and this kind of microstructure in the prepared scaffold is highly desirable for tissue engineering application. Using the technique of near-field electrospinning layer-wise deposition of HAp/PCL scaffold possessing uniform and narrow pore size distribution was executed [135]. Both pore size and the degradation rate of the fabricated scaffolds could be tailored by varying the PCL-to-HAp volume % ratio. The fabricated scaffolds exhibited no cytotoxicity as cultured MC3T3-E1 cells were found to adhere, multiply, and differentiate effectively in vitro. Bio-mimetically deposited nano-HAp onto near-field electrospun PCL scaffold was also tested for bone tissue engineering [136]. The prepared scaffold exhibited a pore size distribution between 50–100 μm, with a strand diameter of 10 μm. MC3T3-E1 cells cultured onto it, found ideal microenvironment as cells committed to adhere and proliferate to support bone tissue regeneration and repair. In a separate study, the electro-hydrodynamic printing technique was utilized by Kim et al. [137] to produce 3D microfibrous PCL scaffolds with a very high load of TCP nanoparticles. The electro-hydrodynamic printing technique is similar to the near-field direct-write electrospinning in principle, and this case was effectively employed to fabricate layer-by-layer ceramic struts entangled with PCL microfibers. Unlike other types of near-field electrospinning-based scaffolds containing a regular microfibrous structure, the struts in the fabricated scaffolds exhibited a diameter of 500 μm, resembling a rough microporous structure composed of numerous curly PCL microfibers and TCP particles. Process parameters such as flow rate, nozzle size, applied electric field, bioceramic phase content were tailored to optimize the properties of a fabricated scaffold. This newly designed scaffold elicited considerably higher mineralization capacity and osteogenic properties as evident from cellular activities of cultured pre-osteoblasts onto the scaffolds.

9.13.5 Synthetic Natural Polymer- and Inorganic-Based Composites for Bone Tissue Regeneration

Bone regeneration is a complex process, which requires incorporating a number of molecular, cellular, biochemical, and mechanical stimuli. Hence, for inducing bone regeneration, porous bone tissue engineering scaffolds with the right shape, pore size, porosity, degradability, biocompatibility, mechanical properties, and cellular responses are essential [138–139]. Polyesters, which are biocompatible, biodegradable, and bioresorbable, play an important role in the 3D printing of polymeric scaffolds [140]. These polyesters can be dissolved in an organic/aqueous solvent to allow micro-extrusion-based 3D printing at room/low temperatures or processed into wires, pellets, or even powders to enable 3D printing of polymer scaffolds with the help of high-temperature melting extrusion followed by sintering [141]. Davila *et al.* [142] reported the fabrication of composite scaffolds containing β-TCP/PCL via micro-screw extrusion-based 3D printing in which β-TCP was used as a nucleating agent, which allows a proper arrangement of polymeric chains of PCL, and resulted in increased crystallinity of the polymeric matrix. The authors reported that the addition of β-TCP enhances the mechanical and hydrophilic properties of the scaffold. Biological surface functionalization of bioceramics/polymeric scaffolds enhances the bioactivity of the composite scaffolds. Goncalves et. al. [143] reported a unique 3D-printed composite scaffold that consists of nano HA, carbon nanotubes, and PCL matrix by using FDM for bone tissue regeneration. The constructed 3D-printed scaffolds exhibited an interconnected network of square pores of about 450–700 µm, and the best balance of mechanical strength and electrical conductivity was found in scaffolds with 2 wt% of carbon nanotubes with compressive strength of 4 MPa.

9.14   VAT PHOTOPOLYMERIZATION TECHNIQUES

The most common vat photopolymerization (VPP) process is stereolithography (SLA). Dr. Hideo Kodama of Nagoya Municipal Industrial Research Institute released his research of a working rapid prototyping system employing photopolymers in 1981, which launched the SLA method. Charles (Chuck) W. Hull made 3D-printing history by developing SLA and cofounding the 3D Systems Corporation to commercialize technology 3 years later, in 1984. SLA refers to a group of AM techniques in which a liquid resin is turned into a solid product by exposing it to a light source that selectively initiates the polymerization of the material. To build a solid 3D model, an older technique uses a vat of liquid photopolymer resin cured by a UV laser. A computer-controlled mirror directs the UV laser beam onto the surface of the photopolymer resin to draw one cross section of the CAD model of the part. The building platform is lowered into the vat when one layer is completed, and the laser beam–tracing procedure is repeated. A blade is typically used to create a smooth resin layer. The technique is repeated layer by layer until the part's manufacture is complete. The platform lifts out of the vat once the model is finished, and the leftover resin is drained. In order to satisfy the material's requisite strength, the model is then removed from the platform and placed in a UV oven for final curing. After that, the supports are ultimately removed. Because the object is constructed upside-down, another SLA system is known as inverted SLA [91, 97, 144]. Although two-photon polymerization is a type of VPP, it isn't used in bone tissue engineering. Indeed, the build space is restricted, the fabrication speed is slow, and the materials that can be used are limited. Photosensitive polymers and ceramic scaffolds can be printed using SLA and digital light processing (DLP) [145–147]. The materials cannot be printed without a photoinitiator; this condition excludes ceramics and metals alone. The printing is multifunctional, with an approximately 25-µm resolution and ±0.1-mm precision. However, because the resin might be cytotoxic, it is not often employed in bone tissue engineering [97, 148–149]. Furthermore, even though the machines are compact and simple to operate, it is rather costly. Models or molds for cranial surgical implants, bespoke heart valves, ear-shaped implants, and aortas have all been created using a combination of medical imaging and SLA. Thanks to the development of biodegradable macromers and resins, dental applications and tissue engineering scaffold production are on the rise [150–158].

9.15   CLINICAL APPLICATIONS

Orthopedic surgeons often insert artificial components inside the body to support bone structurally [159]. In the case of joint arthroplasty, people suffering from severe osteoarthritis and other trauma undergo hip, knee, ankle, and shoulder replacements by artificial components, such as joint prostheses possessing low-friction-bearing surfaces [160]. In the case of fixation of a fracture, bone fragments generated due to simple and complex fracture or because of large bone voids are typically stabilized and achieve structural support by artificial implants [161]. Large bone voids can also originate from removal surgery of bony sections suffering from bone tumors or infection-related complications. As compared to patients requiring fracture fixation or joint replacements, patients in need of revision surgery or tumors resection to cure large bone voids are few in number, but the latter case may turn out to be very challenging to treat [162]. Other important orthopedic applications of artificial implants are joint arthrodesis and reconstruction of soft tissue, among others. However, osteophytes or poor-quality bone may also require to be removed during normal surgical processes. And this necessitates an improvement of AM technologies to endow the capability of capturing and processing 3D imaging data within a short clinical timeline. The potential of AM implants in each of these procedures is discussed further in the following sections.

9.15.1   PATIENT VARIABILITY

Orthopedic patients possess a variable structure in the anatomy in their musculoskeletal organ that AM techniques necessarily have to meet to produce patient-specific implants and prostheses. First, variability in bone anatomy is very common across healthy individuals. There exists macroscale variability in bone shape [163], soft tissues geometry, and interconnects among tissues [164]. For example, in healthy individuals, the glenoid version, that is, the angular disposition of the shoulder socket with the horizontal plane, exhibits a variation of at least 20° [165]. Moreover, depending on the height and weight of an individual, different sections of the bone organ experience different lengths and sizes. There also exists variation in morphology and mechanical properties of individual bone at the microscale. Denser trabecular bones, thicker cortical tissues with stronger average mechanical strength, and higher Young's modulus are evident in younger men than those in older females.

9.15.2   SHOULDER AND OTHER JOINT REPLACEMENTS

The replacement of one or both sides of a joint with synthetic articulated joints and components with low friction and wear is termed *joint arthroplasty*. The degeneration of cartilage and subchondral bone is the most probable cause for joint arthroplasty, and the associated disease with such an inflammatory condition is known as osteoarthritis. However, there may be other reasons for joint replacements, such as symptoms due to rheumatoid arthritis, arthritis due to posttraumatic injury, avascular necrosis, and so on. Joint replacement on account of hip and knee arthritis is more frequently observed clinically than that due to the malfunctioning of the shoulder, ankle, or other joints. Recently, a dramatically increasing trend has been observed in joint arthroplasty for each type of bone joint [166].

9.15.3 Fracture Fixation

Bone injury mechanisms vary widely due to complexity in fracture mechanics in bone and the nature of accident and thus, depending on these factors' characteristic features of those bone fractures, differ on a case-to-case basis. For instance, injuries due to higher energy impact usually result in more complex with multiple separate pieces of bone fragments [167]. By mere visual inspection of the fracture, pattern categorization and classification of fracture phenomena have been tried, but in fact, it has been found that no two fractures exactly resemble each other. Moreover, as discussed before, bone qualities, body types, healing capacity, activity levels, and so on vary from one individual to other. In addition, to offer efficient patient-specific solutions in fracture fixation, AM techniques need to address numerous acute trauma cases that require quicker execution of precise implant design and fabrication processes to reasonably meet clinical demand within hours or days but not weeks. Fixing SS, titanium alloy, or other bio-metals to the fragmented bony pieces using screws and needles is a general surgical practice for guided bone tissue regeneration to heal the fractured bony site to preoperative anatomy. Two major types of implants, such as plate and screw/nail are most commonly used for fixation of a bone fracture. Generally, plates are fixed outside the bone cortex with the help of screw/nails that are drilled within the cortex, down to the intramedullary canal of long bones. The commercial availability of AM-derived straight and pre-contoured anatomic plates and screws are observed in the market to meet the demand for fracture fixation at different musculoskeletal sites. The metallic plates and the screws or nails are of the same type of material in order to avoid galvanic corrosion.

9.15.4 Large Bone Defects

Large bone defects occur in patients because of various complications; trauma and cancerous and infectious bone surgery play a major role in them. With surgical advancement, radiation therapy, and chemotherapy, survival tenure for cancerous patients with osteosarcoma has enhanced dramatically, such as from 20% to 70% for individuals with a cancerous distal femur. With the evolution of limb salvage surgeries, the biomechanical functioning of a limb has been restored by incorporating an implant together with regeneration of the surrounding soft tissue. Unfortunately, in pediatric patients especially, amputations cannot still be avoided. Since most of the implants are predesigned for adult patients, even an 8-year-old pediatric patient suffering from a primary malignant bone tumor is recommended for amputation because of a lack of availability of implants at the pediatric scale. In addition, amputations can often result in severe complications, such as wound care, neuromas, chronic pain, poor residual limb padding, recurrent ulceration, and impaired limb function [168]. The advancement in AM technology has now enabled us to provide a design perfectly compatible with the specific anatomy of a patient. For example, the perfect conjugation of the implant with a patient's medullary canal is possible to produce a "press fit design". A patient-specific implant as delivered by AM technology can minimize strain associated with implant loosening, fracture history, and dislocations.

9.15.5 SURGICAL GUIDES

Unlike traditional methods, AM techniques can be utilized in fabricating patient-specific surgical guides for proper planning before carrying out surgery. Richard Bibb et al. reported the first maxillofacial osteotomy guide utilizing an AM technique [169]. This is a case involving distraction osteogenesis in which two precision locator devices were mounted to displace the maxilla gradually with respect to the rest of the skull. In addition, two separate cuts were produced across the maxilla under the nose to get rid of some bone from the skull. For each cut, the designed surgical guides were created using FreeForm software and manufactured using L-PBF. The surgeon experienced better control in the course of surgery with the help of the designed surgical guides [170]. Today, companies producing AM-derived orthopedic implants provide support for knee replacement surgery for supplying a "patient-specific instrumentation" guide. Although there has been potential advancement in surgical procedures using customized surgical guides, further investigation is necessary to promote the surgical planning design for AM-mediated production of patient-specific guides.

9.16   RESEARCH DIRECTION AND FUTURE SCOPE

AM techniques with enhanced capability for product customization will appear in the future, and that will be associated with its application at a reasonable cost. All traditional tools and techniques for fabricating medical devices and models will become obsolete as patient-specific medical implants with specific geometrical dimensions will be available within a reasonable time frame with the help of AM techniques. It will open new horizons in surgical planning as the implant models generated by AM techniques will provide visual aids for surgical and physical teams for better planning at the surgical sites. AM techniques have the capability to produce customized fixtures and implants even with complex shapes and architectures within a short time. AM techniques are quite adept at designing and fabricating bio-models, implants, surgical-aid tools, and different scaffolds for tissue engineering applications. AM will also be helpful in developing multiple devices of medical origin and different models related to surgical training. Collaboration and cooperation between medical teams and AM researchers are imminent in the near future to produce medical products commercially.

9.17 SUMMARY

This chapter presented a review of existing AM technologies, materials used for fabricating bone implants, and a survey of reported orthopedic applications of such developed products. Over the past two decades, research on AM-based 3D-printing technologies has achieved significant momentum because of their capability in fabricating products with desirable shapes, tailored geometries and architectures, tunable compositions, and the like; they have been especially useful in the biomedical sector such as for orthopedic applications. Patient-specific implants are more necessary for the purpose of tailor-made medical care in orthopedic tissue engineering because bone shape, size, geometry, and the nature of the bone ECM vary from individual to individual. That is why the possibility of fabricating patient-specific 3D-printed scaffolds via AM technology soon may bring about a great promise in the field of bone tissue engineering. With a specific surface design, the possibility of minimizing the deleterious effects of stress shielding by tailoring the porosity, and hence Young's modulus, features like guiding cell migration in order to regenerate bone ECM, bone scaffolds fabricated by AM technologies can nearly meet the specific needs of bone tissue repair and regeneration. Despite recent advancements in the development of AM for orthopedic implants, several challenges still need to be overcome for its widespread application in orthopedics. First, natural bone tissue is composed of a hierarchical organization of collagen fibril and apatite nanoparticles from the nanoscale to macroscale, and 3D-printed orthopedic scaffolds are expected to mimic that hierarchical structure of human bone tissue in a precise manner. However, most of the AM technologies suffer from inadequate printing resolution and can only replicate the hierarchical structure at a far lower resolution. Therefore, the advanced level of actuation and the introduction of extrusion nozzle at a micron scale should be associated with AM processes for fabricating bone scaffolds with much higher resolution. Second, defected bone tissue shows a heterogeneous structure with a gradient combination of cortical and cancellous bone; hence, it exhibits FGM properties. However, integrated bone scaffolds with varying mechanical properties along both the longitudinal and transverse directions are difficult to fabricate with currently existing AM technologies, and hence, better 3D-printing strategies with complex features must be developed. Third, it is essential to stimulate regeneration of vascularized tissues surrounding the areas of bone regeneration for effective transport of nutrients, oxygen, and metabolic waste products to and from living tissues, but few AM-derived scaffolds can promote the required vascularization of neobone tissues. In this respect, scaffolds fabricated with AM technologies are needed to be endowed with capacity to release angiogenic agents in controlled and sustained manner and formation of vascular-like capillary channel in its microporous architecture. Fourth, especially for repairing defects with a critical size, incorporating cells into 3D-printed scaffolds promises to be a more powerful strategy. Although 3D-printing technology exists for producing cell-incorporated hydrogel scaffolds, technology is needed to improve and enhance cell viability in the fabricated scaffolds. For this reason, inventing superior AM printing techniques is required to successfully achieve both scaffold fabrication and cell incorporation attributes. Finally, AM-derived scaffolds are required to be fortified with antibacterial or anticancer capabilities to overcome threats from bone infection– and tumor-related diseases at the surgical sites. Thus, AM-printed 3D scaffolds are required to be precisely designed to satisfy the best bone regeneration condition at the surgical site under the physiological environment. In this regard, researchers can benefit from postoperative follow-up, with valuable input from previous cases, for the further development of AM-derived orthopedic implants.

REFERENCES

1. M. Lipian, M. Kulak, M. Stepien, Fast track integration of computational methods with experiments in small wind turbine development, *Energies*. 12 (2019) 1625.
2. K. Altaf, J.A. Qayyum, A.M.A. Rani, F. Ahmad, P.S.M. Megat-Yusoff, M. Baharom, A.R.A. Aziz, M. Jahanzaib, R.M. German, Performance analysis of enhanced 3D printed polymer molds for metal injection molding process, *Met.* 8 (2018). https://doi.org/10.3390/met8060433.
3. C.N. Kelly, A.T. Miller, S.J. Hollister, R.E. Guldberg, K. Gall, Design and structure—function characterization of 3D printed synthetic porous biomaterials for tissue engineering, *Adv. Healthc. Mater.* 7 (2018) 1701095.
4. Y.W.D. Tay, B. Panda, S.C. Paul, N.A. Noor Mohamed, M.J. Tan, K.F. Leong, 3D printing trends in building and construction industry: A review, *Virtual Phys. Prototyp.* 12 (2017) 261–276. https://doi.org/10.1080/17452759.2017.1326724.
5. S. Bose, S. Vahabzadeh, A. Bandyopadhyay, Bone tissue engineering using 3D printing, *Mater. Today.* (2013). https://doi.org/10.1016/j.mattod.2013.11.017.
6. C.M.B. Ho, S.H. Ng, K.H.H. Li, Y.-J. Yoon, 3D printed microfluidics for biological applications, *Lab Chip.* 15 (2015) 3627–3637. https://doi.org/10.1039/C5LC00685F.
7. S. V Murphy, A. Atala, 3D bioprinting of tissues and organs, *Nat. Biotechnol.* 32 (2014) 773–785. https://doi.org/10.1038/nbt.2958.
8. J.-F. Xing, M.-L. Zheng, X.-M. Duan, Two-photon polymerization microfabrication of hydrogels: An advanced 3D printing technology for tissue engineering and drug delivery, *Chem. Soc. Rev.* 44 (2015) 5031–5039. https://doi.org/10.1039/C5CS00278H.
9. K. Hölzl, S. Lin, L. Tytgat, S. Van Vlierberghe, L. Gu, A. Ovsianikov, Bioink properties before, during and after 3D bioprinting, *Biofabrication.* 8 (2016) 32002.
10. D.W. Hutmacher, State of the art and future directions of scaffold-based bone engineering from a biomaterials perspective, *J. Tissue Eng. Regen. Med.* (2007) 245–260. https://doi.org/10.1002/term.
11. I. Denry, L.T. Kuhn, Design and characterization of calcium phosphate ceramic scaffolds for bone tissue engineering, *Dent. Mater.* 32 (2016) 43–53.
12. A. Kumar, S. Mandal, S. Barui, R. Vasireddi, U. Gbureck, M. Gelinsky, B. Basu, Low temperature additive manufacturing of three dimensional scaffolds for bone-tissue engineering applications: Processing related challenges and property assessment, *Mater. Sci. Eng. R Reports.* 103 (2016) 1–39. https://doi.org/10.1016/j.mser.2016.01.001.
13. F.J. Martínez-Vázquez, M. V. Cabañas, J.L. Paris, D. Lozano, M. Vallet-Regí, Fabrication of novel Si-doped hydroxyapatite/gelatine scaffolds by rapid prototyping for drug delivery and bone regeneration, *Acta Biomater.* 15 (2015) 200–209. https://doi.org/10.1016/j.actbio.2014.12.021.
14. I. Astm, ASTM52900–15 standard terminology for additive manufacturing—general principles—terminology, *ASTM Int. West Conshohocken, PA.* 3 (2015) 5.
15. E. Sachs, M. Cima, J. Cornie, D. Brancazio, J. Bredt, A. Curodeau, M. Esterman, T. Fan, C. Harris, K. Kremmin, S.J. Lee, B. Pruitt, P. Williams, Dimensional printing: Rapid tooling and prototypes directly from CAD representation, *Int. Solid Free. Fabr. Symp.* (1990) 27–47.

16. C.R. Deckard, Method and apparatus for producing parts by selective sintering (1989). US Patent US4863538A.

17. S.S. Crump, Apparatus and method for creating three-dimensional objects (1992). US Patent No. US5121329A.

18. W.E. Masters, Computer automated manufacturing process and system (1987). Patent No. US4665492A.

19. P.K. Wu, B.R. Ringeisen, J. Callahan, M. Brooks, D.M. Bubb, H.D. Wu, A. Piqué, B. Spargo, R.A. McGill, D.B. Chrisey, The deposition, structure, pattern deposition, and activity of biomaterial thin-films by matrix-assisted pulsed-laser evaporation (MAPLE) and MAPLE direct write, *Thin Solid Films* 399 (2001, Nov 1) 607–614.

20. T. Ghidini, Regenerative medicine and 3D bioprinting for human space exploration and planet colonisation 10 (2018) 2363–2375. https://doi.org/10.21037/jtd.2018.03.19.

21. X. Cui, T. Boland, Biomaterials human microvasculature fabrication using thermal ink-jet printing technology, *Biomaterials*. 30 (2009) 6221–6227. https://doi.org/10.1016/j.biomaterials.2009.07.056.

22. J. Stringer, B. Derby, Formation and stability of lines produced by inkjet printing 26 (2010) 10365–10372. https://doi.org/10.1021/la101296e.

23. X. Cui, D. Dean, Z.M. Ruggeri, T. Boland, Cell damage evaluation of thermal inkjet printed Chinese hamster ovary cells, *Biotechnol. Bioeng.* 106 (2010) 963–969. https://doi.org/https://doi.org/10.1002/bit.22762.

24. C.W. Hull, Apparatus for production of three-dimensional objects by stereolithography, United States Patent, Appl., No. 638905, Filed. (1984).

25. M. Feygin, S.S. Pak, Laminated object manufacturing apparatus and method (1999). US Patent No. US5876550A.

26. A. Biswas, I.S. Bayer, A.S. Biris, T. Wang, E. Dervishi, F. Faupel, Advances in top—down and bottom—up surface nanofabrication: Techniques, applications & future prospects 170 (2012) 2–27. https://doi.org/10.1016/j.cis.2011.11.001.

27. E. Ruiz-Hitzky, P. Aranda, M. Darder, M. Ogawa, Hybrid and biohybrid silicate based materials: Molecular vs. block-assembling bottom—up processes, *Chem. Soc. Rev.* 40 (2011) 801–828.

28. Y. Yang, G. Wang, H. Liang, C. Gao, S. Peng, L. Shen, C. Shuai, Additive manufacturing of bone scaffolds, *Int. J. Bioprinting*. (2019). https://doi.org/10.18063/IJB.v5i1.148.

29. X.Y. Zhang, G. Fang, J. Zhou, Additively manufactured scaffolds for bone tissue engineering and the prediction of their mechanical behavior: A review, *Materials (Basel)*. (2017). https://doi.org/10.3390/ma10010050.

30. S. Ma, Q. Tang, Q. Feng, J. Song, X. Han, F. Guo, Mechanical behaviours and mass transport properties of bone-mimicking scaffolds consisted of gyroid structures manufactured using selective laser melting, *J. Mech. Behav. Biomed. Mater*. (2019). https://doi.org/10.1016/j.jmbbm.2019.01.023.

31. D. Carluccio, A.G. Demir, L. Caprio, B. Previtali, M.J. Bermingham, M.S. Dargusch, The influence of laser processing parameters on the densification and surface morphology of pure Fe and Fe-35Mn scaffolds produced by selective laser melting, *J. Manuf. Process*. (2019). https://doi.org/10.1016/j.jmapro.2019.03.018.

32. T. Habijan, C. Haberland, H. Meier, J. Frenzel, J. Wittsiepe, C. Wuwer, C. Greulich, T.A. Schildhauer, M. Köller, The biocompatibility of dense and porous Nickel-Titanium produced by selective laser melting, *Mater. Sci. Eng. C*. (2013). https://doi.org/10.1016/j.msec.2012.09.008.

33. P. Caravaggi, E. Liverani, A. Leardini, A. Fortunato, C. Belvedere, F. Baruffaldi, M. Fini, A. Parrilli, M. Mattioli-Belmonte, L. Tomesani, S. Pagani, CoCr porous scaffolds manufactured via selective laser melting in orthopedics: Topographical, mechanical, and biological characterization, *J. Biomed. Mater. Res.—Part B Appl. Biomater*. (2019). https://doi.org/10.1002/jbm.b.34328.

34. C. Herlin, M. Koppe, J.L. Béziat, A. Gleizal, Rapid prototyping in craniofacial surgery: Using a positioning guide after zygomatic osteotomy—A case report, *J. Cranio-Maxillofacial Surg.* 39 (2011) 376–379. https://doi.org/10.1016/J.JCMS.2010.07.003.

35. E. Berry, J.M. Brown, M. Connell, C.M. Craven, N.D. Efford, A. Radjenovic, M.A. Smith, Preliminary experience with medical applications of rapid prototyping by selective laser sintering, *Med. Eng. Phys.* 19 (1997) 90–96. https://doi.org/10.1016/S1350-4533(96)00039-2.

36. I. Shishkovsky, V. Scherbakov, Selective laser sintering of biopolymers with micro and nano ceramic additives for medicine, *Phys. Procedia.* 39 (2012) 491–499. https://doi.org/10.1016/J.PHPRO.2012.10.065.

37. C.K. Chua, K.F. Leong, K.H. Tan, F.E. Wiria, C.M. Cheah, Development of tissue scaffolds using selective laser sintering of polyvinyl alcohol/hydroxyapatite biocomposite for craniofacial and joint defects, *J. Mater. Sci. Mater. Med.* (2004). https://doi.org/10.1023/B:JMSM.0000046393.81449.a5.

38. K.H. Tan, C.K. Chua, K.F. Leong, C.M. Cheah, P. Cheang, M.S. Abu Bakar, S.W. Cha, Scaffold development using selective laser sintering of polyetheretherketone-hydroxyapatite biocomposite blends, *Biomaterials.* (2003). https://doi.org/10.1016/S0142-9612(03)00131-5.

39. C. Adamzyk, P. Kachel, M. Hoss, F. Gremse, A. Modabber, F. Hölzle, R. Tolba, S. Neuss, B. Lethaus, Bone tissue engineering using polyetherketoneketone scaffolds combined with autologous mesenchymal stem cells in a sheep calvarial defect model, *J. Cranio-Maxillofacial Surg.* (2016). https://doi.org/10.1016/j.jcms.2016.04.012.

40. W.Y. Zhou, S.H. Lee, M. Wang, W.L. Cheung, W.Y. Ip, Selective laser sintering of porous tissue engineering scaffolds from poly(L-lactide)/carbonated hydroxyapatite nanocomposite microspheres, *J. Mater. Sci. Mater. Med.* (2008). https://doi.org/10.1007/s10856-007-3089-3.

41. R.L. Simpson, F.E. Wiria, A.A. Amis, C.K. Chua, K.F. Leong, U.N. Hansen, M. Chandrasekaran, M.W. Lee, Development of a 95/5 poly(L-lactide-co-glycolide)/hydroxylapatite and β-tricalcium phosphate scaffold as bone replacement material via selective laser sintering, *J. Biomed. Mater. Res.—Part B Appl. Biomater.* (2008). https://doi.org/10.1002/jbm.b.30839.

42. F. Calignano, G. Cattano, D. Manfredi, Manufacturing of thin wall structures in AlSi10Mg alloy by laser powder bed fusion through process parameters, *J. Mater. Process. Technol.* (2018). https://doi.org/10.1016/j.jmatprotec.2018.01.029.

43. F. Trevisan, F. Calignano, A. Aversa, G. Marchese, M. Lombardi, S. Biamino, D. Ugues, D. Manfredi, Additive manufacturing of titanium alloys in the biomedical field: Processes, properties and applications, *J. Appl. Biomater. Funct. Mater.* (2018). https://doi.org/10.5301/jabfm.5000371.

44. F.A. Shah, O. Omar, F. Suska, A. Snis, A. Matic, L. Emanuelsson, B. Norlindh, J. Lausmaa, P. Thomsen, A. Palmquist, Long-term osseointegration of 3D printed CoCr constructs with an interconnected open-pore architecture prepared by electron beam melting, *Acta Biomater.* (2016). https://doi.org/10.1016/j.actbio.2016.03.033.

45. M. Galati, L. Iuliano, A literature review of powder-based electron beam melting focusing on numerical simulations, *Addit. Manuf.* (2018). https://doi.org/10.1016/j.addma.2017.11.001.

46. S. Biamino, A. Penna, U. Ackelid, S. Sabbadini, O. Tassa, P. Fino, M. Pavese, P. Gennaro, C. Badini, Electron beam melting of Ti-48Al-2Cr-2Nb alloy: Microstructure and mechanical properties investigation, *Intermetallics.* (2011). https://doi.org/10.1016/j.intermet.2010.11.017.

47. O.L.A. Harrysson, O. Cansizoglu, D.J. Marcellin-Little, D.R. Cormier, H.A. West, Direct metal fabrication of titanium implants with tailored materials and mechanical properties using electron beam melting technology, *Mater. Sci. Eng. C.* (2008). https://doi.org/10.1016/j.msec.2007.04.022.

48. A. Palmquist, A. Snis, L. Emanuelsson, M. Browne, P. Thomsen, Long-term biocompatibility and osseointegration of electron beam melted, free-form—fabricated solid and porous titanium alloy: Experimental studies in sheep, *J. Biomater. Appl.* (2013). https://doi.org/10.1177/0885328211431857.
49. P. Heinl, A. Rottmair, C. Körner, R.F. Singer, Cellular titanium by selective electron beam melting, *Adv. Eng. Mater.* (2007). https://doi.org/10.1002/adem.200700025.
50. P. Thomsen, J. Malmström, L. Emanuelsson, M. René, A. Snis, Electron beam-melted, free-form-fabricated titanium alloy implants: Material surface characterization and early bone response in rabbits, *J. Biomed. Mater. Res.—Part B Appl. Biomater.* (2009). https://doi.org/10.1002/jbm.b.31250.
51. J. Parthasarathy, B. Starly, S. Raman, A. Christensen, Mechanical evaluation of porous titanium (Ti6Al4V) structures with electron beam melting (EBM), *J. Mech. Behav. Biomed. Mater.* (2010). https://doi.org/10.1016/j.jmbbm.2009.10.006.
52. X. Li, Y.F. Feng, C.T. Wang, G.C. Li, W. Lei, Z.Y. Zhang, L. Wang, Evaluation of biological properties of electron beam melted Ti6Al4V implant with biomimetic coating in vitro and in vivo, *PLoS One.* (2012). https://doi.org/10.1371/journal.pone.0052049.
53. R. Wauthle, J. Van Der Stok, S.A. Yavari, J. Van Humbeeck, J.P. Kruth, A.A. Zadpoor, H. Weinans, M. Mulier, J. Schrooten, Additively manufactured porous tantalum implants, *Acta Biomater.* (2015). https://doi.org/10.1016/j.actbio.2014.12.003.
54. K.S. Munir, Y. Li, C. Wen, Metallic scaffolds manufactured by selective laser melting for biomedical applications, *Met. Foam Bone Process. Modif. Charact. Prop.* (2017). https://doi.org/10.1016/B978-0-08-101289-5.00001-9.
55. L. Yuan, S. Ding, C. Wen, Additive manufacturing technology for porous metal implant applications and triple minimal surface structures: A review, *Bioact. Mater.* (2019). https://doi.org/10.1016/j.bioactmat.2018.12.003.
56. A. Ataee, Y. Li, D. Fraser, G. Song, C. Wen, Anisotropic Ti-6Al-4V gyroid scaffolds manufactured by electron beam melting (EBM) for bone implant applications, *Mater. Des.* (2018). https://doi.org/10.1016/j.matdes.2017.10.040.
57. A. Biesiekierski, J. Lin, K. Munir, S. Ozan, Y. Li, C. Wen, An investigation of the mechanical and microstructural evolution of a TiNbZr alloy with varied ageing time, *Sci. Rep.* (2018). https://doi.org/10.1038/s41598-018-24155-y.
58. A. Ataee, Y. Li, M. Brandt, C. Wen, Ultrahigh-strength titanium gyroid scaffolds manufactured by selective laser melting (SLM) for bone implant applications, *Acta Mater.* (2018). https://doi.org/10.1016/j.actamat.2018.08.005.
59. G. Poumarat, P. Squire, Comparison of mechanical properties of human, bovine bone and a new processed bone xenograft, *Biomaterials.* (1993). https://doi.org/10.1016/0142-9612(93)90051-3.
60. M. Brandt, S. Sun, M. Leary, S. Feih, J. Elambasseril, Q. Liu, High-value SLM aerospace components: From design to manufacture, *Adv. Mater. Res.* (2013). https://doi.org/10.4028/www.scientific.net/AMR.633.135.
61. C. Zhu, Y. Lv, C. Qian, H. Qian, T. Jiao, L. Wang, F. Zhang, Proliferation and osteogenic differentiation of rat BMSCs on a novel Ti/SiC metal matrix nanocomposite modified by friction stir processing, *Sci. Rep.* (2016). https://doi.org/10.1038/srep38875.
62. Z. Yang, H. Gu, G. Sha, W. Lu, W. Yu, W. Zhang, Y. Fu, K. Wang, L. Wang, TC4/Ag metal matrix nanocomposites modified by friction stir processing: Surface characterization, antibacterial property, and cytotoxicity in vitro, *ACS Appl. Mater. Interfaces.* (2018). https://doi.org/10.1021/acsami.8b16343.
63. Y. Lv, Z. Ding, X. Sun, L. Li, G. Sha, R. Liu, L. Wang, Gradient microstructures and mechanical properties of Ti-6Al-4V/Zn composite prepared by friction stir processing, *Materials (Basel).* (2019). https://doi.org/10.3390/ma12172795.
64. A. Cheng, A. Humayun, D.J. Cohen, B.D. Boyan, Z. Schwartz, Additively manufactured 3D porous Ti-6Al-4V constructs mimic trabecular bone structure and regulate osteoblast proliferation, differentiation and local factor production in a

porosity and surface roughness dependent manner, *Biofabrication*. (2014). https://doi.org/10.1088/1758-5082/6/4/045007.

65. S. Amin Yavari, L. Loozen, F.L. Paganelli, S. Bakhshandeh, K. Lietaert, J.A. Groot, A.C. Fluit, C.H.E. Boel, J. Alblas, H.C. Vogely, H. Weinans, A.A. Zadpoor, Antibacterial behavior of additively manufactured porous titanium with nanotubular surfaces releasing silver ions, *ACS Appl. Mater. Interfaces*. (2016). https://doi.org/10.1021/acsami.6b03152.

66. J. Liu, J. Liu, S. Attarilar, C. Wang, M. Tamaddon, C. Yang, K. Xie, J. Yao, L. Wang, C. Liu, Y. Tang, Nano-modified titanium implant materials: A way toward improved antibacterial properties, *Front. Bioeng. Biotechnol*. (2020). https://doi.org/10.3389/fbioe.2020.576969.

67. J.P. Luo, Y.J. Huang, J.Y. Xu, J.F. Sun, M.S. Dargusch, C.H. Hou, L. Ren, R.Z. Wang, T. Ebel, M. Yan, Additively manufactured biomedical Ti-Nb-Ta-Zr lattices with tunable Young's modulus: Mechanical property, biocompatibility, and proteomics analysis, *Mater. Sci. Eng. C*. (2020). https://doi.org/10.1016/j.msec.2020.110903.

68. M. Speirs, B. Van Hooreweder, J. Van Humbeeck, J.P. Kruth, Fatigue behaviour of NiTi shape memory alloy scaffolds produced by SLM, a unit cell design comparison, *J. Mech. Behav. Biomed. Mater*. (2017). https://doi.org/10.1016/j.jmbbm.2017.01.016.

69. Z. Lin, L. Wang, X. Xue, W. Lu, J. Qin, D. Zhang, Microstructure evolution and mechanical properties of a Ti-35Nb-3Zr-2Ta biomedical alloy processed by equal channel angular pressing (ECAP), *Mater. Sci. Eng. C*. (2013). https://doi.org/10.1016/j.msec.2013.07.010.

70. J. Čapek, M. Machová, M. Fousová, J. Kubásek, D. Vojtěch, J. Fojt, E. Jablonská, J. Lipov, T. Ruml, Highly porous, low elastic modulus 316L stainless steel scaffold prepared by selective laser melting, *Mater. Sci. Eng. C*. (2016). https://doi.org/10.1016/j.msec.2016.07.027.

71. A. Yamamoto, Y. Kohyama, D. Kuroda, T. Hanawa, Cytocompatibility evaluation of Ni-free stainless steel manufactured by nitrogen adsorption treatment, *Mater. Sci. Eng. C*. (2004). https://doi.org/10.1016/j.msec.2004.08.017.

72. L. Wang, C. Wang, L.C. Zhang, L. Chen, W. Lu, D. Zhang, Phase transformation and deformation behavior of NiTi-Nb eutectic joined NiTi wires, *Sci. Rep*. (2016). https://doi.org/10.1038/srep23905.

73. S. Liu, S. Han, L. Wang, J. Liu, H. Tang, Effects of Nb on the microstructure and compressive properties of an As-Cast Ni44Ti44Nb12 eutectic alloy, *Materials (Basel)*. (2019). https://doi.org/10.3390/ma12244118.

74. L. Baldwin, J.A. Hunt, Host inflammatory response to NiCr, CoCr, and Ti in a soft tissue implantation model, *J. Biomed. Mater. Res.—Part A*. (2006). https://doi.org/10.1002/jbm.a.30856.

75. C. Castellani, R.A. Lindtner, P. Hausbrandt, E. Tschegg, S.E. Stanzl-Tschegg, G. Zanoni, S. Beck, A.M. Weinberg, Bone-implant interface strength and osseointegration: Biodegradable magnesium alloy versus standard titanium control, *Acta Biomater*. (2011). https://doi.org/10.1016/j.actbio.2010.08.020.

76. Y. Chen, Z. Xu, C. Smith, J. Sankar, Recent advances on the development of magnesium alloys for biodegradable implants, *Acta Biomater*. (2014). https://doi.org/10.1016/j.actbio.2014.07.005.

77. N.T. Kirkland, N. Birbilis, M.P. Staiger, Assessing the corrosion of biodegradable magnesium implants: A critical review of current methodologies and their limitations, *Acta Biomater*. (2012). https://doi.org/10.1016/j.actbio.2011.11.014.

78. F. Witte, Reprint of: The history of biodegradable magnesium implants: A review, *Acta Biomater*. (2015). https://doi.org/10.1016/j.actbio.2015.07.017.

79. P. Li, C. Schille, E. Schweizer, F. Rupp, A. Heiss, C. Legner, U.E. Klotz, J.G. Gerstorfer, L. Scheideler, Mechanical characteristics, in vitro degradation, cytotoxicity, and

antibacterial evaluation of Zn-4.0Ag alloy as a biodegradable material, *Int. J. Mol. Sci.* (2018). https://doi.org/10.3390/ijms19030755.

80. Y. Li, H. Jahr, K. Lietaert, P. Pavanram, A. Yilmaz, L.I. Fockaert, M.A. Leeflang, B. Pouran, Y. Gonzalez-Garcia, H. Weinans, J.M.C. Mol, J. Zhou, A.A. Zadpoor, Additively manufactured biodegradable porous iron, *Acta Biomater.* (2018). https://doi.org/10.1016/j.actbio.2018.07.011.
81. Y. Li, P. Pavanram, J. Zhou, K. Lietaert, P. Taheri, W. Li, H. San, M.A. Leeflang, J.M.C. Mol, H. Jahr, A.A. Zadpoor, Additively manufactured biodegradable porous zinc, *Acta Biomater.* (2020). https://doi.org/10.1016/j.actbio.2019.10.034.
82. Y. Li, H. Jahr, P. Pavanram, F.S.L. Bobbert, U. Puggi, X.Y. Zhang, B. Pouran, M.A. Leeflang, H. Weinans, J. Zhou, A.A. Zadpoor, Additively manufactured functionally graded biodegradable porous iron, *Acta Biomater.* (2019). https://doi.org/10.1016/j.actbio.2019.07.013.
83. Y. Su, I. Cockerill, Y. Wang, Y.X. Qin, L. Chang, Y. Zheng, D. Zhu, Zinc-based biomaterials for regeneration and therapy, *Trends Biotechnol.* (2019). https://doi.org/10.1016/j.tibtech.2018.10.009.
84. J. Fu, Y. Su, Y.X. Qin, Y. Zheng, Y. Wang, D. Zhu, Evolution of metallic cardiovascular stent materials: A comparative study among stainless steel, magnesium and zinc, *Biomaterials.* (2020). https://doi.org/10.1016/j.biomaterials.2019.119641.
85. N. Ma, S. Liu, W. Liu, L. Xie, D. Wei, L. Wang, L. Li, B. Zhao, Y. Wang, Research progress of titanium-based high entropy alloy: Methods, properties, and applications, *Front. Bioeng. Biotechnol.* (2020). https://doi.org/10.3389/fbioe.2020.603522.
86. E. Vorndran, M. Klarner, U. Klammert, L.M. Grover, S. Patel, J.E. Barralet, U. Gbureck, 3D powder printing of β-tricalcium phosphate ceramics using different strategies, *Adv. Eng. Mater.* (2008). https://doi.org/10.1002/adem.200800179.
87. E. Mancuso, N. Alharbi, O.A. Bretcanu, M. Marshall, M.A. Birch, A.W. McCaskie, K.W. Dalgarno, Three-dimensional printing of porous load-bearing bioceramic scaffolds, *Proc. Inst. Mech. Eng. Part H J. Eng. Med.* (2017). https://doi.org/10.1177/0954411916682984.
88. A. Zocca, P. Colombo, C.M. Gomes, J. Günster, Additive manufacturing of ceramics: Issues, potentialities, and opportunities, *J. Am. Ceram. Soc.* (2015). https://doi.org/10.1111/jace.13700.
89. U. Klammert, U. Gbureck, E. Vorndran, J. Rödiger, P. Meyer-Marcotty, A.C. Kübler, 3D powder printed calcium phosphate implants for reconstruction of cranial and maxillofacial defects, *J. Cranio-Maxillofacial Surg.* (2010). https://doi.org/10.1016/j.jcms.2010.01.009.
90. G.A. Fielding, A. Bandyopadhyay, S. Bose, Effects of silica and zinc oxide doping on mechanical and biological properties of 3D printed tricalcium phosphate tissue engineering scaffolds, *Dent. Mater.* (2012). https://doi.org/10.1016/j.dental.2011.09.010.
91. A. Wubneh, E.K. Tsekoura, C. Ayranci, H. Uludağ, Current state of fabrication technologies and materials for bone tissue engineering, *Acta Biomater.* (2018). https://doi.org/10.1016/j.actbio.2018.09.031.
92. S.K. Lan Levengood, S.J. Polak, M.B. Wheeler, A.J. Maki, S.G. Clark, R.D. Jamison, A.J. Wagoner Johnson, Multiscale osteointegration as a new paradigm for the design of calcium phosphate scaffolds for bone regeneration, *Biomaterials.* (2010). https://doi.org/10.1016/j.biomaterials.2010.01.052.
93. S. Wang, Z. Zhao, Y. Yang, A.G. Mikos, Z. Qiu, T. Song, F. Cui, X. Wang, C. Zhang, A high-strength mineralized collagen bone scaffold for large-sized cranial bone defect repair in sheep, *Regen. Biomater.* (2018). https://doi.org/10.1093/rb/rby020.
94. G. Monaco, R. Cholas, L. Salvatore, M. Madaghiele, A. Sannino, Sterilization of collagen scaffolds designed for peripheral nerve regeneration: Effect on microstructure, degradation and cellular colonization, *Mater. Sci. Eng. C.* (2017). https://doi.org/10.1016/j.msec.2016.10.030.

95. N.P. Tipnis, D.J. Burgess, Sterilization of implantable polymer-based medical devices: A review, *Int. J. Pharm.* (2018). https://doi.org/10.1016/j.ijpharm.2017.12.003.

96. C.C. Chen, J.Y. Chueh, H. Tseng, H.M. Huang, S.Y. Lee, Preparation and characterization of biodegradable PLA polymeric blends, *Biomaterials.* (2003). https://doi.org/10.1016/S0142-9612(02)00466-0.

97. P. Rider, Ž.P. Kačarević, S. Alkildani, S. Retnasingh, R. Schnettler, M. Barbeck, Additive manufacturing for guided bone regeneration: A perspective for alveolar ridge augmentation, *Int. J. Mol. Sci.* (2018). https://doi.org/10.3390/ijms19113308.

98. Y. Zhang, X. Liu, L. Zeng, J. Zhang, J. Zuo, J. Zou, J. Ding, X. Chen, Polymer fiber scaffolds for bone and cartilage tissue engineering, *Adv. Funct. Mater.* (2019). https://doi.org/10.1002/adfm.201903279.

99. H. Huang, X. Zhang, X. Hu, L. Dai, J. Zhu, Z. Man, H. Chen, C. Zhou, Y. Ao, Directing chondrogenic differentiation of mesenchymal stem cells with a solid-supported chitosan thermogel for cartilage tissue engineering, *Biomed. Mater.* 9 (2014). https://doi.org/10.1088/1748-6041/9/3/035008.

100. J.M. Williams, A. Adewunmi, R.M. Schek, C.L. Flanagan, P.H. Krebsbach, S.E. Feinberg, S.J. Hollister, S. Das, Bone tissue engineering using polycaprolactone scaffolds fabricated via selective laser sintering, *Biomaterials.* (2005). https://doi.org/10.1016/j.biomaterials.2004.11.057.

101. C.-G. Liu, Y.-T. Zeng, R.K. Kankala, S.-S. Zhang, A.-Z. Chen, S.-B. Wang, Characterization and preliminary biological evaluation of 3D-printed porous scaffolds for engineering bone tissues, *Materials (Basel).* 11 (2018) 1832.

102. A. Kopp, T. Derra, M. Müther, L. Jauer, J.H. Schleifenbaum, M. Voshage, O. Jung, R. Smeets, N. Kröger, Influence of design and postprocessing parameters on the degradation behavior and mechanical properties of additively manufactured magnesium scaffolds, *Acta Biomater.* (2019). https://doi.org/10.1016/j.actbio.2019.04.012.

103. M. Seidenstuecker, S. Lange, S. Esslinger, S.H. Latorre, R. Krastey, R. Gadow, H.O. Mayr, A. Bernstein, Inversely 3D-printed β-TCP scaffolds for bone replacement, *Materials.* 12(20) (2019, Jan): 3417.

104. X. Song, H. Tetik, T. Jirakittsonthon, P. Parandoush, G. Yang, D. Lee, S. Ryu, S. Lei, M.L. Weiss, D. Lin, Biomimetic 3D printing of hierarchical and interconnected porous hydroxyapatite structures with high mechanical strength for bone cell culture, *Adv. Eng. Mater.* 21 (2019) 1800678. https://doi.org/https://doi.org/10.1002/adem.201800678.

105. L. Chen, C. Deng, J. Li, Q. Yao, J. Chang, L. Wang, C. Wu, Biomaterials 3D printing of a lithium-calcium-silicate crystal bioscaffold with dual bioactivities for osteochondral interface reconstruction, *Biomaterials.* 196 (2019) 138–150.

106. H. Wang, K. Su, L. Su, P. Liang, P. Ji, C. Wang, Comparison of 3D-printed porous tantalum and titanium scaffolds on osteointegration and osteogenesis, *Mater. Sci. Eng. C.* (2019). https://doi.org/10.1016/j.msec.2019.109908.

107. Y. Song, K. Lin, S. He, C. Wang, S. Zhang, D. Li, J. Wang, T. Cao, L. Bi, G. Pei, Nano-biphasic calcium phosphate/polyvinyl alcohol composites with enhanced bioactivity for bone repair via low-temperature three-dimensional printing and loading with platelet-rich fibrin, *Int. J. Nanomedicine.* 13 (2018) 505–523.

108. J.C. Boga, S.P. Miguel, D. de Melo-Diogo, A.G. Mendonca, R.O. Louro, I.J. Correia, In vitro characterization of 3D printed scaffolds aimed at bone tissue regeneration, *Colloids Surf. B: Biointerfaces.* 165 (2018, May 1) 207–218.

109. M. Touri, F. Moztarzadeh, N.A. Osman, M.M. Dehghan, M. Mozafari, 3D—printed biphasic calcium phosphate scaffolds coated with an oxygen generating system for enhancing engineered tissue survival, *Mater. Sci. Eng. C.* 84 (2018, Mar 1) 236–242.

110. B.S. Kim, S.S. Yang, C.S. Kim, Incorporation of BMP-2 nanoparticles on the surface of a 3D-printed hydroxyapatite scaffold using an ε-polycaprolactone polymer emulsion coating method for bone tissue engineering, *Colloids Surf. B: Biointerfaces.* 170 (2018) 421–429.

111. A. Motallebzadeh, N.S. Peighambardoust, S. Sheikh, H. Murakami, S. Guo, D. Canadinc, Microstructural, mechanical and electrochemical characterization of TiZrTaHfNb and Ti1.5ZrTa0.5Hf0.5Nb0.5 refractory high-entropy alloys for biomedical applications, *Intermetallics*. (2019). https://doi.org/10.1016/j.intermet.2019.106572.

112. H. Kim, G.H. Yang, C.H. Choi, Y.S. Cho, G. Kim, Gelatin/PVA scaffolds fabricated using a 3D-printing process employed with a low-temperature plate for hard tissue regeneration: Fabrication and characterizations, *Int. J. Biol. Macromol.* 120 (2018, Dec 1) 119–127.

113. H. Lee, G.H. Yang, M. Kim, J. Lee, J. Huh, G. Kim, Fabrication of micro/nanoporous collagen/dECM/silk-fibroin biocomposite scaffolds using a low temperature 3D printing process for bone tissue regeneration, *Mater. Sci. Eng. C*. 84 (2018, Mar 1) 140–147.

114. F. Gao, Z. Xu, Q. Liang, B. Liu, H. Li, Y. Wu, Y. Zhang, Direct 3D printing of high strength biohybrid gradient hydrogel scaffolds for efficient repair of osteochondral defect *Adv. Funct. Mater*. 28 (2018) 1706644. https://doi.org/10.1002/adfm.201706644.

115. Y. Luo, Y. Li, X. Qin, Q. Wa, 3D printing of concentrated alginate/gelatin scaffolds with homogeneous nano apatite coating for bone tissue engineering, *Mater. Des*. 146 (2018) 12–19.

116. Y. Luo, G. Luo, M. Gelinsky, P. Huang, C. Ruan, 3D bioprinting scaffold using alginate/polyvinyl alcohol bioinks, *Mater. Lett*. 189 (2017, Feb 15) 295–298.

117. E.Y. Heo, N.R. Ko, M.S. Bae, S.J. Lee, B.-J. Choi, J.H. Kim, H.K. Kim, S.A. Park, I.K. Kwon, Novel 3D printed alginate—BFP1 hybrid scaffolds for enhanced bone regeneration, *J. Ind. Eng. Chem*. 45 (2017) 61–67.

118. X. Zhai, C. Ruan, Y. Ma, D. Cheng, M. Wu, W. Liu, X. Zhao, H. Pan, W.W. Lu, 3D-bioprinted osteoblast-laden nanocomposite hydrogel constructs with induced microenvironments promote cell viability, differentiation, and osteogenesis both in vitro and in vivo, *Adv. Sci*. 5 (2018) 1700550.

119. T.T. Demirtaş, G. Irmak, M. Gümüşderelioğlu, A bioprintable form of chitosan hydrogel for bone tissue engineering, *Biofabrication*. 9 (2017) 35003.

120. L.S. Bertol, R. Schabbach, L.A. Loureiro dos Santos, Different post-processing conditions for 3D bioprinted α-tricalcium phosphate scaffolds, *J. Mater. Sci. Mater. Med*. (2017). https://doi.org/10.1007/s10856-017-5989-1.

121. C.F.L. Santos, A.P. Silva, L. Lopes, I. Pires, I.J. Correia, Design and production of sintered β-tricalcium phosphate 3D scaffolds for bone tissue regeneration, *Mater. Sci. Eng. C*. (2012). https://doi.org/10.1016/j.msec.2012.04.010.

122. A. Grémare, V. Guduric, R. Bareille, V. Heroguez, S. Latour, N. L'heureux, J. Fricain, S. Catros, D. Le Nihouannen, Characterization of printed PLA scaffolds for bone tissue engineering, *J. Biomed. Mater. Res. Part A*. 106 (2018) 887–894.

123. H. Seitz, W. Rieder, S. Irsen, B. Leukers, C. Tille, Three-dimensional printing of porous ceramic scaffolds for bone tissue engineering, *J. Biomed. Mater. Res.—Part B Appl. Biomater*. (2005). https://doi.org/10.1002/jbm.b.30291.

124. W. Wang, G. Caetano, W.S. Ambler, J.J. Blaker, M.A. Frade, P. Mandal, C. Diver, P. Bártolo, Enhancing the hydrophilicity and cell attachment of 3D printed PCL/graphene scaffolds for bone tissue engineering, *Materials (Basel)*. 9 (2016) 992.

125. A. Kosik-Kozioł, E. Graham, J. Jaroszewicz, A. Chlanda, P.T.S. Kumar, S. Ivanovski, W. Swieszkowski, C. Vaquette, Surface modification of 3D printed polycaprolactone constructs via a solvent treatment: Impact on physical and osteogenic properties, *ACS Biomater. Sci. Eng*. 5 (2018) 318–328.

126. S.A. Park, S.J. Lee, J.M. Seok, J.H. Lee, W.D. Kim, I.K. Kwon, Fabrication of 3D printed PCL/PEG polyblend scaffold using rapid prototyping system for bone tissue engineering application, *J. Bionic Eng*. 15 (2018) 435–442.

127. B.N. Teixeira, P. Aprile, R.H. Mendonca, D.J. Kelly, R.M. da S.M. Thiré, Evaluation of bone marrow stem cell response to PLA scaffolds manufactured by 3D printing and coated with polydopamine and type I collagen, *J. Biomed. Mater. Res. Part B Appl. Biomater*. 107 (2019) 37–49.

128. U. Ritz, R. Gerke, H. Götz, S. Stein, P.M. Rommens, A new bone substitute developed from 3D-prints of polylactide (PLA) loaded with collagen I: An in vitro study, *Int. J. Mol. Sci.* 18 (2017) 2569.

129. H. Liang, D. Zhao, X. Feng, L. Ma, X. Deng, C. Han, Q. Wei, C. Yang, 3D-printed porous titanium scaffolds incorporating niobium for high bone regeneration capacity, *Mater. Des.* (2020). https://doi.org/10.1016/j.matdes.2020.108890.

130. J.I. Kim, C.S. Kim, Nanoscale resolution 3D printing with pin-modified electrified ink-jets for tailorable nano/macrohybrid constructs for tissue engineering, *ACS Appl. Mater. Interfaces.* 10 (2018) 12390–12405.

131. C. Wang, Y. Zhou, M. Wang, In situ delivery of rhBMP-2 in surface porous shape memory scaffolds developed through cryogenic 3D plotting, *Mater. Lett.* 189 (2017) 140–143.

132. T. Yang, Y. Hu, C. Wang, B.P. Binks, Fabrication of hierarchical macroporous biocom-patible scaffolds by combining pickering high internal phase emulsion templates with three-dimensional printing, *ACS Appl. Mater. Interfaces.* 9 (2017) 22950–22958.

133. P. Habibovic, U. Gbureck, C.J. Doillon, D.C. Bassett, C.A. van Blitterswijk, J.E. Bar-ralet, Osteoconduction and osteoinduction of low-temperature 3D printed bioceramic implants, *Biomaterials.* (2008). https://doi.org/10.1016/j.biomaterials.2007.10.023.

134. N. Ristovski, N. Bock, S. Liao, S.K. Powell, J. Ren, G.T.S. Kirby, K.A. Blackwood, M.A. Woodruff, Improved fabrication of melt electrospun tissue engineering scaffolds using direct writing and advanced electric field control, *Biointerphases.* 10 (2015) 11006.

135. F.-L. He, D.-W. Li, J. He, Y.-Y. Liu, F. Ahmad, Y.-L. Liu, X. Deng, Y.-J. Ye, D.-C. Yin, A novel layer-structured scaffold with large pore sizes suitable for 3D cell culture pre-pared by near-field electrospinning, *Mater. Sci. Eng. C.* 86 (2018) 18–27.

136. X. Qu, P. Xia, J. He, D. Li, Microscale electrohydrodynamic printing of biomimetic PCL/nHA composite scaffolds for bone tissue engineering, *Mater. Lett.* 185 (2016) 554–557.

137. M. Kim, H. Yun, G.H. Kim, Electric-field assisted 3D-fibrous bioceramic-based scaf-folds for bone tissue regeneration: Fabrication, characterization, and in vitro cellular activities, *Sci. Rep.* 7 (2017) 1–13.

138. M. Asadi-Eydivand, M. Solati-Hashjin, A. Farzad, N.A. Abu Osman, Effect of technical parameters on porous structure and strength of 3D printed calcium sulfate prototypes, *Robot. Comput. Integr. Manuf.* (2016). https://doi.org/10.1016/j.rcim.2015.06.005.

139. M. Vaezi, C.K. Chua, Effects of layer thickness and binder saturation level parame-ters on 3D printing process, *Int. J. Adv. Manuf. Technol.* (2011). https://doi.org/10.1007/s00170-010-2821-1.

140. Z. Zhou, F. Buchanan, C. Mitchell, N. Dunne, Printability of calcium phosphate: Calcium sulfate powders for the application of tissue engineered bone scaffolds using the 3D print-ing technique, *Mater. Sci. Eng. C.* (2014). https://doi.org/10.1016/j.msec.2014.01.027.

141. M. Castilho, C. Moseke, A. Ewald, U. Gbureck, J. Groll, I. Pires, J. Teßmar, E. Vorndran, Direct 3D powder printing of biphasic calcium phosphate scaffolds for substitution of complex bone defects, *Biofabrication.* (2014). https://doi.org/10.1088/1758-5082/6/1/015006.

142. J.L. Dávila, M.S.D. Freitas, P. Inforçatti Neto, Z.D.C. Silveira, J. Silva, M.A. d'Ávila, Fabrication of PCL/β-TCP scaffolds by 3D mini-screw extrusion printing, *J. Appl. Polym. Sci.* 133 (2016).

143. E.M. Goncalves, F.J. Oliveira, R.F. Silva, M.A. Neto, M.H. Fernandes, M. Amaral, M. Vallet-Regí, M. Vila, Three-dimensional printed PCL-hydroxyapatite scaffolds filled with CNT s for bone cell growth stimulation, *J. Biomed. Mater. Res. Part B Appl. Bio-mater.* 104 (2016) 1210–1219.

144. F. Calignano, M. Galati, L. Iuliano, P. Minetola, Design of additively manufactured structures for biomedical applications: A review of the additive manufacturing processes applied to the biomedical sector, *J. Healthc. Eng.* 2019 (2019). https://doi.org/10.1155/2019/9748212.

145. J. Brie, T. Chartier, C. Chaput, C. Delage, B. Pradeau, F. Caire, M.-P. Boncoeur, J.-J. Moreau, A new custom made bioceramic implant for the repair of large and complex craniofacial bone defects, *J. Cranio-Maxillofacial Surg.* 41 (2013) 403–407.

146. J.-W. Kim, B.-E. Yang, S.-J. Hong, H.-G. Choi, S.-J. Byeon, H.-K. Lim, S.-M. Chung, J.-H. Lee, S.-H. Byun, Bone regeneration capability of 3D printed ceramic scaffolds, *Int. J. Mol. Sci.* 21 (2020) 4837.

147. F. Xu, H. Ren, M. Zheng, X. Shao, T. Dai, Y. Wu, L. Tian, Y. Liu, B. Liu, J. Gunster, Development of biodegradable bioactive glass ceramics by DLP printed containing EPCs/BMSCs for bone tissue engineering of rabbit mandible defects, *J. Mech. Behav. Biomed. Mater.* 103 (2020) 103532.

148. J. Babilotte, V. Guduric, D. Le Nihouannen, A. Naveau, J. Fricain, S. Catros, 3D printed polymer—mineral composite biomaterials for bone tissue engineering: Fabrication and characterization, *J. Biomed. Mater. Res. Part B Appl. Biomater.* 107 (2019) 2579–2595.

149. S. Kreß, R. Schaller-Ammann, J. Feiel, J. Priedl, C. Kasper, D. Egger, 3D printing of cell culture devices: Assessment and prevention of the cytotoxicity of photopolymers for stereolithography, *Materials (Basel).* 13 (2020) 3011.

150. J.H.P. Pallari, K.W. Dalgarno, J. Woodburn, Mass customization of foot orthoses for rheumatoid arthritis using selective laser sintering, *IEEE Trans. Biomed. Eng.* 57 (2010) 1750–1756.

151. P.S. D'Urso, D.J. Effeney, W.J. Earwaker, T.M. Barker, M.J. Redmond, R.G. Thompson, F.H. Tomlinson, Custom cranioplasty using stereolithography and acrylic, *Br. J. Plast. Surg.* 53 (2000) 200–204.

152. G. Wurm, B. Tomancok, K. Holl, J. Trenkler, Prospective study on cranioplasty with individual carbon fiber reinforced polymere (CFRP) implants produced by means of stereolithography, *Surg. Neurol.* 62 (2004) 510–521.

153. R. Sodian, M. Loebe, A. Hein, D.P. Martin, S.P. Hoerstrup, E. V Potapov, H. Hausmann, T. Lueth, R. Hetzer, Application of stereolithography for scaffold fabrication for tissue engineered heart valves, *ASAIO J.* 48 (2002) 12–16.

154. A. Naumann, J. Aigner, R. Staudenmaier, M. Seemann, R. Bruening, K.H. Englmeier, G. Kadegge, E. Pavesio, E. Kastenbauer, A. Berghaus, Clinical aspects and strategy for biomaterial engineering of an auricle based on three-dimensional stereolithography, *Eur. Arch. Oto-Rhino-Laryngology.* 260 (2003) 568–575.

155. A. Dawood, B.M. Marti, V. Sauret-Jackson, A. Darwood, 3D printing in dentistry, *Br. Dent. J.* 219 (2015) 521–529.

156. J. Wallace, M.O. Wang, P. Thompson, M. Busso, V. Belle, N. Mammoser, K. Kim, J.P. Fisher, A. Siblani, Y. Xu, Validating continuous digital light processing (cDLP) additive manufacturing accuracy and tissue engineering utility of a dye-initiator package, *Biofabrication.* 6 (2014) 15003.

157. D. Dean, J. Wallace, A. Siblani, M.O. Wang, K. Kim, A.G. Mikos, J.P. Fisher, Continuous digital light processing (cDLP): Highly accurate additive manufacturing of tissue engineered bone scaffolds: This paper highlights the main issues regarding the application of Continuous Digital Light Processing (cDLP) for the production of hig, *Virtual Phys. Prototyp.* 7 (2012) 13–24.

158. R. Sodian, P. Fu, C. Lueders, D. Szymanski, C. Fritsche, M. Gutberlet, S.P. Hoerstrup, H. Hausmann, T. Lueth, R. Hetzer, Tissue engineering of vascular conduits: Fabrication of custom-made scaffolds using rapid prototyping techniques, *Thorac. Cardiovasc. Surg.* 53 (2005) 144–149.

159. A. Khalyfa, S. Vogt, J. Weisser, G. Grimm, A. Rechtenbach, W. Meyer, M. Schnabelrauch, Development of a new calcium phosphate powder-binder system for the 3D printing of patient specific implants, *J. Mater. Sci. Mater. Med.* (2007). https://doi.org/10.1007/s10856-006-0073-2.

160. T. Nagase, Y. Iijima, A. Matsugaki, K. Ameyama, T. Nakano, Design and fabrication of Ti—Zr-Hf-Cr-Mo and Ti—Zr-Hf-Co-Cr-Mo high-entropy alloys as metallic biomaterials, *Mater. Sci. Eng. C.* (2020). https://doi.org/10.1016/j.msec.2019.110322.

161. M. Castilho, M. Dias, U. Gbureck, J. Groll, P. Fernandes, I. Pires, B. Gouveia, J. Rodrigues, E. Vorndran, Fabrication of computationally designed scaffolds by low temperature 3D printing, *Biofabrication.* (2013). https://doi.org/10.1088/1758-5082/5/3/035012.

162. M. Vlasea, E. Toyserkani, R. Pilliar, Effect of gray scale binder levels on additive manufacturing of porous scaffolds with heterogeneous properties, *Int. J. Appl. Ceram. Technol.* (2015). https://doi.org/10.1111/ijac.12316.

163. P.C. Noble, J.W. Alexander, L.J. Lindahl, D.T. Yew, W.M. Granberry, H.S. Tullos, The anatomic basis of femoral component design, *Clin. Orthop. Relat. Res.* (1988) 148–165.

164. G.N. Duda, D. Brand, S. Freitag, W. Lierse, E. Schneider, Variability of femoral muscle attachments, *J. Biomech.* 29 (1996) 1185–1190.

165. R.S. Churchill, J.J. Brems, H. Kotschi, Glenoid size, inclination, and version: An anatomic study, *J. Shoulder Elb. Surg.* 10 (2001) 327–332.

166. S.H. Kim, B.L. Wise, Y. Zhang, R.M. Szabo, Increasing incidence of shoulder arthroplasty in the United States, *JBJS.* 93 (2011) 2249–2254.

167. D.D. Anderson, T. Mosqueda, T. Thomas, E.L. Hermanson, T.D. Brown, J.L. Marsh, Quantifying tibial plafond fracture severity: Absorbed energy and fragment displacement agree with clinical rank ordering, *J. Orthop. Res.* 26 (2008) 1046–1052.

168. R.C. Andersen, G.P. Nanos, M.S. Pinzur, B.K. Potter, *Amputations in Trauma, Skelet. Trauma* (5th ed.). Philadelphia, PA: Elsevier Saunders. (2015) 2513–2534.

169. R. Bibb, D. Eggbeer, P. Evans, A. Bocca, A. Sugar, Rapid manufacture of custom-fitting surgical guides, *Rapid Prototyp. J.* (2009).

170. D.M. Dines, L. Gulotta, E. V Craig, J.S. Dines, Novel solution for massive glenoid defects in shoulder arthroplasty: A patient-specific glenoid vault reconstruction system, *Am J Orthop.* 46 (2017) 104–108.

10 Role of 3D Printing and Chitosan-Hydrogel-Based Modifiers in Drug Delivery

Lalita Chopra¹ and Jasgurpreet Singh Chohan¹
¹ Chandigarh University, Mohali, India

CONTENTS

10.1   Introduction 205
10.2   Extraction of Chitosan 207
10.3   Chitosan as a Biomedical Agent 208
10.4   Drug Uptake and Release Studies 210
10.5   Drug Release Kinetics 211
10.6   Swelling Controlled Drug Release Systems 211
10.7   Diffusion Controlled Drug Release Systems 212
10.8   Erosion Controlled Drug Release Systems 212
10.9   Drug Release Kinetic Models 213
10.10 Zero-Order Drug Release 213
10.11 First-Order Drug Release Model 213
10.12 Fick's Law 214
10.13 Higuchi Release Model 215
10.14 Hixson–Crowell Release Model 215
10.15 3D Printing of Chitosan Hydrogels 217
10.16 Conclusion 217
References 219

10.1 INTRODUCTION

Polymers have become an indispensable part of human life in the contemporary world due to their unique and vast range of properties. It is demarcated as a large macromolecule made up of the repetition of its building blocks that are a monomer in a specific and repetitive manner [1–2]. The term *polymer* has been initially employed in 1866 by a Chemical Society of France Bulletin, stating as *"styrolene* (styrene), *heated at 200° during a few hours, transforms itself into a resinous polymer"* [3].

The origin of polymers can be natural as well as artificially manufactured as per requirement. Polymers such as proteins, carbohydrates, dextrin, guar gum, chitin,

DOI: 10.1201/9781003217961-10

and others originate from nature and hence are called biopolymers. In contrast, polymers such as polythene, PVC, Teflon, polystyrene, and the like are prepared in the laboratory and, therefore, are called artificial [4–5]. The local applications of the polymers were have been vastly exhausted. Still, apart from fabricated polymers, the polymers of bio-origin attracted interest globally due to the multiple functionalities available. Biopolymers are one of the leading categories of polymers with a wide horizon of application everywhere one can see or utilize [6–8]. The applications can be industrial, such as dye sorption, metal ion removal, green technologies, environmental solutions. In the biomedical field, biopolymers are used for the construction of dialysis membrane, cytotoxicity, mucoadhesive properties, lipid dispersion, anti-ulcer effects (as food tested on rats), ophthalmology, chemotherapy, neurology, anticoagulants, skin engineering, tissue engineering, drug delivery vehicles, and the like [9–11]. Figure 10.1 shows the diverse applications of biopolymers.

The sustainable/controlled/slow/steady release of the loaded drug offers one of the foremost quarters of biomedical science [12–13]. A number of biopolymers studied showed that their hydrogel, due to their tendency to absorb, hold a considerable quantity of water compared to their dry weight. These hydrogels and their modified versions have been well exhausted as stimuli-responsive drug delivery devices [14–15]. The biopolymers have been chemically modified to introduce chosen functionalities to advance their employability [16–17]. There are a vast number of biopolymers that can be derived from the natural biomass or animals or agro-waste, such as starch [18], cellulose [19], chitin, chitosan [20], guar gum [21], agar-agar [22], and others. Cellulose polymers have the highest natural abundance; hence, they are the most utilized or exhausted polymer. After cellulose, chitin is second in the natural abundance [23–24]. Chitin can be obtained from various sources, such as exoskeletons of marine creatures, such as arthropods, crabs, prawns, insects, scorpions, spiders, ants, cockroaches, microbes such as yeast, fungus, brown algae, and more [25–26].

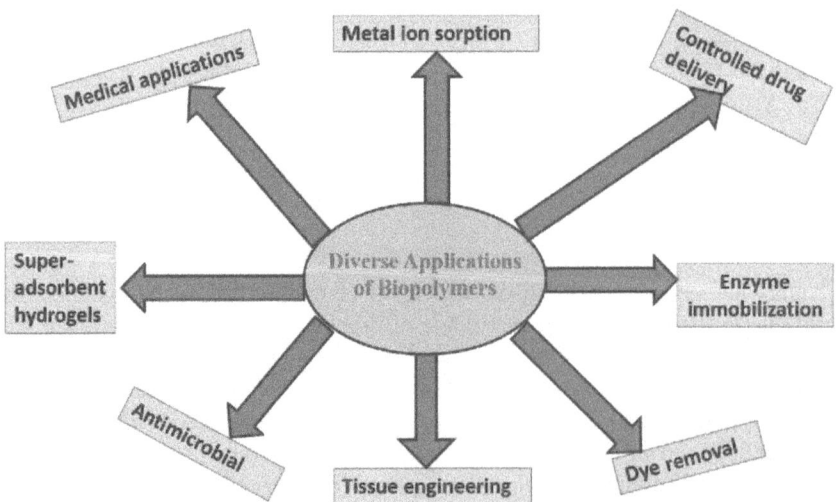

FIGURE 10.1   Diversified employability of biopolymers.

10.2 EXTRACTION OF CHITOSAN

Biopolymer chitin is a basic polysaccharide, otherwise commonly known as polysaccharides, such as cellulose, dextrin, and guar gum, which are acidic. The pure form of chitin is insoluble in an aqueous solution and in other common solvents, and this property has resulted in the limitation of its employability. Chitosan can be obtained from chitin by deacetylation by reacting with concentrated NaOH at 90–120 °C for 2–4 hours [27–28], as shown in Figure 10.2. Researchers have isolated and optimized them from Omani shrimp shells for industrial applications. The isolation was carried out chemically from shrimp waste by using demineralization, deproteinization, discoloration, and deacetylation without using chlorine. The yield of the product was satisfactory, concluding that shrimp waste can serve as a most significant natural reservoir for the preparation of these polysaccharides [29].

In chitosan, due to deacetylation, an amine group is introduced, giving it basic properties and making it unique from the commonly known acidic biopolymers [30–31]. The deacetylation degree may vary from 60–100%, and this is dependent on the source of chitin as well as the experimental conditions and procedures. With a 50% deacetylation product, chitosan becomes soluble in an aqueous media. This conversion also led to the lowering of the molecular weight. The commercially available chitosan has a molecular weight in the range of 3800–20,000 Daltons [32].

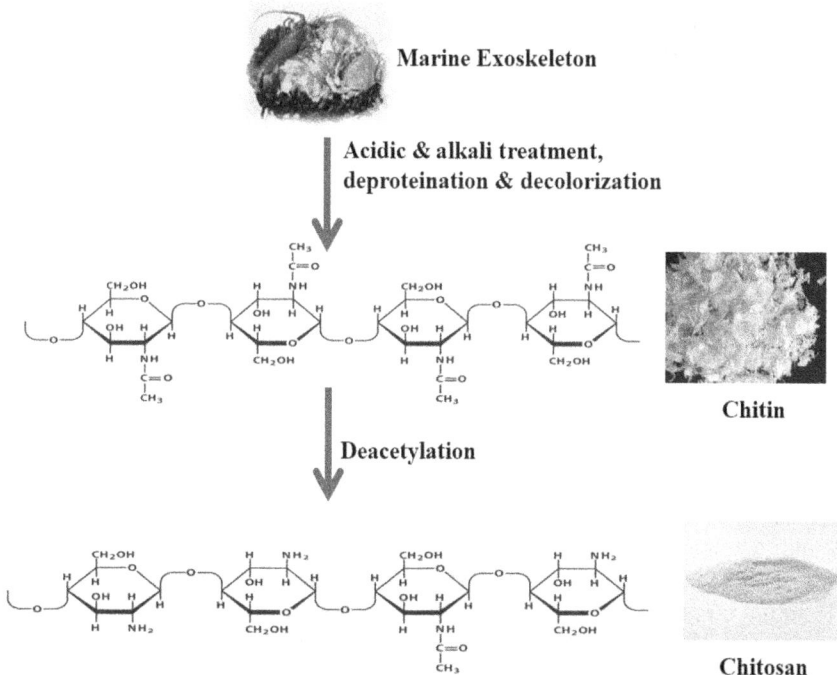

FIGURE 10.2 Extraction of chitosan.

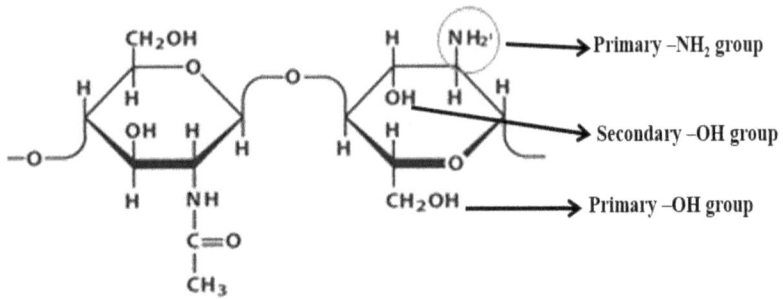

FIGURE 10.3   Functionalities of chitosan.

Chitosan is an alkaline hydrolytic derivative of chitin that has improved solubility and less crystallinity. It has dual functionality of –OH and –NH$_2$ groups and is amenable to chemical modifications of any functional group to enhance its activity [33–34]. This property added to the versatility of Chitosan as compared to chitin. Chitosan is a linear polyamine having acidic (–OH; primary or secondary) and basic (–NH$_2$) function groups (NH$_2$ group at C$_2$ position) as shown in Figure 10.3. Chitosan can be derivatized to get desirable properties by modifying the –OH (primary or secondary) and –NH$_2$ groups. There are various techniques of modification, such as graft copolymerization [35–36].

10.3   CHITOSAN AS A BIOMEDICAL AGENT

The distinct characteristics of chitosan such as biodegradability, absorbability to a biosystem, non-bioaccumulation, and nontoxicity make it safe for utilization in the health sector [37–39]. The literature survey revealed that pristine, as well as its modified, derivatives have biomedical status in the building of dialysis membrane [40], treatment of cytotoxicity [41], neurology [42], anticoagulants [43], mucoadhesive surfaces [44], lipid dispersion properties [45], anti-ulcer impacts (as food tested on rats) [46], chemotherapy [47], skin engineering, tissue engineering, and more [48].

At a low pH, the –NH$_2$ group of chitosan gets protonated, resulting in cationic polysaccharides that induce bio-adhesion properties, as shown in Figure 10.4. Bio-adhesive compounds tend to ascribe two surfaces collectively where at least one surface must be living tissue [49]. S. M. Luna and coworkers in 2011 investigated cell adhesion mechanism by the membranes based on chitosan materials by plasma treatment [50].

Antimicrobial properties are also exhibited by chitosan and its derivatives, because of which these can be proficiently labored in wound-healing applications in hospitals [51]. In the literature, modified forms of chitosan were exhausted for antimicrobial properties against *Pseudomonas aeruginosa*, *Bacillus subtilis*, and *Fusarium solani*, respectively [52–54].

Low pH

NH_2

NH_3^+

High pH

Insoluble chitosan

Soluble chitosan

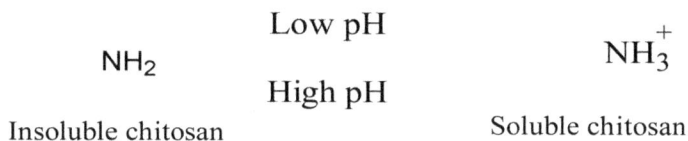

FIGURE 10.4 Effect of pH variation on chitosan solubility.

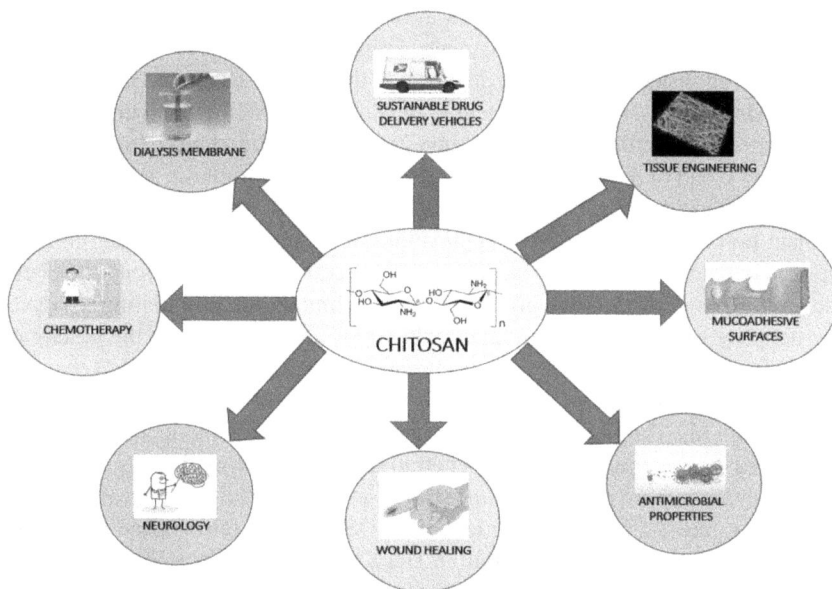

FIGURE 10.5 Employability of chitosan in the health sector.

The applicability of chitosan in various domains of the biomedical field and health care industry is shown in Figure 10.5. The literature survey also revealed that chitosan powder in pristine, as well as modified, form presented as a promising means of transport for the triggered delivery of a vast number of biomolecules, such as peptides, lipids, nucleic acids, and vaccines in the biosystems, and the activity could be enhanced by fabricating desired functionalities on it by chemical modifications [55–60]. Alex et al. worked on spermine-grafted galactosylated chitosan nanoparticles for the delivery of genes [61].

Tissue engineering connects technology with health care, and it is one of the practices growing the most in the arena of bioengineering. This has been defined as a multidisciplinary approach that utilizes the principles of therapeutic science with procedures of engineering. The chitosan-supported polymers were well-known applicants for tissue scaffolds due to their properties, such as nontoxicity, biocompatibility, porosity, and biodegradability of the systems when fresh tissues are formed, thus giving no waste in the body [62–63]. Researchers examined the calcium–phosphate–chitosan composite scaffolds and reported nano-hydroxyapatite of chitosan support with thermoresponsive monomers (NPAM) for tissue engineering applications [64–66].

The controlled and sustainable release of any therapeutic drug to the biosystem signifies some major domains of medicinal chemistry that involve multidisciplinary slant of science and technology together in the arena of medical science [67]. The target-oriented/stimuli-responsive drug delivery vehicle delivers at the rate determined by a human's requirement for a definite time period and on an exact target [68]. Sustainable drug delivery devices allow slow or controlled drug release in a definite cell, tissue, organ, or bloodstream. Drug delivery devices work by incorporating the drug inside a biopolymer network so that this incorporated or absorbed or adsorbed drug diffuses into the system at the target in a well-defined and controlled manner [69–70]. The literature survey investigated that drug delivery structures had a boundless blend of their widespread hydrophobic and hydrophilic apparatuses [71]. The bi-polymeric hydrogels/matrices/nanomaterials had great functionalities, making them potent for drug delivery applications. The uploading of a drug into polymeric matrices/hydrogels/nanoparticles with several hydrophilic groups for better drug–polymer interaction has proved to be a technique for formulating a targeted drug delivery vehicle [72]. These materials are of great interest for the sustainable release of an enormous number of drugs because of their unique and green characteristics like bioactivity, biodegradability, pH and temperature sensitivity, nontoxicity, and the like. [73]. The literature survey reveals that chitosan and its modified forms (crosslinked graft copolymers, interpenetrating polymer network (IPN), semi-IPN, graft copolymers) were exploited in the stimuli-targeted sustainable release of a variety of drugs like 5-FU, ibuprofen, fenbufen, DS, Insulin, tetracycline and methotrexate, nifidifine (NFD), pentoxifylline (PTX), indomethacin (IM), vancomycin, ketoprofen, berberine, verapamil, and others [74–77].

10.4   DRUG UPTAKE AND RELEASE STUDIES

In one study, a sample's known weight was immersed in a known amount of drug solution to study the drug release from the biopolymeric matrices. A stock solution of the drug with the available concentration was prepared and scanned at a wavelength range by a Thermo ultraviolet (UV)-visible spectrophotometer. The calibration curve was prepared for the drug solution between absorbance versus wavelength in order to get the λ_{max}. Drug solutions of different concentrations were manufactured at λ_{max} [78]. For drug uploading, a measured mass of polymeric samples was placed in a 10.00-mL drug solution of a particular concentration for 24 hours for the maximum drug uptake and was investigated for the concentration of drug left in the supernatant by Thermo UV-Visible spectrophotometer [79–80]. The amount of the drug absorbed by the polymeric sample was calculated by deducting the concentration of the drug left in the filtrate from the initial drug concentration taken into the solution. The drug-uploaded samples were then dried for 3–4 days at room temperature until its weight was constant. The drug release can be studied with variations in stimuli such as pH, temperature, and ionic concentration [81–82]. Kinetic factors, such as the percentage of drug uptake and the percentage of drug release, were analyzed for the drug diffusion and studied with respect to time [82]; they can be expressed as follows:

$$\text{Percent Drug Uptake} = \frac{\text{Total drug taken in solution} - \text{Drug left in supernatant}}{\text{Total drug taken in solution}} \times 100$$

$$\text{Percent Drug Release} = \frac{\text{Concentration of drug in solution}}{\text{Total drug taken in solution}} \times 100$$

10.5 DRUG RELEASE KINETICS

Drug release from the biopolymeric-based system represents a process through which the drug entrapped within leave the product as shown in Figure 10.6. The drug release kinetics reveal the rate at which a drug is diffused out to the system, drug dissolution, drug erosion, and the type of diffusion it follows. Various mathematical models for the drug release process were applied to study the kinetics of the release of a drug. The release of a drug from the biopolymeric matrices can be derived by three factors, such as swelling controlled drug release [83–84].

10.6 SWELLING CONTROLLED DRUG RELEASE SYSTEMS

The biopolymers proved to be excellent candidates for hydrogel studies as these will allow a huge quantity of water to penetrate them, and they have the capacity to hold it. This will be due to the number of pores present on the surface and may be due to the large number of hydrophilic functionalities present on them. When a dry polymeric sample is placed in water, it will absorb water [85]. Figure 10.7 shows the process of swelling a hydrogel from dried hydrogel.

The percentage of water uptake or the percentage of swelling can be calculated [86] by using the following expression:

$$P_s = \frac{W_s - W_d}{W_d} \times 100$$

where, P_s represents the percentage of swelling and W_s and W_d signify the weight of the swollen and dry polymer, respectively.

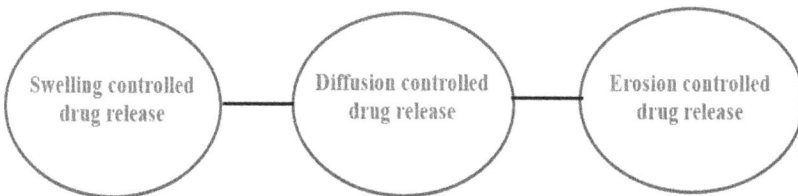

FIGURE 10.6 Drug release systems.

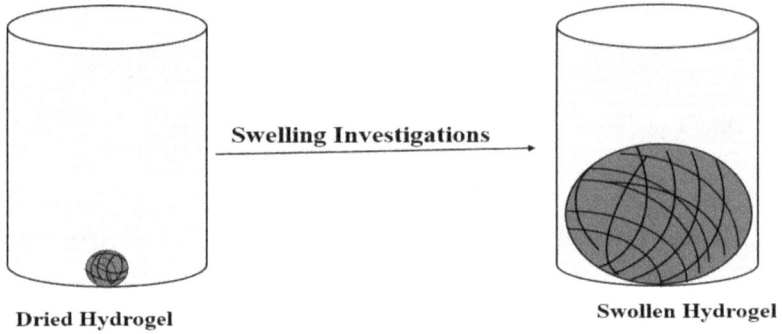

FIGURE 10.7 Swelling investigations of hydrogels.

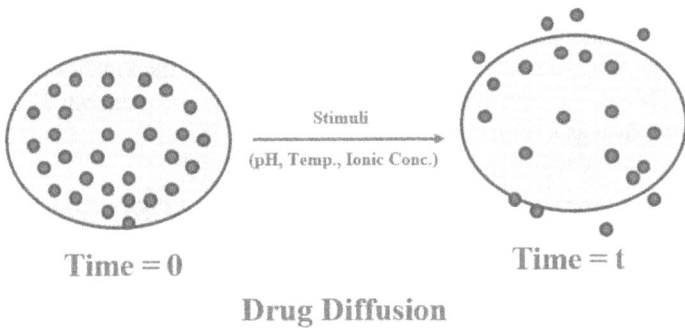

FIGURE 10.8 Drug diffusion from the polymeric matrix.

10.7 DIFFUSION CONTROLLED DRUG RELEASE SYSTEMS

Some drug devices release drugs at a controlled rate, and the diffusion of the drug out of the polymeric matrix is controlled by the type and rate of diffusion. Figure 10.8 shows the drug diffusion after the effect of stimuli such as pH, temperature, and ionic concentration. The diffusion of the drug entrapped within the biopolymeric sample depends on the size of the drug molecules, drug–polymer interactions, and drug–solvent interactions. In these kinds of release reactions, the rate-determining step is the diffusion of the drug through a biopolymeric matrix. The rate and the type of drug diffusion that occurs can be understood with the help of Fick's law [87].

10.8 EROSION CONTROLLED DRUG RELEASE SYSTEMS

In an eroding drug delivery system, the drug release mechanism occurs by erosion. Erosion of the biopolymeric matrix can take place at the bulk level or only at the surface level. In this process, the biopolymeric matrix are degraded, and during this process, the drug entrapped gets to escape. In the case of surface erosion, only the surface of the matrix gets degraded; at the bulk level, drug molecules entrapped due to adsorption escape easily whereas those entrapped in the bulk will take more time for the case of bulk erosion, the system as a whole degrades and lets the drug diffuse completely at a faster rate [88].

10.9   DRUG RELEASE KINETIC MODELS

A number of mathematical models were given to study drug release from different models. Models are based on various mathematical functions in order to describe the drug release rate from the observed system [89]. Researchers have tried to modelized the particular drug release under investigation through various mathematical models so as to find out which drug release model will suit to their process or formulation of dosage in the best way.

10.10   ZERO-ORDER DRUG RELEASE

The formula for this case is defined as when the rate of release of the drug does not depend on the concentration of the drug entrapped in the sample under investigation. A graph (Figure 10.9) when plotted between cumulative drug release (CDR) at time t (Q_t) versus time (t) should be a straight line. K_0 value is obtained from the slope, and Q_0 can be obtained from the intercept of the curve [90].

10.11   FIRST-ORDER DRUG RELEASE MODEL

According to the first-order rate model for drug release, drug release depends on the first order of the concentration of the drug inside the biopolymeric sample. With a greater the concentration of the drug entrapped, more of it will be released. Therefore, this mathematical model follows linear kinetics [91]. A curve when plotted between log Q_t versus time (t) will give straight line with a slope equal to $K/2.303$ and an intercept equal to log Q_0 as shown in Figure 10.10.

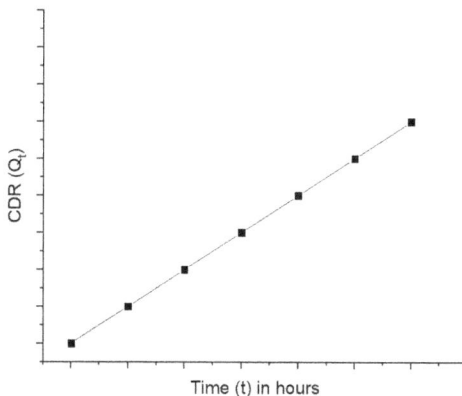

FIGURE 10.9   Change in CDR with time.

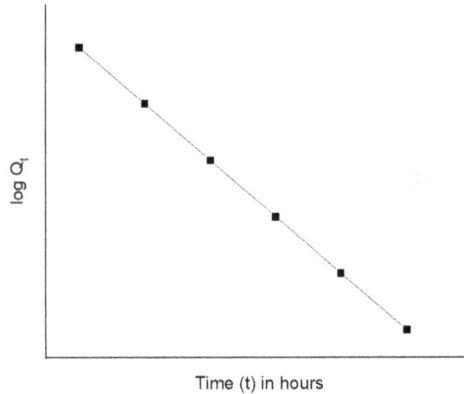

FIGURE 10.10   Change in Q_t with time.

10.12   FICK'S LAW

Korsmeyer-Peppas gave a kinetic model unfolding the relationship between drug diffusion with respect to time from the biopolymeric sample. The equation assisted with discovering the mechanism of drug release. Drug diffusion from the biopolymeric samples can take place by Fickian or non-Fickian types of diffusion. For Fickian diffusion, the transportation of the drug from the sample occurs in such a way that the polymer relaxation time (t_r) is significantly higher than the diffusion time (t_d), whereas in non-Fickian diffusion, $t_r \approx t_d$. Hence, it follows zero-order drug release kinetics, showing that the rate is constant [92–93]. According to Fick's law, the portion of drug release at a particular time t was given by the following equation:

$$F = \frac{M_t}{M_\infty} = kt^n$$

Taking log on both sides, we get

$$log \frac{M_t}{M_\infty} = logk + nlogt$$

when a graph is plotted between $log \dfrac{M_t}{M_\infty}$ verses $log\ t$, it will be a linear regression curve. This phenomenon is represented in Figure 10.11. The value of n is calculated from the slope of the curve whereas the value of k has to be calculated from the crossing point of the plot.

The curve statistics giving the value of r must approach unity, which represents that the release of the drug from the polymeric material must follow a linear release pattern [94]. With respect to variation in the value of the n, the type of drug diffusion varies.

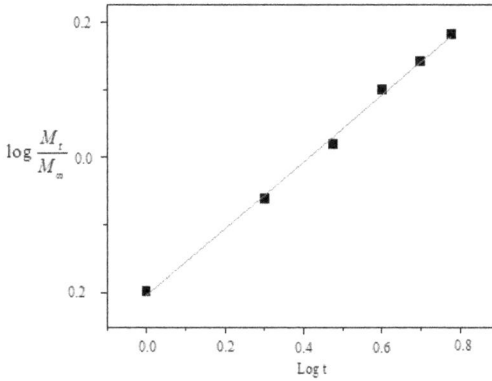

FIGURE 10.11 Linear regression curve for fraction of drug.

10.13 HIGUCHI RELEASE MODEL

Higuchi drug release kinetic model describes the release of drugs from biopolymeric samples dependent on the square root of time and follows Fick's law. The model worked well for water-soluble drugs and poorly for soluble drugs [95–96]. The model may be applicable to a number of insoluble matrices that can be solid as well as semisolid. The Higuchi release equation for drug release through the matrix can be expressed as

$$Q = K_H t^{1/n}$$

In the preceding expressed equation,
Q = CDR (cumulative drug release at time t),
K_H = Higuchi's constant, and
t = time in hours.

If a curve, when plotted between Q (CDR %age) versus square root of time, goes linear, with $r2$ approaching to unity, it shows the applicability of the kinetic model to the release as shown in Figure 10.12.

10.14 HIXSON–CROWELL RELEASE MODEL

The Hixson–Crowell release model describes that the release of the entrapped drug from the insoluble biopolymeric matrices took place by the dissolution-controlled mechanism. According to the model, the rate of release of drug is dependent on the surface area of the solvent, with the increase of which the drug release gets enhanced indeed [97–98]. The Hixson–Crowell equation can be expressed as

$$\sqrt[3]{Q_0} - \sqrt[3]{\theta_t} = Kt$$

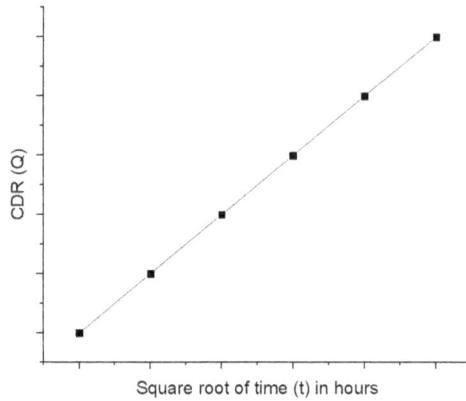

FIGURE 10.12   Change in CDR with the square root of time.

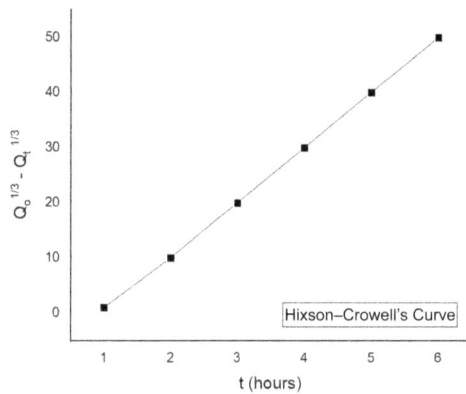

FIGURE 10.13   Change in the Hixson–Crowell equation with time.

where
Q_0 = initial concentration of the drug,
θ_t = cumulative release of drug (CDR) at time t,
K = Hixson–Crowell constant, and
t = time in hours.

Hixson–Crowell's cube root equation/model of the drug release investigations suits erodible polymeric nanomaterials, microspheres, mesosphere, matrices, and others the best. When a graph is plotted between $\sqrt[3]{Q_0} - \sqrt[3]{\theta_t}$ versus time t, it will be a straight line curve with the value of Hixson–Crowell constant K obtained from the slope of the curve as shown in Figure 10.13.

10.15   3D PRINTING OF CHITOSAN HYDROGELS

Three-dimensional (3D) printing technologies emerged in the late 1980s due to enormous growth in computer-aided design and manufacturing (CAD and CAM, respectively). *Three-dimensional printing* is a generic term used for a number of technologies that enable the fabrication of physical objects directly from CAD data. Among several techniques, the first demonstration was made by stereolithography apparatus (SLA) that was pioneered by 3D Systems Corporation in the United States in 1988. Since then, the continuous progression and refinements through several generations lead to the development of more than 25 AM techniques. Selective laser sintering (SLS), laminated object manufacturing (LOM), fused deposition modeling (FDM), multijet modeling (MJM) and additive manufacturing (AM) are some of the most widely used AM techniques [99].

The implementation of 3D printing in tissue engineering and drug delivery research has been intensified in the areas of biomedical science and engineering. Tissue engineering researchers frequently contemplate cells, scaffolds, and growth aspects to be the most important mechanisms. A 3D assembly filled with cells that are regulated enables customized cell dispersion, resulting in better cell proliferation and tissue regeneration. To that purpose, 3D printing, also known as AM, has been utilized to create 3D structures that imitate the characteristics of tissue, and it is currently one of the most exciting study subjects in the biomedical and tissue engineering sectors. The 3D printing using bio-inks through a pneumatic piston–driven mechanisms [100] is demonstrated in Figure 10.14.

The scientometric analysis has been performed to ascertain recent research trends in the area of 3D printing and chitosan hydrogels (see Figure 10.15). A keyword analysis was performed using the Vosviewer analytical tool for the interrelationship between 3D printing and chitosan hydrogels. The research trends indicate that intensive research has been performed in the last 5 years in this domain. Chitosan has been extensively utilized for tissue engineering applications since 2018 as per the Scopus database. However, there is a scope for research and analysis of mechanical properties, in vitro studies, and extracellular matrices of chitosan hydrogels.

10.16   CONCLUSION

In this comprehensive review study, novel stimuli-responsive biopolymeric materials, such as mesopores, whiskers, nanomaterials, copolymers, matrices, and more, based on chitosan support were discussed regarding their employment in the health industry as potential candidates for controlled/slow/sustainable in vitro release of numerous drugs. Chitosan is a natural, semisynthetic, nontoxic, biocompatible, and biodegradable polymer derived from chitin (the second-most abundant biopolymer on earth after cellulose). The incidence of cationic $-NH_2$ groups on chitosan makes it a unique cationic polymer compared to others and increases its potential with respect to biomedical applications. The dual functionality of chitosan is susceptible to being fabricated as per the requirements of the study. The polymeric samples/materials/matrices were capable of swelling to different extents in response to various biological stimuli, such as pH, temperature, ionic strength, and so on; swelling helps

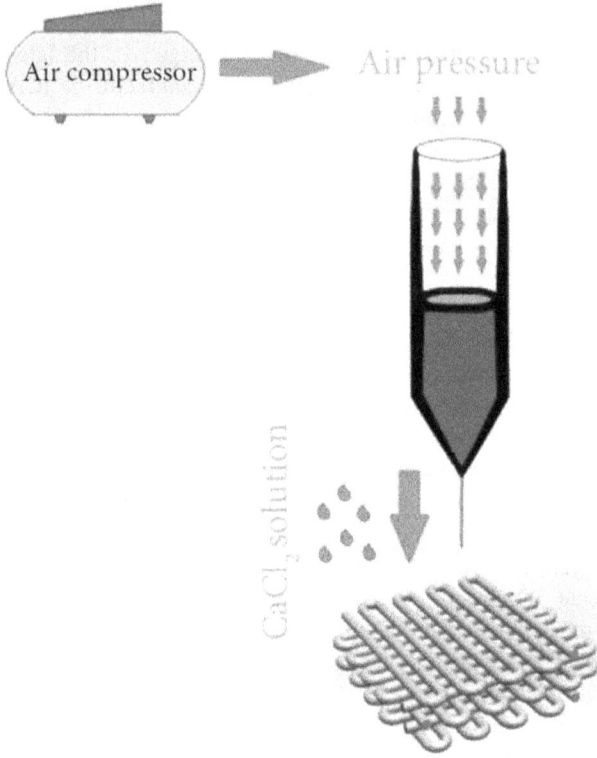

FIGURE 10.14   3D printing of hydrogels [100].

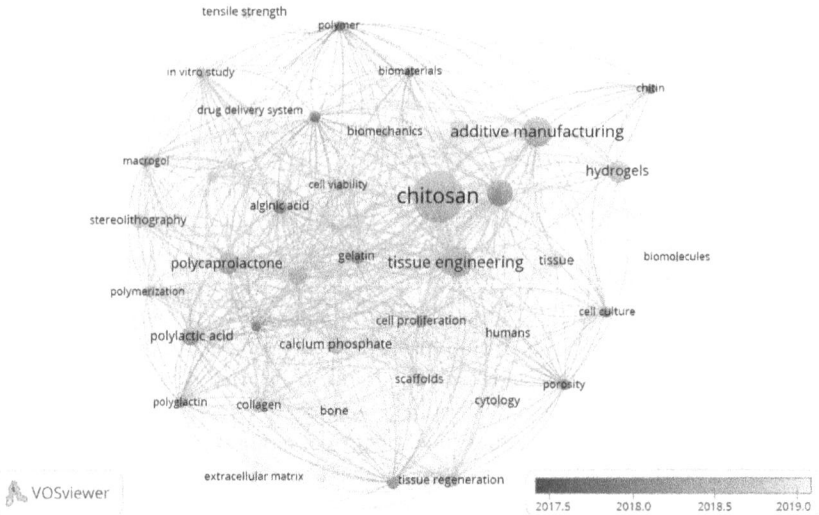

FIGURE 10.15   Scientometric analysis chart.

the drug molecules diffuse into (drug uptake) and out (drug release) of polymeric samples. Due to these swelling properties, these materials were well exhausted as drug delivery vehicles. Applying different kinetic models on the drug release will help with investigating the rate, as well as the mechanism, of the release of the drug. Drug release investigations should be done with various kinetic drug release models, and models that well suit specific drug releases from specific formulations should be considered.

Today, scholars are exploring new isolation techniques of 3D bioprinting of hydrogels using digital manufacturing techniques. This has enabled the customization of biomaterials using bio-inks and has helped with drug delivery. With respect to the preceding discussion, upcoming research efforts should emphasize new opportunities for utilizing a number of potent samples for in vivo performance of drug release and applying the models to the drug under investigation to observe the drug release profile and do a comparison of the various keratin models and their suitability in that specific situation to have distinct view about dealings among drugs and their carriers.

REFERENCES

1. Chandra, R. U. S. T. G. I., & Rustgi, R. (1998). Biodegradable polymers. *Progress in Polymer Science*, 23(7), 1273–1335.
2. Young, R. J., & Lovell, P. A. (2011). *Introduction to Polymers*. CRC Press.
3. Rasmussen, S. C. (2018). Revisiting the early history of synthetic polymers: Critiques and new insights. *Ambix*, 65(4), 356–372.
4. Olatunji, O. (2016). Classification of natural polymers. In *Natural Polymers* (pp. 1–17). Springer.
5. Massy, J. (2017). *A Little Book about BIG Chemistry: The Story of Man-Made Polymers*. Springer.
6. Liu, H., Qing, H., Li, Z., Han, Y. L., Lin, M., Yang, H., . . . Xu, F. (2017). A promising material for human-friendly functional wearable electronics. *Materials Science and Engineering: R: Reports*, 112, 1–22.
7. Niaounakis, M. (2015). *Biopolymers: Applications and Trends*. William Andrew.
8. Van de Velde, K., & Kiekens, P. (2002). Biopolymers: Overview of several properties and consequences on their applications. *Polymer Testing*, 21(4), 433–442.
9. Kalia, S., & Averous, L. (2011). *Biopolymers: Biomedical and Environmental Applications* (Vol. 70). John Wiley & Sons.
10. Sahana, T. G., & Rekha, P. D. (2018). Biopolymers: Applications in wound healing and skin tissue engineering. *Molecular Biology Reports*, 45(6), 2857–2867.
11. Chilkoti, A., Christensen, T., & MacKay, J. A. (2006). Stimulus responsive elastin biopolymers: Applications in medicine and biotechnology. *Current Opinion in Chemical Biology*, 10(6), 652–657.
12. Narayanaswamy, R., & Torchilin, V. P. (2019). Hydrogels and their applications in targeted drug delivery. *Molecules*, 24(3), 603.
13. Jantzen, G. M., & Robinson, J. R. (2002). Sustained and controlled-release drug delivery systems. *Modern Pharmaceutics*, 4, 501–502.
14. Malachowski, K., Breger, J., Kwag, H. R., Wang, M. O., Fisher, J. P., Selaru, F. M., & Gracias, D. H. (2014). Stimuli-responsive theragrippers for chemomechanical controlled release. *Angewandte Chemie International Edition*, 53(31), 8045–8049.
15. Wang, S. (2009). Ordered mesoporous materials for drug delivery. *Microporous and Mesoporous Materials*, 117(1–2), 1–9.

16. Zhang, Q., Li, Y., Lin, Z. Y. W., Wong, K. K., Lin, M., Yildirimer, L., & Zhao, X. (2017). Electrospun polymeric micro/nanofibrous scaffolds for long-term drug release and their biomedical applications. *Drug Discovery Today*, 22(9), 1351–1366.

17. Bhattarai, N., Ramay, H. R., Gunn, J., Matsen, F. A., & Zhang, M. (2005). PEG-grafted chitosan as an injectable thermosensitive hydrogel for sustained protein release. *Journal of Controlled Release*, 103(3), 609–624.

18. López, O. V., Versino, F., Villar, M. A., & Garcia, M. A. (2015). Agro-industrial residue from starch extraction of Pachyrhizus ahipa as filler of thermoplastic corn starch films. *Carbohydrate Polymers*, 134, 324–332.

19. Menon, M. P., Selvakumar, R., & Ramakrishna, S. (2017). Extraction and modification of cellulose nanofibers derived from biomass for environmental application. *RSC Advances*, 7(68), 42750–42773.

20. El Knidri, H., Belaabed, R., Addaou, A., Laajeb, A., & Lahsini, A. (2018). Extraction, chemical modification and characterization of chitin and Chitosan. *International Journal of Biological Macromolecules*, 120, 1181–1189.

21. George, A., Shah, P. A., & Shrivastav, P. S. (2019). Guar gum: Versatile natural polymer for drug delivery applications. *European Polymer Journal*, 112, 722–735.

22. Vuai, S. A. H., & Mpatani, F. (2019). Optimization of agar extraction from local seaweed species, Gracilaria salicornia in Tanzania. *Phycological Research*, 67(4), 261–266.

23. Shaghaleh, H., Xu, X., & Wang, S. (2018). Current progress in production of biopolymeric materials based on cellulose, cellulose nanofibers, and cellulose derivatives. *RSC Advances*, 8(2), 825–842.

24. Motaung, T. E., & Linganiso, L. Z. (2018). Critical review on agrowaste cellulose applications for biopolymers. *International Journal of Plastics Technology*, 22(2), 185–216.

25. Zhao, X., Zhang, J., & Zhu, K. Y. (2019). Chito-protein matrices in arthropod exoskeletons and peritrophic matrices. In *Extracellular Sugar-Based Biopolymers Matrices* (pp. 3–56). Springer.

26. Ibitoye, E. B., Lokman, I. H., Hezmee, M. N. M., Goh, Y. M., Zuki, A. B. Z., & Jimoh, A. A. (2018). Extraction and physicochemical characterization of chitin and Chitosan isolated from house cricket. *Biomedical Materials*, 13(2), 025009.

27. Mohan, K., Ganesan, A. R., Muralisankar, T., Jayakumar, R., Sathishkumar, P., Uthayakumar, V., Chandirasekar, R., Revathi, N. (2020, Nov 1). Recent insights into the extraction, characterization, and bioactivities of chitin and chitosan from insects. *Trends in Food Science & Technology*, 105, 17–42.

28. Santos, V. P., Marques, N. S., Maia, P. C., Lima, M. A. B. D., Franco, L. D. O., & Campos-Takaki, G. M. D. (2020). Seafood waste as attractive source of chitin and chitosan production and their applications. *International Journal of Molecular Sciences*, 21(12), 4290.

29. Al Hoqani, H. A. S., Noura, A. S., Hossain, M. A., & Al Sibani, M. A. (2020). Isolation and optimization of the method for industrial production of chitin and Chitosan from Omani shrimp shell. *Carbohydrate Research*, 492, 108001.

30. Lizardi-Mendoza, J., Monal, W. M. A., & Valencia, F. M. G. (2016). Chemical characteristics and functional properties of Chitosan. In *Chitosan in the Preservation of Agricultural Commodities* (pp. 3–31). Academic Press.

31. Muxika, A., Etxabide, A., Uranga, J., Guerrero, P., & De La Caba, K. (2017). Chitosan as a bioactive polymer: Processing, properties and applications. *International Journal of Biological Macromolecules*, 105, 1358–1368.

32. Zhao, D., Yu, S., Sun, B., Gao, S., Guo, S., & Zhao, K. (2018). Biomedical applications of Chitosan and its derivative nanoparticles. *Polymers*, 10(4), 462.

33. Paul, P., Kolesinska, B., & Sujka, W. (2019). Chitosan and its derivatives-biomaterials with diverse biological activity for manifold applications. *Mini Reviews in Medicinal Chemistry*, 19(9), 737–750.

34. Li, Q., Dunn, E. T., Grandmaison, E. W., & Goosen, M. F. (2020). Applications and properties of Chitosan. In *Applications of Chitin and Chitosan* (pp. 3–29). CRC Press, Taylor and Francis.

35. Thakur VK, Thakur MK. Recent advances in graft copolymerization and applications of chitosan: a review. *ACS Sustainable Chemistry & Engineering*. 2014 Dec 1;2(12):2637–52.

36. Bodnar, M., Hartmann, J. F., & Borbely, J. (2005). Preparation and characterization of chitosan-based nanoparticles. *Biomacromolecules*, 6(5), 2521–2527.

37. Vunain, E., Mishra, A. K., & Mamba, B. B. (2017). Fundamentals of Chitosan for biomedical applications. In *Chitosan Based Biomaterials* (Vol. 1, pp. 3–30). Woodhead Publishing.

38. Alves, N. M., & Mano, J. F. (2008). Chitosan derivatives obtained by chemical modifications for biomedical and environmental applications. *International Journal of Biological Macromolecules*, 43(5), 401–414.

39. Szymańska, E., & Winnicka, K. (2015). Stability of chitosan—a challenge for pharmaceutical and biomedical applications. *Marine Drugs*, 13(4), 1819–1846.

40. Wahid, A., Sridhar, B. K., & Shivakumar, S. (2008). Preparation and evaluation of transdermal drug delivery system of etoricoxib using modified Chitosan. *Indian Journal of Pharmaceutical Sciences*, 70(4), 455.

41. Loutfy, S. A., El-Din, H. M. A., Elberry, M. H., Allam, N. G., Hasanin, M. T. M., & Abdellah, A. M. (2016). Synthesis, characterization and cytotoxic evaluation of chitosan nanoparticles: In vitro liver cancer model. *Advances in Natural Sciences: Nanoscience and Nanotechnology*, 7(3), 035008.

42. Lara-Velazquez, M. A., Al-kharboosh, R. M., Norton, E. S., Ramirez-Loera, C., Freeman, W. D., Guerrero-Cazares, H., . . . Sarabia Estrada, R. (2020). Chitosan-based non-viral gene and drug delivery systems for brain cancer. *Frontiers in Neurology*, 11, 740.

43. Jayakumar, R., Nagahama, H., Furuike, T., & Tamura, H. (2008). Synthesis of phosphorylated Chitosan by novel method and its characterization. *International Journal of Biological Macromolecules*, 42(4), 335–339.

44. Chaiyasan, W., Srinivas, S. P., & Tiyaboonchai, W. (2013). Mucoadhesive Chitosan—dextran sulfate nanoparticles for sustained drug delivery to the ocular surface. *Journal of Ocular Pharmacology and Therapeutics*, 29(2), 200–207.

45. Pereda, M., Amica, G., & Marcovich, N. E. (2012). Development and characterization of edible chitosan/olive oil emulsion films. *Carbohydrate Polymers*, 87(2), 1318–1325.

46. Abd El Hady, W. E., Mohamed, E. A., Soliman, O. A. E. A., & El-Sabbagh, H. M. (2019). In vitro—in vivo evaluation of chitosan-PLGA nanoparticles for potentiated gastric retention and anti-ulcer activity of diosmin. *International Journal of Nanomedicine*, 14, 7191.

47. Rahimi, M., Shafiei-Irannejad, V., Safa, K. D., & Salehi, R. (2018). Multi-branched ionic liquid-chitosan as a smart and biocompatible nano-vehicle for combination chemotherapy with stealth and targeted properties. *Carbohydrate Polymers*, 196, 299–312.

48. Pandey, A. R., Singh, U. S., Momin, M., & Bhavsar, C. (2017). Chitosan: Application in tissue engineering and skin grafting. *Journal of Polymer Research*, 24(8), 1–22.

49. Carvalho, C. R., López-Cebral, R., Silva-Correia, J., Silva, J. M., Mano, J. F., Silva, T. H., . . . Oliveira, J. M. (2017). Investigation of cell adhesion in chitosan membranes for peripheral nerve regeneration. *Materials Science and Engineering: C*, 71, 1122–1134.

50. Luna, S. M., Silva, S. S., Gomes, M. E., Mano, J. F., & Reis, R. L. (2011). Cell adhesion and proliferation onto chitosan-based membranes treated by plasma surface modification. *Journal of Biomaterials Applications*, 26(1), 101–116.

51. Divya, K., Vijayan, S., George, T. K., & Jisha, M. S. (2017). Antimicrobial properties of chitosan nanoparticles: Mode of action and factors affecting activity. *Fibers and Polymers*, 18(2), 221–230.

52. Ghosh, S., Singh, B. P., & Webster, T. J. (2021). Nanoparticle-impregnated biopolymers as novel antimicrobial nanofilms. In *Biopolymer-Based Nano Films* (pp. 269–309). Elsevier.
53. Huang, H. F., & Peng, C. F. (2015). Antibacterial and antifungal activity of alkylsulfonated Chitosan. *Biomarkers and Genomic Medicine*, 7(2), 83–86.
54. Lim, S. H., & Hudson, S. M. (2003). Review of Chitosan and its derivatives as antimicrobial agents and their uses as textile chemicals. *Journal of Macromolecular Science, Part C: Polymer Reviews*, 43(2), 223–269.
55. Liu, W. G., & De Yao, K. (2002). Chitosan and its derivatives—a promising non-viral vector for gene transfection. *Journal of Controlled Release*, 83(1), 1–11.
56. Rathor, S., Bhatt, D. C., Aamir, S., Singh, S. K., & Kumar, V. (2017). A comprehensive review on role of nanoparticles in therapeutic delivery of medicine. *Pharmaceutical Nanotechnology*, 5(4), 263–275.
57. Nevagi, R. J., Khalil, Z. G., Hussein, W. M., Powell, J., Batzloff, M. R., Capon, R. J., . . . Toth, I. (2018). Polyglutamic acid-trimethyl chitosan-based intranasal peptide nano-vaccine induces potent immune responses against group a streptococcus. *Acta Biomaterialia*, 80, 278–287.
58. Kumar, C. S., Thangam, R., Mary, S. A., Kannan, P. R., Arun, G., & Madhan, B. (2020). Targeted delivery and apoptosis induction of trans-resveratrol-ferulic acid loaded Chitosan coated folic acid conjugate solid lipid nanoparticles in colon cancer cells. *Carbohydrate Polymers*, 231, 115682.
59. Lai, W. F., & Lin, M. C. M. (2009). Nucleic acid delivery with Chitosan and its derivatives. *Journal of Controlled Release*, 134(3), 158–168.
60. Li, J., Cai, C., Li, J., Li, J., Li, J., Sun, T., . . . Yu, G. (2018). Chitosan-based nanomaterials for drug delivery. *Molecules*, 23(10), 2661.
61. Alex, S. M., Rekha, M. R., & Sharma, C. P. (2011). Spermine grafted galactosylated Chitosan for improved nanoparticle mediated gene delivery. *International Journal of Pharmaceutics*, 410(1–2), 125–137.
62. Croisier, F., & Jérôme, C. (2013). Chitosan-based biomaterials for tissue engineering. *European Polymer Journal*, 49(4), 780–792.
63. Kim, I. Y., Seo, S. J., Moon, H. S., Yoo, M. K., Park, I. Y., Kim, B. C., & Cho, C. S. (2008). Chitosan and its derivatives for tissue engineering applications. *Biotechnology Advances*, 26(1), 1–21.
64. Zhang, Y., Ni, M., Zhang, M., & Ratner, B. (2003). Calcium phosphate—chitosan composite scaffolds for bone tissue engineering. *Tissue Engineering*, 9(2), 337–345.
65. Yu, Y., Zhang, H., Sun, H., Xing, D., & Yao, F. (2013). Nano-hydroxyapatite formation via co-precipitation with chitosan-g-poly (N-isopropylacrylamide) in coil and globule states for tissue engineering application. *Frontiers of Chemical Science and Engineering*, 7(4), 388–400.
66. Li, Z., Ramay, H. R., Hauch, K. D., Xiao, D., & Zhang, M. (2005). Chitosan—alginate hybrid scaffolds for bone tissue engineering. *Biomaterials*, 26(18), 3919–3928.
67. Ciechanska, D. (2004). Multifunctional bacterial cellulose/chitosan composite materials for medical applications. *Fibres and Textiles in Eastern Europe*, 12(4), 69–72.
68. Liu, H., Liu, J., Xie, X., & Li, X. (2020). Development of photo-magnetic drug delivery system by facile-designed dual stimuli-responsive modified biopolymeric Chitosan capped nano-vesicle to improve efficiency in the anesthetic effect and its biological investigations. *Journal of Photochemistry and Photobiology B: Biology*, 202, 111716.
69. Verestiuc, L., Ivanov, C., Barbu, E., & Tsibouklis, J. (2004). Dual-stimuli-responsive hydrogels based on poly (N-isopropylacrylamide)/chitosan semi-interpenetrating networks. *International Journal of Pharmaceutics*, 269(1), 185–194.
70. Harris, M., Ahmed, H., Barr, B., LeVine, D., Pace, L., Mohapatra, A., . . . Jennings, J. A. (2017). Magnetic stimuli-responsive chitosan-based drug delivery biocomposite for multiple triggered release. *International Journal of Biological Macromolecules*, 104, 1407–1414.

71. Pourjavadi, A., Bagherifard, M., & Doroudian, M. (2020). Synthesis of micelles based on Chitosan functionalized with gold nanorods as a light sensitive drug delivery vehicle. *International Journal of Biological Macromolecules*, 149, 809–818.

72. Sabourian, P., Tavakolian, M., Yazdani, H., Frounchi, M., van de Ven, T. G., Maysinger, D., & Kakkar, A. (2020). Stimuli-responsive Chitosan as an advantageous platform for efficient delivery of bioactive agents. *Journal of Controlled Release*, 317, 216–231.

73. Nisar, S., Pandit, A. H., Wang, L. F., & Rattan, S. (2020). Strategy to design a smart photocleavable and pH sensitive chitosan-based hydrogel through a novel crosslinker: A potential vehicle for controlled drug delivery. *RSC Advances*, 10(25), 14694–14704.

74. Nagarwal, R. C., Kumar, R., & Pandit, J. K. (2012). Chitosan coated sodium alginate—chitosan nanoparticles loaded with 5-FU for ocular delivery: In vitro characterization and in vivo study in rabbit eye. *European Journal of Pharmaceutical Sciences*, 47(4), 678–685.

75. Pereira, A. K. D. S., Reis, D. T., Barbosa, K. M., Scheidt, G. N., da Costa, L. S., & Santos, L. S. S. (2020). Antibacterial effects and ibuprofen release potential using chitosan microspheres loaded with silver nanoparticles. *Carbohydrate Research*, 488, 107891.

76. Patel, M. P., Patel, R. R., & Patel, J. K. (2010). Chitosan mediated targeted drug delivery system: A review. *Journal of Pharmacy & Pharmaceutical Sciences*, 13(4), 536–557.

77. Safdar, R., Omar, A. A., Arunagiri, A., Regupathi, I., & Thanabalan, M. (2019). Potential of Chitosan and its derivatives for controlled drug release applications—A review. *Journal of Drug Delivery Science and Technology*, 49, 642–659.

78. Kono, H., & Teshirogi, T. (2015). Cyclodextrin-grafted chitosan hydrogels for controlled drug delivery. *International Journal of Biological Macromolecules*, 72, 299–308.

79. Varaprasad, K., Vimala, K., Ravindra, S., Reddy, N. N., Reddy, G. S. M., & Raju, K. M. (2012). Biodegradable chitosan hydrogels for in vitro drug release studies of 5-flurouracil an anticancer drug. *Journal of Polymers and the Environment*, 20(2), 573–582.

80. Shim, J. W., & Nho, Y. C. (2003). Preparation of poly (acrylic acid)—chitosan hydrogels by gamma irradiation and in vitro drug release. *Journal of Applied Polymer Science*, 90(13), 3660–3667.

81. Das, D., Ghosh, P., Ghosh, A., Haldar, C., Dhara, S., Panda, A. B., & Pal, S. (2015). Stimulus-responsive, biodegradable, biocompatible, covalently cross-linked hydrogel based on dextrin and poly (N-isopropylacrylamide) for in vitro/in vivo controlled drug release. *ACS Applied Materials & Interfaces*, 7(26), 14338–14351.

82. Varaprasad, K., Vimala, K., Ravindra, S., Reddy, N. N., Reddy, G. S. M., & Raju, K. M. (2012). Biodegradable chitosan hydrogels for in vitro drug release studies of 5-flurouracil an anticancer drug. *Journal of Polymers and the Environment*, 20(2), 573–582.

83. Sharma, R. K., Singh, A. P., & Chauhan, G. S. (2014). Grafting of GMA and some comonomers onto Chitosan for controlled release of diclofenac sodium. *International Journal of Biological Macromolecules*, 64, 368–376.

84. Fu, Y., & Kao, W. J. (2010). Drug release kinetics and transport mechanisms of non-degradable and degradable polymeric delivery systems. *Expert Opinion on Drug Delivery*, 7(4), 429–444.

85. Ferrero, C., Massuelle, D., & Doelker, E. (2010). Towards elucidation of the drug release mechanism from compressed hydrophilic matrices made of cellulose ethers. II. Evaluation of a possible swelling-controlled drug release mechanism using dimensionless analysis. *Journal of Controlled Release*, 141(2), 223–233.

86. Rao, K. R., & Devi, K. P. (1988). Swelling controlled-release systems: Recent developments and applications. *International Journal of Pharmaceutics*, 48(1–3), 1–13.

87. Siepmann, J., Lecomte, F., & Bodmeier, R. (1999). Diffusion-controlled drug delivery systems: Calculation of the required composition to achieve desired release profiles. *Journal of Controlled Release*, 60(2–3), 379–389.

88. Efentakis, M., & Politis, S. (2006). Comparative evaluation of various structures in polymer-controlled drug delivery systems and the effect of their morphology and characteristics on drug release. *European Polymer Journal*, 42(5), 1183–1195.

89. Yadav, G., Bansal, M., Thakur, N., Khare, S., & Khare, P. (2013). Multilayer tablets and their drug release kinetic models for oral controlled drug delivery system. *Middle-East Journal of Scientific Research*, 16, 782–795.

90. Huanbutta, K., & Sangnim, T. (2019). Design and development of zero-order drug release gastroretentive floating tablets fabricated by 3D printing technology. *Journal of Drug Delivery Science and Technology*, 52, 831–837.

91. Schwartz, J. B., Simonelli, A. P., & Higuchi, W. I. (1968). Drug release from wax matrices I. Analysis of data with first-order kinetics and with the diffusion-controlled model. *Journal of Pharmaceutical Sciences*, 57(2), 274–277.

92. Caccavo, D., Cascone, S., Lamberti, G., & Barba, A. A. (2015). Modeling the drug release from hydrogel-based matrices. *Molecular Pharmaceutics*, 12(2), 474–483.

93. Gouda, R., Baishya, H., & Qing, Z. (2017). Application of mathematical models in drug release kinetics of carbidopa and levodopa ER tablets. *Journal of Developing Drugs*, 6(02), 1–8.

94. Siepmann, J., & Peppas, N. A. (2012). Modeling of drug release from delivery systems based on hydroxypropyl methylcellulose (HPMC). *Advanced Drug Delivery Reviews*, 64, 163–174.

95. Paul, D. R. (2011). Elaborations on the Higuchi model for drug delivery. *International Journal of Pharmaceutics*, 418(1), 13–17.

96. Siepmann, J., & Peppas, N. A. (2011). Higuchi equation: Derivation, applications, use and misuse. *International Journal of Pharmaceutics*, 418(1), 6–12.

97. Singhvi, G., & Singh, M. (2011). In-vitro drug release characterization models. *International Journal of Pharmaceutical Sciences and Research*, 2(1), 77–84.

98. Paarakh, M. P., Jose, P. A., Setty, C., & Christoper, G. P. (2018). Release kinetics—concepts and applications. *International Journal of Pharmacy Research & Technology*, 8(1), 12–20.

99. Mohamed OA, Masood SH, Bhowmik JL. Optimization of fused deposition modeling process parameters: a review of current research and future prospects. *Advances in manufacturing*. 2015 Mar;3(1):42–53.

100. Chohan, J. S., & Singh, R. (2017). Pre and post processing techniques to improve surface characteristics of FDM parts: A state of art review and future applications. *Rapid Prototyping Journal*, 23(3), 495–513.

Index

Note: Page numbers in *italic* indicate a figure and page numbers in **bold** indicate a table on the corresponding page.

A

additive manufacturing, 66, 81
aerosols, 75
antimicrobial, 75
artificial livers, 144
artificial muscles, 108
auricular prostheses, 131

B

binder jetting, 147
biocompatibility, biomedical, 104
biomanufacturing, 118
biomaterials, 171
biomolecules, 82
biopolymeric matrix, *212*
bioprinting, bioinks, 81
bioresorbable, biodegradable, 188
braces, 124

C

cancellous bone, 174
capsules, 126
carbon nanotubes, 189
cardiac surgeries, 120
cardiovascular, 144
cell-based printing, 170
cells, 82
cephalometry, 119
chambers, 75
chitosan, *207*
clinical, composite, 155
clubfoot, *52*
compressive strength, ceramics, 104
computational fluid dynamics, *177*
computed tomography, 53
computer-aided manufacturing, *50*
congenital issues, 82
corrosion rate, 176
cost-effective, 144
COVID-19, 65, *67*
curing, 189
customization, crowns, 124
cyber-physical system, 133

D

dental, 132
dentistry, 118
dialysis membrane, 206
diffusion, *212*
digital imaging, 122
digital information, 166
directed energy deposition, 147
droplets, *75*
drop-on-demand, 170
drug delivery, 125
durability, 133

E

elastic modulus, 175
electrospinning, 188
embryonic stem cells, 82
epidemic, **68**
exoskeletons, *206*

F

face mask, face shield, *70*
feedstock, 172
flexibility, 104
foot orthosis, *49*
fully functional organ, 81
functional polymers, 105
fused deposition modelling, 48

G

gastrointestinal tract, 126
general medical model, *150*
guar gum, *207*
gypsum-based powders, 155

H

Hixson–Crowell release model, 215
hydrogel, 105
hydrophilic, 210
hydroxyapatite, 178

I

implant design, 118
inkjet technology, 170
intravenous Catheters, 127
in vitro, 120

J

jet ability, 104
jewellery, 84
joint replacement, 191
just-in-time production, 148

K

kinetics, 15
knee replacements, 31
knowledge base, 19

L

layer by layer, 132
liquid bonding, 104

M

macro/micro-porous characteristics, 166
magnetic resonance imaging, 53
maxilla, 192
maxillofacial prostheses, 118
mechanical properties, 132
medical Education, 122
medicines, medical devices, 108
membrane, 170
metals, 104
microfibers, 188
microfluidic devices, 144
microstructures, 174
MIMICS, *62*
mitral valve, 121
multimaterial, 155

N

nanofabrication, 171
natural bone, 144
next-generation, 166
non-bioaccumulation, 208

O

organs, 82
orthosis, 48, *61*
oral Medications, 126
orthodontic aligners, *151*
orthopedic implants, 144

osseointegration, 174
oxidization, 172

P

pandemic, **68**, *69*
patient-specific medical implants, 192
personal protection equipment, 66
pharmacodynamics, 125
photopolymerization, printability, 104
physiology, 150
plaster of paris, *58*
poly-lactic acid, *71*
polymer matrix composites, 105
polymers, *69*
polystyrene, *206*
porous, 174
powder flowability, 172
presurgical or preoperative planning, 120
prostheses, *109*
prosthetic foot, 131
prototyping, *61*

Q

quality, 154
quicker, *7*

R

rapid prototype (RP), 48
regenerative medicine, 82
rehabilitation, *49*, 128
respiratory valves, *73*, *74*
rheumatoid arthritis, 191

S

scaffolds, 82
selective laser melting, selective laser sintering, 118
snorkel mask, *71*
specific gravity, **57**
stainless steel, 174
stents, skin, 108
stereolithography, 104
sterilizing, 151
strength, *51*
subtractive manufacturing, *69*
surgical guides, 133
surgical planning, 122

T

teflon, 206
tensile strength, 104
thermoplastic, 105

thermoresponsive monomers, 210
tissue compatibility, *150*
tissue engineering, 108
tissues, 82
titanium, 174
transdermal drug delivery, 127

U

unidirectional blood flow, 121
unique designs, 166

V

vacuum chamber, *59*
vaginal and rectal medicine, **126**
vat photopolymerization, 104
vitro models, 76

W

water adsorption, 179
wear resistance, 176
wettability, water-soluble, 186

X

x-ray, 42, 119, 122

Y

young's moduli, 174

Z

zero-order drug release, 213

For Product Safety Concerns and Information please contact our EU
representative GPSR@taylorandfrancis.com
Taylor & Francis Verlag GmbH, Kaufingerstraße 24, 80331 München, Germany

www.ingramcontent.com/pod-product-compliance
Lightning Source LLC
Chambersburg PA
CBHW060403220326
41598CB00023B/3003